SIXTH EDITION

Handbook of
Psychiatric
Drug Therapy

SIXTH EDITION

Handbook of Psychiatric Drug Therapy

Lawrence A. Labbate, MD
Chief, Inpatient Mental Health Services
Central Arkansas Veterans Healthcare System
Professor of Psychiatry
University of Arkansas

Maurizio Fava, MD
Executive Vice Chair, Department of Psychiatry
Director, Depression Clinical and Research
    Program
Executive Director, MGH Clinical Trials
    Network and Institute
Massachusetts General Hospital
Professor of Psychiatry
Harvard Medical School

Jerrold F. Rosenbaum, M.D
Chief of Psychiatry, Massachusetts
General Hospital Stanley Cobb Professor of
    Psychiatry,
Harvard Medical School

George W. Arana, MD
Chief Medical Officer
VA New England Healthcare Network
    (VISN 1)
Professor of Psychiatry
Vanderbilt University School of Medicine

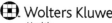 Wolters Kluwer | Lippincott Williams & Wilkins
Health
Philadelphia • Baltimore • New York • London
Buenos Aires • Hong Kong • Sydney • Tokyo

Acquisitions Editor: Lisa McAllister
Product Manager: Tom Gibbons
Manufacturing Manager: Benjamin Rivera
Marketing Manager: Brian Freiland
Cover Designer: Theresa Mallon
Production Service: Aptara, Inc.
Printer: Strategic Content Imaging

Library of Congress Cataloging-in-Publication Data
Handbook of psychiatric drug therapy / Lawrence A. Labbate . . . [et al.].
— 6th ed.
     p. ; cm.
  Includes bibliographical references and index.
  ISBN-13: 978-0-7817-7486-4
  ISBN-10: 0-7817-7486-1
  1. Mental illness—Chemotherapy—Handbooks, manuals, etc. 2.
Psychopharmacology—Handbooks, manuals, etc. I. Labbate, Lawrence A.
  [DNLM: 1. Mental Disorders—drug therapy. 2. Psychotropic
Drugs—pharmacology. WM 402 H2366 2010]
  RC483.A73 2010
  616.89'18—dc22   2009015472

Care has been taken to confirm the accuracy of the information presented and to describe generally accepted practices. However, the authors, editors, and publisher are not responsible for errors or omissions or for any consequences from application of the
information in this book and make no warranty, expressed or implied, with respect to the
currency, completeness, or accuracy of the contents of the publication. Application of the information in a particular situation remains the professional responsibility of the practitioner.
     The authors, editors, and publisher have exerted every effort to ensure that drug se-
lection and dosage set forth in this text are in accordance with current recommendations
and practice at the time of publication. However, in view of ongoing research, changes in
government regulations, and the constant flow of information relating to drug therapy
and drug reactions, the reader is urged to check the package insert for each drug for any
change in indications and dosage and for added warnings and precautions. This is particularly important when the recommended agent is a new or infrequently employed drug.
     Some drugs and medical devices presented in the publication have Food and Drug
Administration (FDA) clearance for limited use in restricted research settings. It is the responsibility of the health care provider to ascertain the FDA status of each drug or device
planned for use in their clinical practice.
     For a complete list of all the relevant disclosures of Dr. Fava and Dr. Rosenbaum,
please go to: www.mghacademy.org, and click on Psychiatry.

To purchase additional copies of this book, call our customer service department at (800)
638-3030 or fax orders to (301) 223-2320. International customers should call (301) 223-2300.

Visit Lippincott Williams & Wilkins on the Internet: at LWW.com. Lippincott Williams &
Wilkins customer service representatives are available from 8:30 am to 6 pm, EST.

15 14 13 12 11 10

To our colleagues and their patients to do
the best with the therapeutics that are available,
to be encouraged by the number of options, and to be
unrelenting in the pursuit of the best outcomes.

CONTENTS

DISEASE-SPECIFIC TABLE OF CONTENTS

This table provides the reader with easy access to major places in the book that discuss the indications for medications in specific disorders or clinical situations. The major pages on which a disorder is discussed are given in bold. This table does not contain every citation; that purpose is served by the subject index.

This volume from its earliest iterations was inspired by the unique and extraordinary vision and knowledge of Steve Hyman: psychiatrist, neuroscientist, former NIMH Director, and current Harvard Provost. Committed to the advance of the field through science and evidence but pragmatic and savvy about the realities of clinical practice, he intended and ensured that this volume would be underpinned by data but be useful in the mission of delivering treatments to individual patients. As Steve has determined that this edition is the moment to step down from authorship, we acknowledge with pride and admiration our association with him and our gratitude for the enduring wisdom that this work retains from his years of input.

LAL

MF

JFR

GWA

PREFACE TO THE FIFTH EDITION

This handbook is a guide to the use of modern psychotherapeutic drugs. Some scientific background is presented, but this is, above all, meant to be a practical volume. It is intended to be useful not only for psychiatrists but also for primary care providers and for other health professionals who are involved in the management of patients with mental disorders. We have avoided an encyclopedic approach and focused on the major classes of drugs used in clinical practice. In the interest of brevity and practicality, we have excluded those drugs whose use has largely been superseded (e.g., some of the older sedative-hypnotics). We have attempted to delineate what is known on the basis of controlled clinical trials, but in the areas where adequate systematic evidence is lacking, we have tried to identify the best clinical practices. Above all, the authors hope that this volume can contribute to the successful care of patients.

JFR
GWA
SEH
LAL
MF

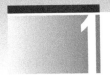

Psychiatric Drug Therapy

The practice of psychopharmacology is challenging. Psychiatric disorders frequently have unpredictable courses, complicating comorbid psychiatric or medical disorders are common, and symptoms of psychiatric disorders may interfere with treatment adherence (e.g., denial of illness in mania, suspiciousness in many psychotic disorders, and a pattern of interpersonal turmoil in certain personality disorders that does not spare caregivers). In addition, current medications are **not fully effective** in many patients. Although in some illnesses, such as major depression and panic disorder, available therapies help most patients, many patients respond only incompletely, and a substantial minority prove to be treatment refractory. In bipolar disorder, polypharmacy is the rule and, nonetheless, many patients have residual symptoms. For other disorders, such as schizophrenia, the current treatments are only palliative, leaving the patient with many disabling symptoms, such as cognitive deficits. It takes great skill for the practitioner to maintain the right balance between pharmacologic and psychological approaches to therapy. Skilled use of the psychiatric drugs currently available can result in good outcomes for many patients who would otherwise suffer severe morbidity or even death.

Although pharmacologic interventions are effective treatments for many psychiatric disorders, cognitive behavioral therapies or other symptom-focused **psychotherapies** have been shown to be effective in clinical trials for a variety of disorders. For many patients, the benefits of medication and psychotherapy are additive and occasionally synergistic. For example, some patients who have panic disorder with agoraphobia may recover from their panic attacks with drug therapy but remain disabled by agoraphobia unless they participate in cognitive behavioral therapy. Major depression responds well to pharmacotherapy, but many patients are optimally treated when medication and psychotherapy are combined. Patients with bipolar disorder and other complex illnesses benefit from education and support. On the other hand, there are situations, such as acute mania, in which psychotherapy might be counterproductive, until the acute symptoms abate.

In general, an ideologic preference for either pharmacologic or psychosocial treatment, as opposed to reliance on the best available information derived from controlled studies, has no place in successful psychiatric practice. An ideologic preference for one form of treatment over another—which may be caricatured as "Here is the treatment, now tell me the problem"—serves patients' needs poorly. The standard of care for psychiatric disorders requires a careful diagnostic assessment before the introduction of therapy, and the therapy chosen must have documented efficacy for the patient's condition. This standard leaves much room for clinical judgment. The clinician must recognize that available controlled studies are as yet an incomplete guide to actual clinical situations. Subjects eligible for clinical studies are a small subset of patients requiring treatment. They are typically relatively young, taking no other medications, lacking serious comorbidity, and willing to be on a placebo for several weeks. Useful clinical trials data for children and elderly people are particularly lacking.

We have relied on data from well-designed clinical trials where possible, but in the spirit of practicality we also offer information, with explicit caveats, that has guided our practice in situations in which systematic data are lacking. Here we offer certain principles that have been useful in guiding our approaches to treatment.

BEFORE INITIATING MEDICATIONS

1. Before prescribing psychotropic medication, it is important to be **clear about the diagnosis.** If the diagnosis has not been determined, a clear set of diagnostic hypotheses should be established, and a systematic approach to clarifying the diagnosis should be outlined. For example, depressive or psychotic states may result from medical or psychiatric illness or from drug abuse, or they may represent an adverse reaction to antipsychotic drugs.

2. Before prescribing psychotropic medications, it is important to be aware of medical problems or drug interactions that could (a) be responsible for the patient's psychiatric symptoms, (b) increase the toxicity of prescribed drugs (e.g., diuretics or nonsteroidal antiinflammatory agents may increase lithium levels), or (c) decrease the effectiveness of the planned therapy (e.g., carbamazepine could hasten the metabolism of certain tricyclic antidepressants).

3. Be aware of the possibility of **alcohol or drug abuse,** which might confound treatment. Unless symptoms are so severe as to demand immediate intervention, it is recommended that patients first be detoxified from alcohol or drugs before attempting treatment of a presumed psychiatric disorder (e.g., depression) during ongoing substance abuse.

4. Before prescribing a psychiatric medication, it is imperative to **identify target symptoms** (e.g., sleep disturbance, panic attacks, or hallucinations) that can be followed during the course of therapy to monitor the success of treatment. It is also important to monitor changes in the patient's quality of life (e.g., satisfaction with home and family life, functioning at work, and overall sense of well-being). An alternative for patients who cannot report their own symptoms (e.g., those with dementia or psychosis) is to ask patients' families to rate their behavior (e.g., a simple daily rating on a scale of 1 to 10 points). The use of identified target symptoms and quality-of-life assessment is especially important when the medication is being given as an **empirical trial** in a patient whose diagnosis is unclear.

5. Suggestions for optimal drug selection are presented throughout this handbook. However, if a medication was previously effective and well tolerated by a patient, it is a reasonable clinical judgment to use that medication again even if newer drugs are now available for the patient's condition.

6. When there is significant doubt about the correct diagnosis or therapy, consultation should be sought. The clinician's response to the consultant's recommendations (including agreement or disagreement) should be documented.

ADMINISTRATION OF MEDICATIONS

1. Once a drug is chosen, **administer a full trial with adequate doses and duration of treatment** so that if the target symptoms do not improve, there will be no need to return to that agent. **Inadequate dosing and duration are the main reasons for failure of antidepressant trials** in well-diagnosed patients.

2. Be aware of side effects, and **warn patients in advance** if appropriate (e.g., about sedation early in the course of daytime benzodiazepine use or sexual side effects with selective serotonin reuptake inhibitors). Develop a clear idea of which toxicities require reassurance (e.g., dry mouth), treatment (e.g., antipsychotic drug–induced extrapyramidal effects), or drug

discontinuation (e.g., prolongation of the Q-T interval on the electrocardiogram). Examine patients when appropriate (e.g., for rigidity or oral dyskinesia). Recall that the side effects of some psychotropic agents may mimic symptoms of the disorder being treated (e.g., selective serotonin reuptake inhibitor–induced agitation may mimic agitated depression).

3. Keep regimens as simple as possible both to improve adherence and to avoid additive toxicity. Adherence is often enhanced if regimens and dosing schedules are kept simple (e.g., lithium once or twice daily instead of three or four times daily).

4. Engage patients in a dialog about the time course of expected improvement. Take concerns about side effects seriously.

5. Patients who are psychotic, demented, or retarded need careful supervision from family or other caregivers to adhere to their regimens.

6. **Readjust the dosage of medication** to determine the lowest effective dose for the particular stage of the patient's illness because, for psychotic disorders in particular, dosage requirements often change over time. For example, in schizophrenia, the dosage of antipsychotic medication needed to treat acute exacerbations is generally higher than that for long-term maintenance.

7. In elderly patients, it is prudent to initiate treatment with lower doses of medication. Dosage changes should be less frequent in elderly patients than in younger patients because the time required for drugs to achieve steady-state levels is often prolonged.

8. Follow-up care includes evaluating efficacy of treatment; monitoring and managing side effects, treatment-relevant intercurrent life events, and comorbid medical and psychiatric conditions; obtaining and evaluating appropriate laboratory data; and, when necessary, planning changes in the treatment regimen.

DISCONTINUATION OF MEDICATIONS

1. **All too often ineffective medications are continued indefinitely** and multiple medications accumulate in the patient's regimen, leading to unnecessary costs and side effects. Adjunctive and combination therapies may be appropriate for certain conditions; however, when medications no longer prove useful to the treatment regimen, it is critical to discontinue them. It may be difficult to determine that a medication has failed unless the physician has kept track of objective target symptoms from the beginning of the trial.

2. Even after apparent therapeutic success, criteria for discontinuation of psychotropic drugs in most clinical situations are ill defined. When discontinuing psychotropic medications, it is best to taper dosages slowly, which can help prevent **rebound or withdrawal** symptoms. Because they have different therapeutic implications, it is important to distinguish among temporary symptom rebound (as frequently occurs after discontinuing short-acting benzodiazepines), which is brief and transient but can be severe; recurrence of the disorder, in which original symptoms return long-term; and withdrawal, in which new symptoms characteristic of withdrawal from the particular drug appear. In general, conditions that have been **chronic** before treatment, **recurrent,** or have emerged late in life are more likely to require **long-term maintenance treatment.**

OTHER ISSUES IN PSYCHOPHARMACOLOGY

1. To optimize clinical management of complicated illnesses, it is important to document observations of the patient (including mental status at

baseline and changes with treatment), clinical reasoning, and side effects. Particular attention should be given to documenting risk of suicide or violence and educating the patient (and, where appropriate, family) about the risk of serious side effects such as tardive dyskinesia with certain antipsychotic drugs or the risk of suicidal behaviors with initiation of antidepressant treatment in children. It is also important for the record to indicate that the patient understands the reason for treatment, its risks and benefits, alternative treatments, and the risks of no treatment. If the competence of the patient to make his or her own decisions fluctuates or is questionable, the clinician should obtain the patient's permission to include the family in important treatment decisions. If the patient is clearly not competent to make decisions, a formal legal mechanism for substituted judgment must be used.

2. Many of the drugs discussed in this book have not yet been approved by the U.S. Food and Drug Administration for the particular indication discussed. However, a physician is free to choose any approved drug for non-approved indications (so-called off-label use). The record should reflect the basis for this clinical decision, which ideally should reflect appreciation and understanding of the available evidence.

3. The **cost of therapeutic drugs is an important issue** in treatment selection. If treatment adherence and safety are enhanced and risk of relapse diminished, an initially more costly drug may ultimately prove to be the most cost-effective choice. Thus, a narrow focus on drug costs alone is not a good practice. On the other hand, when drugs are equally safe and effective, cost is a valid basis for selection.

2

Drugs for the Treatment of Psychotic Disorders

SCHIZOPHRENIA

Schizophrenia is a chronic psychotic illness that typically begins early in adulthood. Some cases begin with a **prodromal** period of several years, characterized by nonspecific symptoms (depression, social withdrawal, and subtle perceptual changes), that is followed by the eventual development of acute, frank psychosis (i.e., hallucinations, delusions, or disorganized thinking or behavior). Other cases have a more abrupt onset of psychosis. Often, the illness course shows periods of less florid psychosis, punctuated by acute exacerbations. Unfortunately, the overall course of this illness generally leads to a diminished plateau of function and an inability to maintain an active and productive life. Symptoms of schizophrenia are often divided into **positive symptoms** (i.e., symptoms that are not present in normal human cognitions, perceptions, or affect, such as hallucinations, delusions, and thought disorder), negative or **deficit symptoms** (i.e., loss of qualities normally present in healthy individuals, such as impoverishment of thought, blunted affect, and lack of initiative and motivation), and **cognitive symptoms** (particularly impairment in executive function and verbal memory). The cognitive impairment and the negative symptoms are essential features of the illness in that they underlie the poor functioning that is typical for many patients.

Many patients also have co-occurring **anxiety** disorders (e.g., obsessive-compulsive disorder or panic disorder) and depression. Suicide is the leading cause of death. Substance abuse occurs in approximately half of the patients. These co-occurring disorders worsen the course of the illness and complicate treatment. Stimulant use and alcohol binges often lead to psychosis exacerbation. Nicotine dependence is highly prevalent, and while cigarette smoking may help improve attention (by partially correcting the so-called sensory gating deficit) and provide some pleasure, it clearly contributes to cardiovascular and pulmonary diseases frequently experienced by these patients.

Patients with schizophrenia often neglect their health and avoid getting medical and dental treatment. They frequently have **untreated medical conditions,** including hypertension, coronary artery disease, diabetes, chronic obstructive pulmonary disease, and dyslipidemia. Unfortunately, even when patients have laboratory evidence of medical conditions such as diabetes, they frequently go undertreated or untreated. Patients with schizophrenia die young—10 to 15 years younger than the general population, on average. Cardiovascular disease is the most common medical cause of death. Several of the second-generation antipsychotics, unfortunately, may contribute to cardiovascular morbidity because of their propensity to cause weight gain, dyslipidemia, and insulin resistance.

Even though antipsychotics are critical for illness treatment, these drugs **do not treat the full syndrome** of schizophrenia, and rarely does drug treatment alone lead to patients regaining their premorbid function. Antipsychotics are frequently helpful for the positive symptoms of schizophrenia, but they provide only limited to no benefit for primary negative and cognitive symptoms. Other psychosocial treatments including social skills and vocational training, case management, and cognitive behavioral therapy are necessary adjuncts to achieve the best possible satisfactory outcomes.

OTHER PRIMARY PSYCHOTIC DISORDERS

In addition to schizophrenia, several other closely related psychotic conditions such as **schizophreniform** disorder, **schizoaffective disorder**, or **delusional disorder** may be amenable to antipsychotic treatment. Schizoaffective disorder probably represents a heterogeneous group of diseases rather than a single disease entity. The diagnosis is applied to patients who have periods of major manic or depressive symptoms or both but who have prominent psychotic symptoms **which meet criteria for schizophrenia**, even at times when they are relatively free of affective symptoms. Clinically, affective symptoms sometimes respond to lithium, antidepressants, or an anticonvulsant. Psychotic symptoms, especially those that occur between episodes of mood disorder, generally require treatment with antipsychotic medication. The dosages of antipsychotic medication for both acute florid symptoms and chronic maintenance are the same as those for the analogous stages of schizophrenia. All second-generation compounds are likely to be effective for schizoaffective disorder, although more study is warranted.

Schizophreniform disorder involves overt psychotic symptoms of less than 6 months' duration, with return to the premorbid level of functioning. The onset of symptoms tends to be rapid, rather than insidious, and patients may demonstrate confusion or perplexity at the height of their syndrome. Many, but not all, patients lack the flat affect of typical schizophrenia. Schizophreniform patients represent a heterogeneous group. Depending on the population studied, some investigators predominantly find mood disorders represented, whereas others find heterogeneity, with perhaps half of them going on to manifest schizophrenia over time. The early stages of treatment of schizophreniform disorder are the same as for any acute psychosis (see later section on therapeutic use). Given that the long-term prognosis for recovery of many of these patients is good, after the first episode an attempt can be made to taper and discontinue antipsychotic drugs entirely if symptoms fully remit and remain in remission for 6 months to a year. Many patients who meet criteria for schizophreniform disorder will also benefit from lithium or anticonvulsants (see Chapter 4) if symptoms of bipolar disorder emerge.

Delusional disorder entails the presence of delusions without hallucinations or language impairment. This condition is considerably less common than schizophrenia, and usually starts in middle age. The most common types include paranoid delusions, but some patients may experience delusional jealousy, erotomania, or somatic delusions. Patients with delusional disorder are often difficult to treat because of illness denial, and their pervasive suspiciousness often extends to physicians and medical personnel. As a result, they are often brought to treatment by others and are often nonadherent to treatment. If medication is introduced to the patient as a means of helping cope with anxiety, stress, or other complaints rather than explicitly confronting delusions, the initiation of treatment may be more acceptable. Nonetheless, over time, it is best if the patient can be helped to develop insight into the distortions and misperceptions.

Antipsychotic drugs are effective in some patients with delusional disorder, especially in those whose symptoms are of recent onset. As with other psychotic disorders, the agents of choice are the atypical antipsychotics. For patients with chronic, systematized delusions, the response rate may be lower than for those with a more recent onset. Pending systematic studies of this clinical population, dosing guidelines should follow those for treating schizophrenia, while considering the possibility that lower doses may be adequate for some patients. If first-generation drugs are tried, low doses should be used initially (e.g., haloperidol 2 to 5 mg per day or the equivalent) to minimize side effects and to enhance compliance. Consideration should be given to a trial of antidepressants or lithium if affective symptoms are apparent or if there is a family history of mood disorder.

GENERAL COMMENTS ABOUT ANTIPSYCHOTICS

The antipsychotic drugs are the cornerstone of treatment of schizophrenia and other psychotic disorders, such as schizoaffective disorder. Antipsychotic drugs have been in clinical use since the 1950s, when chlorpromazine, a phenothiazine derivative that was developed as an antihistamine, was found to have antipsychotic properties. The key observation was that chlorpromazine and later antipsychotic drugs were not acting as nonspecific sedatives but were ameliorating core psychotic symptoms such as hallucinations and delusions.

Chlorpromazine provided a model for the development of a wide variety of chemically distinct compounds effective for the psychoses, but all of these first-generation compounds (with the exception of clozapine) had a liability for causing extrapyramidal symptoms (EPS) by virtue of their major shared property, potent antagonism of the D_2 dopamine receptor. In addition to their antipsychotic properties, these drugs have had other uses on the basis of their ability to block D_2 dopamine receptors (e.g., as antiemetics and in palliation of some movement disorders characterized by excessive movement). The **first-generation** D_2 antagonist antipsychotic drugs have come to be described as typical to contrast them with clozapine and with newer **second-generation** or so-called atypical drugs that have a reduced liability for EPS. The EPS burden also led to use of the term neuroleptic for these older drugs because these drugs could produce neurologic disorders that looked similar to Parkinson's disease or dystonias. In addition, long-term use of these drugs, as is typically required in schizophrenia, posed a high risk of a permanent movement disorder, tardive dyskinesia (TD). Even in the short term, in addition to producing parkinsonian symptoms, first generation antipsychotic drugs produce side effects (e.g., akathisia or akinesia) that could mimic or exacerbate the symptoms for which the drugs were originally prescribed. In short, these older antipsychotic drugs were effective and indeed critically important in the treatment of psychotic disorders for more than 40 years, but at the price of serious motor system problems that could limit therapy. Although the liability for extrapyramidal neurologic side effects is an intrinsic liability of first-generation drugs, as a result of their selective blockade of D_2 dopamine receptors, they were often also administered at **excessive doses**, which markedly exacerbated the problem.

The introduction of risperidone (Consta and Risperdal) in 1993 began a new era in the treatment of psychotic illnesses with the introduction and widespread adoption of a group of compounds that have a reduced liability for producing EPS. These have variously been referred to as "atypical" or **second-generation** antipsychotic drugs. However, this change began with the reintroduction of clozapine, an older drug with very low risk for EPS liability and the greatest efficacy in schizophrenia. Clozapine had not been marketed because it carried approximately a 1% risk of potentially lethal agranulocytosis. Studies that demonstrated the drug's not only very low EPS liability but also greater efficacy for treating schizophrenia than any other antipsychotic drug led to its reintroduction. Because of the risk of agranulocytosis, however, cumbersome and expensive weekly monitoring of white blood cell (WBC) counts became part of any clozapine regimen. In addition, clozapine has its own troublesome side effects (including sedation, weight gain, and a reduction in seizure threshold). However, the benefits of clozapine have been demonstrated to outweigh its risks for many individuals with schizophrenia who respond poorly to other treatments. Although it is still unclear what gives clozapine its enhanced efficacy (it has relatively low affinity for D_2 receptors compared with the other older drugs, exhibits potent antagonism of serotonin 5-HT_{2A} receptors, and interacts with many other receptors), it became a new, if partly mysterious, model for drug development. Since the reintroduction of clozapine, several newer compounds—risperidone, olanzapine (Zyprexa), quetiapine (Seroquel), ziprasidone (Geodon), and aripiprazole (Abilify)—have been shown to be effective for schizophrenia and other psychoses and useful for mania as well, though, unlike clozapine, they are not superior to the older drugs. Because these drugs have reduced EPS liability, have a generally milder side-effect profile than does clozapine, and do not pose a risk of agranulocytosis, they have rapidly become the first-line drugs for the treatment of psychotic disorders. As a group, these drugs have been shown in well-controlled trials of greater than 4 to 20 weeks to be at least as effective as the older typical antipsychotic drugs, although they do not exhibit the clear efficacy advantages of clozapine in the most resistant cases. Moreover, many of these drugs have their own problematic side effects. Recent prospective studies showing similar effectiveness between the old and new drugs have made us question the enthusiasm once accompanying the second-generation antipsychotics.

As noted, a high affinity for D_2 dopamine receptors among the older compounds is clearly associated with their liability for producing EPS. However, the decreased liability for EPS in the newer compounds appears to reflect diverse mechanisms and is still not fully understood. For example, although risperidone has **high affinity for the D_2 receptor**, like haloperidol (Table 2.1), its high affinity for the serotonin 5-HT$_{2A}$ receptor may mitigate its EPS liability when it is given at lower doses (<6 mg per day). In contrast, quetiapine has a lower affinity for the 5-HT$_{2A}$ receptor than haloperidol, but it also has a lower affinity for the D_2 dopamine receptor. As described, clozapine has a relatively low D_2 receptor affinity and a high affinity for the 5-HT$_{2A}$ receptor, but it interacts with so many receptors (Table 2.1) that the basis of its efficacy and atypical side-effect profile remains unclear.

Multiple clinical trials have shown that antipsychotic drugs are effective both for acute exacerbations of schizophrenia and for long-term maintenance. Rigorous studies of clozapine have shown that it may be of particular benefit in chronic schizophrenia refractory to other antipsychotic drugs; case series and anecdotal reports suggest that it also may be effective in refractory atypical psychoses, such as schizoaffective disorder. Clinical trials have not convincingly shown superior efficacy of second-generation antipsychotics, other than clozapine, in schizophrenia when the comparator, most often haloperidol, is administered at appropriately low doses and combined with anticholinergic agents. Use of high doses of haloperidol in several comparison trials creates conditions for newer drugs looking better than they may be.

It has often been stated that traditional antipsychotic drugs are more effective in treating positive symptoms than negative symptoms. However, when examined

TABLE 2.1 Receptor Affinities of Atypical Antipsychotic Drugs Compared with Haloperidol

Drug	D_1	D_2	D_3	D_4	5-HT$_{2A}$	5-HT$_{2C}$	α_1	H_1	ACh
Haloperidol	210	1	2	3	45	>10,000	6	440	5,500
Clozapine	85	160	170	50	16	10	7	1	2
Olanzapine	31	44	50	50	5	11	19	3	2
Quetiapine	460	580	940	1,900	300	5,100	7	11	>1,000
Risperidone	430	2	10	10	0.5	25	1	20	>1,000
Ziprasidone	525	4	7	32	0.4	1	10	50	>1,000
Aripiprazole	410	0.52	7.2	260	20	15	57	61	>1,000

The affinities (dissociation constants) are expressed in nanomoles. The lower the number, the higher the affinity (i.e., the lower concentration to produce half saturation of the receptor).
Adapted with permission from Tamminga CA. Principles of the pharmacotherapy of schizophrenia. In: Charney DS, Nestler EJ, Bunney BS, eds. *Neurobiology of mental illness.* New York: Oxford University Press, 1999:274.

Fluphenazine Same as Haldol profile!

carefully, this generalization is not entirely accurate in that those negative symptoms that occur during an acute exacerbation of schizophrenia often respond well to antipsychotic drugs. Moreover, many patients continue to have some residual positive symptoms, such as hallucinations and delusions, despite the use of antipsychotic medication. The expectation that all positive symptoms should respond to antipsychotic therapy has led to the use of excessive doses in some patients. **Negative symptoms** that characterize the patient's chronic course (i.e., negative symptoms that are present even at times when positive symptoms are minimal) tend to be relatively refractory to antipsychotic drug treatment and appear somewhat more responsive to clozapine. No existing drugs appear to ameliorate executive dysfunction and other core cognitive deficits like impaired verbal memory. These symptoms ultimately contribute substantially to disability even when other symptoms improve.

It is also important to recall that side effects of **first generation** antipsychotic drugs can mimic both positive and negative features of schizophrenia. Akathisia can be indistinguishable from agitation and anxiety (positive symptoms), and EPS effects of antipsychotics (e.g., bradykinesia, akinesia, and masked facies) can masquerade as negative symptoms of the disorder. Indeed, the D_2 dopamine receptor antagonism of antipsychotic drugs, by causing even subtle akinesia, may create a therapeutic ceiling effect vis-à-vis negative symptoms in some patients.

CHEMISTRY

Phenothiazines, the first chemical class of antipsychotic drugs developed, are tricyclic molecules. Three subtypes of phenothiazines are available: aliphatics, piperidines, and piperazines. Those phenothiazines with aliphatic side chains (e.g., chlorpromazine) tend to be low-potency compounds (i.e., higher doses are needed to achieve therapeutic effectiveness). Piperidine substitutions impart anticholinergic properties and a lower incidence of EPS (e.g., thioridazine, mesoridazine). Piperazine phenothiazines (e.g., perphenazine, trifluoperazine, fluphenazine) are among the most potent antipsychotic molecules.

The thioxanthene class of antipsychotic drugs is chemically similar to the phenothiazines. The butyrophenones represent a class of extremely potent antipsychotic drugs. Of these, only haloperidol is currently approved for psychiatric use in the United States. Droperidol, a shorter-acting butyrophenone, is approved for use as a preanesthetic agent.

Several other compounds of varied chemical structures have been approved for the treatment of psychotic and other illnesses in the United States. Pimozide, a diphenylbutylpiperidine approved for Gilles de la Tourette syndrome (but not necessarily superior in efficacy to other antipsychotic drugs for this indication), is also a potent antipsychotic drug with a very long half-life (several days). In addition, there are compounds called dibenzodiazepines that closely resemble the tricyclic antidepressants with a seven-member central ring and a piperazine substitution; this class of antipsychotic drug is represented by the typical antipsychotic drug loxapine, as well as by the atypical drug clozapine. Risperidone is a benzisoxazole derivative that combines high affinity for D_2 dopamine receptors and 5-HT_2 serotonin receptors. Olanzapine is a thienobenzodiazepine agent with greater affinity for the serotonin 5-HT_2 receptors than for dopamine receptors and that, compared with other second-generation antipsychotics, is most like clozapine in its receptor affinities. Quetiapine is a dibenzothiazepine derivative with low affinity for serotonin receptors but weaker activity at dopamine receptors and multiple other receptors. Ziprasidone is a benzisothiazolyl piperazine derivative with greater affinity for serotonin 5-HT_{2A} receptors than for dopamine receptors but higher affinity for D_2 dopamine receptors than does clozapine or quetiapine. In this regard, it is similar to risperidone. Ziprasidone also has relatively low affinity for H_1

histamine receptors and α_1-norepinephrine receptors, which limits its liabilities for sedation and orthostatic hypotension. Aripiprazole is a quinolinone derivative, which like risperidone and ziprasidone, shows higher affinity for serotonin 5-HT$_{2A}$ receptors than for dopamine receptors. In addition, aripiprazole appears to have partial agonist activity at D$_2$ dopamine receptors, although the clinical significance of this effect remains unknown.

PHARMACOLOGY

Potency Versus Efficacy
The distinction between potency and efficacy is helpful to an understanding of the pharmacology of antipsychotic drugs. **Efficacy** refers to the therapeutic **benefits** that can be achieved by a drug, whereas **potency** describes the **amount** of the drug needed to achieve the therapeutic effect. All of the first-generation antipsychotic drugs are equivalent in efficacy, meaning that at an optimal dosage, which differs for each drug (Table 2.2), each of the older drugs has been found to be equally efficacious in treating psychotic disorders. A useful generalization about the older antipsychotic drugs is that those with low potency (which means that they must be given in higher doses) tend to be more sedating, tend to be more anticholinergic, and tend to cause more postural hypotension than the high-potency drugs. The high-potency drugs tend to cause more EPS.

Clozapine is the only drug that has convincingly shown **greater efficacy** than the older drugs. A pivotal trial conducted in patients with schizophrenia who had been unresponsive to at least two different antipsychotic drugs found significant improvement (defined as a modest 20% reduction in the rating scale) in 30% of 126 patients treated with clozapine for 6 weeks compared with only 5% of 141 patients treated with chlorpromazine. Clinical experience and meta-analyses have amply confirmed the results of this well-designed trial; that is, clozapine may effectively treat patients who do not respond to other antipsychotic drugs. For other second-generation drugs, there are both positive and negative trials showing greater efficacy than haloperidol in treatment-refractory patients, but the margin of superiority, if it exists, is not great. The only clear benefit of the second-generation drugs is the relative lack of EPS.

Absorption and Distribution
Traditional antipsychotic drugs are available for both oral and parenteral use, whereas second-generation drugs until recently have only been available for oral use. Parenteral short-acting formulations of second-generation antipsychotic drugs are available for ziprasidone, aripiprazole, and olanzapine and may become available for others (Table 2.3). The pharmacokinetics of the first-generation drugs are well understood only for a few (especially chlorpromazine, thioridazine, and haloperidol), because of the complexity of active and inactive metabolites. Taken orally, the drugs are absorbed adequately, although somewhat variably. Food or antacids may decrease absorption. **Ziprasidone,** however, is to be **taken with food,** which doubles the amount of absorbed drug. Liquid preparations are absorbed more rapidly and reliably than tablets. There is a marked first-pass effect through the liver with oral administration (i.e., a high percentage of the drug is metabolized as it passes through the hepatic portal circulation). The peak effect of an oral dose generally occurs within 2 to 4 hours.

Parenterally administered antipsychotics are rapidly and reliably absorbed. Drug effect is usually apparent within 15 to 20 minutes after intramuscular (i.m.) injection, with peak effect occurring within 30 to 60 minutes. With intravenous (i.v.) administration, some drug effect is apparent within minutes, and peak effect occurs within 20 to 30 minutes. [The i.v. administration of antipsychotic drugs has

TABLE 2.2 First-Generation Antipsychotic Drugs: Relative Potencies and Side-Effect Profiles

Drug	Approximate Dose Equivalent (mg)	Sedative Effect	Hypotensive Effect	Anticholinergic Effect	Extrapyramidal Effect
Phenothiazines					
Aliphatic					
Chlorpromazine (Thorazine)	100	High	High	Medium	Low
Piperidines					
Thioridazine (Mellaril)	95	High	High	High	Low
Piperazines					
Fluphenazine (Prolixin, Permitil)	2	Medium	Low	Low	High
Perphenazine (Trilafon)	8	Low	Low	Low	High
Trifluoperazine (Stelazine)	5	Medium	Low	Low	High
Thioxanthene					
Thiothixene (Navane)	5	Low	Low	Low	High
Dibenzodiazepines					
Loxapine (Loxitane, Daxolin)	10	Medium	Medium	Medium	Medium
Benzisoxazole					
Risperidone (Risperdal)	1–2	Low	Medium	Low	Medium
Butyrophenones					
Droperidol (Inapsin–injection only)	1	Low	Low	Low	High
Haloperidol (Haldol)	2	Low	Low	Low	High
Indolone					
Molindone (Moban)	10	Medium	Low	Medium	High
Diphenylbutylpiperidine					
Pimozide (Orap)	1	Low	Low	Low	High

11

Drug	Tablets (mg)	Capsules (mg)	Sustained Release Forms (mg)	Liquid Concentrate[a]	Liquid Suspension[a] or Elixir	Syrup[a] (mg/5 mL)	Injection[b]
Phenothiazines							
Aliphatics							
Chlorpromazine (Thorazine, generics)	10, 25, 50, 100, 200		30, 75, 150, 200, 300	30 mg/mL, 100 mg/mL		10 mg/5 mL	25 mg/mL, 10 mg/mL
Piperidines							
Thioridazine (Mellaril, generics)	10, 15, 25, 50, 100, 150, 200			30 mg/mL, 100 mg/mL	25 mg/5 mL, 100 mg/5 mL		
Piperazines							
Fluphenazine HCl (Prolixin, Permitil, generics)	1, 2.5, 5, 10			5 mg/mL	0.5 mg/1 mL, 2.5 mg/5 mL		2.5 mg/mL
Fluphenazine enanthate, decanoate (Prolixin)							25 mg/mL, 5 mg/mL
Perphenazine (Trilafon, generics)	2, 4, 8, 16			16 mg/5 mL			5 mg/mL
Trifluoperazine (Stelazine, generics)	1, 2, 5, 10			10 mg/mL			2 mg/mL
Thioxanthene							
Thiothixene (Navane, generics)		1, 2, 5, 10, 20		5 mg/mL			2 mg/mL, 5 mg/mL
Dibenzodiazepines							
Loxapine (Loxitane, generics)		5, 10, 25, 50		25 mg/mL			50 mg/mL
Clozapine (Clozaril)	25, 100						
Benzisoxazole							
Risperidone (Risperdal)	0.25, 0.5, 1, 2, 3, 4				1 mg/mL (oral solution)		
(Risperdal M-tab [oral disintegrating tablet])	0.5, 1, 2						
(Risperdal Consta)		25	37.5 mg				50 mg/2 mL

Class / Generic (Brand)	Tablet/Capsule (mg)	Liquid[a]	Parenteral[b]
Paliperidone (Invega)	3, 6, 9		
Butyrophenone			
Haloperidol (Haldol, generics)	0.5, 1, 2, 5, 10, 20	2 mg/mL	5 mg/mL
Thienobenzodiazepine			
Olanzapine (Zyprexa)	2.5, 5, 7.5, 10, 15, 20		10 mg/mL
(Zyprexa Zydis)	5, 10, 15, 20		
Dibenzothiazepine			
Quetiapine (Seroquel)	25, 50, 100, 200, 300, 400		
Quetiapine XL (Seroquel XL)	200, 300, 400		
Haloperidol decanoate (Haldol)			50 mg/mL, 100 mg/mL
Indolone			
Molindone (Moban)	5, 10, 25, 50, 100	20 mg/mL	
Diphenylbutylpiperidine			
Pimozide (Orap)	2		
Benzisothiazolylpiperazine			
Ziprasidone (Geodon)	20, 40, 60, 80		20 mg/mL
Quinolinone			
Aripiprazole (Abilify)	2, 5, 10, 15, 20, 30	1 mg/mL (150 mL)	9.75 mg/1.3 mL

[a] Liquid form for oral use.
[b] Parenteral form, which is packaged in either vial or ampule.

not been approved by the Food and Drug Administration (FDA). The haloperidol-like drug droperidol is approved for i.v. use for perioperative nausea and vomiting, although it is not marketed as an antipsychotic drug.] Because parenteral administration bypasses the first pass through the portal circulation, it results in a significantly higher serum level of the parent drug than equivalent oral dosages.

Antipsychotic drugs are generally highly protein bound (85% to 90%). Clinicians have traditionally been cautioned when concomitantly treating patients with other medications that are highly protein bound (e.g., warfarin, digoxin) because of the expectation that displacement and competition for these binding sites could increase concentrations of free or unbound antipsychotics and other drugs. Antipsychotics are also highly lipophilic; thus, they readily cross the blood–brain barrier and attain high concentrations in the brain. Indeed, concentrations in the brain appear to be greater than those in blood. Given their high degree of protein and tissue binding, these drugs are not removed efficiently by dialysis.

Metabolism and Elimination

Many antipsychotic drugs are metabolized in the liver to demethylated and hydroxylated forms. These are more water soluble than the parent compounds and thus more readily excreted by the kidneys. The hydroxylated metabolites often are further metabolized by conjugation with glucuronic acid. Many of the hydroxyl and desmethyl metabolites of phenothiazines are active as dopamine receptor antagonists. The hydroxyl metabolite of the butyrophenone antipsychotic drug haloperidol (hydroxyhaloperidol) does not appear to be active. The 9-hydroxyrisperidone metabolite of risperidone, paliperidone (Invega), is marketed as a separate antipsychotic. Much remains unknown about the metabolites of other chemical classes of antipsychotics.

The elimination half-life of most of the first-generation antipsychotic drugs is 18 to 40 hours, but numerous factors, such as genetically determined metabolic rates, age, and the coadministration of other hepatically metabolized drugs, affect the half-life to such a degree that plasma levels may vary among individuals by 10- to 20-fold. The elimination half-life of several of the second-generation antipsychotics (quetiapine, ziprasidone, risperidone) is less than 12 hours, whereas the elimination half-life of **aripiprazole** is approximately **3 days.**

Long-Acting Preparations

Long-acting preparations of **haloperidol** and **fluphenazine** are available in which the active drug is esterified to a lipid side chain. The drug is given as an i.m. injection in an oily vehicle (sesame oil) that slows absorption. The only first-generation preparations currently available in the United States are the decanoate ester of fluphenazine and the decanoate ester of haloperidol. Fluphenazine decanoate has a half-life of 7 to 10 days, allowing administration approximately every 2 weeks, although some patients may tolerate longer spacing of the injections. Haloperidol decanoate has a longer half-life, allowing dosing intervals of 3 to 6 weeks, depending on the individual. Long-acting preparations of second-generation drugs are in development for several drugs, and **risperidone** (Consta) is available in the United States and Europe. This preparation, using microspheres as the vehicle, has a half-life of 7 days, allowing for injections every 2 weeks. A long-acting preparation of olanzapine is under review by the FDA (though will likely be unapproved because of problematic sedation), and a long-acting preparation of paliperidone is being developed.

Blood Levels

Given the marked interindividual differences in plasma levels produced by a given oral dose and the concerns about the consequences of noncompliance among psychotic patients, it would be useful to have some objective measure of drug level to aid in optimizing efficacy and clinical improvement. Specifically, it has been hoped that a range of therapeutic blood levels could be determined for the various antipsychotic drugs. Unfortunately, the measurement of blood levels by various chromatographic techniques and mass spectroscopy has not correlated that well with clinical response, though there is a role for monitoring olanzapine and clozapine. For olanzapine, there is preliminary evidence of a relationship between clinical outcomes and plasma concentrations. A therapeutic range of 20 to 50 ng/mL has been suggested for olanzapine. For clozapine, there appears to be a threshold concentration for response, at approximately 350 ng/mL, although one study found a range of 200 to 300 ng/mL as effective as plasma concentrations above 350 ng/mL. Higher concentrations are associated with more toxicity and electroencephalographic changes. Some antipsychotic drugs have so many active metabolites (e.g., thioridazine) that measurement to assess dose–response relationships is impractical. Thus, clinical observation and documentation of specific symptom changes over time remain the mainstays of assessment of drug efficacy, although plasma levels can still be useful to determine extreme concentrations (close to zero or very high), suggesting either nonadherence or unusual metabolism.

MECHANISM OF ACTION

The therapeutic mechanism of action of the antipsychotic drugs is only partly understood. The first-generation (e.g., haloperidol-like) antipsychotic drugs and the second-generation drugs risperidone, paliperidone, ziprasidone, and aripiprazole are all potent antagonists of D_2 dopamine receptors. On the other hand, clozapine and quetiapine are weak D_2 antagonists, and by positron emission tomography, they show significantly lower levels of D_2 receptor occupancy at effective doses, compared with the haloperidol-like drugs. A common property of second-generation antipsychotic drugs is the ability to block serotonin 5-HT_{2A} receptors. Olanzapine, risperidone, aripiprazole, and ziprasidone do so with high affinity; quetiapine has relatively lower affinity for all its receptor targets (Table 2.1). The second-generation drugs interact with a variety of other serotonin receptors but not with any obvious pattern. All but quetiapine have high affinity for 5-HT_{2C} receptors; all but risperidone have high affinity for 5-HT_6 receptors; risperidone has a particularly high affinity for the 5-HT_7 receptor. All of the second-generation antipsychotics antagonize α_1-adrenergic receptors and histamine H_1 receptors, which may contribute to side effects. Both clozapine and olanzapine are strongly anticholinergic.

This **complex picture of binding properties makes it difficult to pinpoint the mechanism of action.** D_2 receptor antagonism correlates well with both efficacy and EPS liability for the first-generation (haloperidol-like) antipsychotic drugs. In addition, blockade of 5-HT_{2A} receptors appears to correlate with diminished EPS liability. Drugs that antagonize only 5-HT_{2A} receptors, however, do not have antipsychotic properties. Given that clozapine exhibits a high ratio of D_4 antagonism to D_2 antagonism, there was much excitement about a possible role for D_4 antagonists as antipsychotic drugs. However, relatively selective D_4 antagonists, as well as a mixed D_4 and 5-HT_{2A} antagonist (fananserin), have not shown antipsychotic efficacy.

To date it appears that blockade of D_2 receptors in the targets of mesolimbic and mesocortical dopamine projections from the ventral tegmental area is responsible for initiating the therapeutic actions of first-generation antipsychotic drugs and likely for the clozapine-like drugs that exhibit lower D_2 affinity. D_2 blockade in the striatum is responsible for the extrapyramidal effects of the typical antipsychotic drugs (Fig. 2.1). In addition to these midbrain dopamine systems, there is a dopamine projection in the tuberoinfundibular system of the hypothalamus. In this system, dopamine acts as an inhibitor of the synthesis and release of prolactin by pituitary lactotrophs. By antagonizing dopamine in this system, antipsychotic

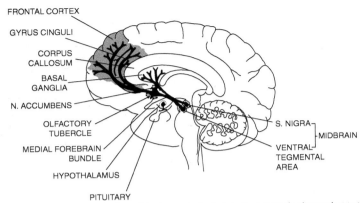

FIGURE 2.1 Dopamine projections of the human brain. Cells in the substantia nigra project to the basal ganglia; cells in the ventral tegmental area of the midbrain project to the frontal cortex and limbic areas. Hypothalamic dopamine neurons project to the pituitary.

drugs with strong D_2 antagonist properties often produce hyperprolactinemia. The key to the increased efficacy of clozapine, despite low affinity for the dopamine D_2 receptors, remains unknown.

The full therapeutic effects of antipsychotic drugs take weeks to accrue (similar to the antidepressants) and are far slower than the time required to block central nervous system (CNS) receptors or, in most cases, to achieve steady-state plasma levels of the drug. Similarly, behavioral effects in patients can last long after serum levels are no longer detectable. Such observations suggest that the therapeutic response to antipsychotic drugs is a **secondary or adaptive response to receptor blockade** with a time course characterized by slower onset and offset than would be predicted by serum or even brain levels. (D_2 receptor occupancy in the human brain may now be measured experimentally from positron emission tomography.) In as much as some initially responsive patients relapse even with apparently adequate serum levels of drugs, other types of adaptations may occur in the brain, reflecting such factors as primary alterations in the disease process, changes in the psychosocial circumstances of the patient's life, intercurrent psychiatric or physical illness, or drug tolerance. The therapeutically relevant delayed-onset neurobiologic effects of antipsychotic drugs remain unknown but are believed to reflect drug-activated changes in **gene expression, protein synthesis, and subsequent synaptic reorganization.** However, there is clearly an early response to antipsychotics as well, and acutely ill patient can show benefit after a few doses. This suggests another hypothesis for the apparent delayed response to antipsychotics. Perhaps once D_2 is sufficiently blocked, psychosis starts to recede. The full resolution of psychosis, however, occurs only if patients deconstruct their psychotic worldview. This psychological process of course takes time and might have led to the somewhat incorrect view that antipsychotics take weeks to show an effect.

In addition to their effects on dopamine receptors, antipsychotic drugs may cause side effects by binding to a variety of other neurotransmitter receptors. For example, low-potency conventional antipsychotic drugs are potent antagonists of muscarinic cholinergic receptors with highest relative affinity for thioridazine followed by chlorpromazine. Among the second-generation drugs, clozapine and olanzapine also have substantial **anticholinergic** potency. As a result, these drugs can produce side effects such as dry mouth and constipation. **Postural hypotension** is produced by antagonism of α_1-adrenergic receptors. Antipsychotic drugs with substantial affinity for this receptor include many first-generation compounds, especially chlorpromazine and thioridazine. Haloperidol, however, has very little propensity for antagonism of α_1-adrenergic receptors. Several of the second-generation antipsychotics, especially risperidone and quetiapine, have substantial affinity for α_1-adrenergic receptors and may cause orthostatic hypotension.

Sedation appears to result from antagonism of several neurotransmitter receptors, including α_1-adrenergic, muscarinic, and histamine H_1 receptors. Because of substantial affinity for these receptor types, low-potency antipsychotics, such as chlorpromazine and thioridazine, and all the second-generation drugs can be sedating (particularly clozapine, olanzapine, and quetiapine). **Weight gain** is a significant consequence of certain second-generation antipsychotics, particularly for clozapine and olanzapine. Weight gain is less problematic with ziprasidone and aripiprazole. The mechanism of weight gain is unknown and may be multifactorial. Blockade of histamine H_1 receptors and increases in plasma leptin or insulin levels are currently being investigated as possible mechanisms. New-onset diabetes or worsening of existing diabetes may occur with clozapine or olanzapine and sometimes with other antipsychotic drugs. In addition, many antipsychotic drugs block certain calcium channels on neurons, cardiac muscle, and smooth muscle.

Glutamate receptors may also be involved in antipsychotics' mechanism of action, though their involvement remains poorly understood. The hypothesized contribution of glutamate to the symptoms of psychosis is largely derived from pharmacologic studies that find that the N-methyl-D-aspartate glutamate antagonist phenylcyclidine induces a clinical syndrome similar to schizophrenia and may exacerbate psychosis in patients with schizophrenia. Because the N-methyl-D-aspartate receptor requires the presence of glutamate and the co-agonist glycine for effective gating, studies have been done with glycine agonists such as D-cycloserine, though these have been disappointing. On the other hand, a recent study of a drug under development finds that a drug (LY 404039) that is an agonist at metabotropic glutamate receptors, but does not antagonize dopamine receptors, was clinically superior to placebo for treating schizophrenia. This drug, however, was less effective than olanzapine in this trial. This promising study may open a new line of investigation into drugs that do not directly affect dopamine receptors.

LONG-TERM TREATMENT OF SCHIZOPHRENIA

Many studies have proven that long-term treatment with antipsychotic drugs increases the time between exacerbations among schizophrenic patients who respond to short-term treatment. The **relapse rate** for schizophrenic patients who are not on maintenance antipsychotic drugs may be as high as 50% at 6 months and 65% to 80% at 12 months, whereas for those maintained on antipsychotic drugs, the relapse rate may be 10% to 15% at 6 months and no higher than 25% at 12 months. Given the disorder's morbidity, most patients with well-diagnosed schizophrenia will have net benefit from long-term maintenance treatment. Intermittent treatment is problematic in patients with chronic psychosis but might be a possibility in selected patients who can recognize the beginning of a new episode. Because long-term treatment with typical antipsychotic drugs brings with it the risk of TD, the clinician should carefully consider the risks and benefits of using the older drugs over time with each patient.

Some patients with refractory symptoms have been treated with high antipsychotic drug doses (more than the equivalent of 20 mg per day of haloperidol), often more reflective of physician frustration than appropriate therapy. There is **no evidence of extra benefit at very high doses** of antipsychotic drugs, although side effects are clearly worsened. Currently, for patients who have failed to respond to adequate doses of several antipsychotic drugs, including atypical drugs, a trial of clozapine is indicated. As described previously, clozapine is the only antipsychotic drug that has been convincingly shown to be effective for substantial numbers of patients with schizophrenia who have proved refractory to other antipsychotic drugs.

THERAPEUTIC USE

Choosing an Antipsychotic Drug

The first-generation antipsychotics provided a breakthrough for previously untreatable psychosis. They, however, presented significant acute neurological side effects and often left patients with the telltale sign of TD. With the second-generation antipsychotics, the problem of neurological toxicity appeared to have been resolved, and these drugs even appeared to be somewhat more effective, but over time it appears that the field's enthusiasm has been premature: **second-generation antipsychotics are probably only as effective as first-generation antipsychotics.** Moreover, some second-generation antipsychotics can cause extrapyramidal side effects, and others often lead to weight gain, hyperlipidemia, and insulin resistance. Hence, despite the near-total switch to the second-generation antipsychotics and the tremendous increase in costs, the overall advantages of the second-generation to the first-generation antipsychotics appear minor.

The second-generation antipsychotics have a lower incidence of EPS symptoms such as dystonia, tremor, stiffness and rigidity, akathisia, and altered affect, as well as greatly diminished risk of neuroleptic malignant syndrome (NMS) and TD. Second-generation antipsychotics are the most commonly used antipsychotics as the initial drug for a first episode, though this practice may be supported by the widespread belief of their superiority rather than by solid evidence confirming their superiority. Indeed, two large-scale effectiveness studies, one in the United States and one in Britain, that compared first- and second-generation antipsychotics found minor effectiveness differences between older and newer antipsychotics in real-world settings. In the British study, second-generation antipsychotics were no better than first-generation antipsychotics over the 1-year study period, and patients failed to express a preference between drug classes. In the U.S. study, perphenazine appeared marginally less effective than olanzapine, and similar to risperidone, ziprasidone, and quetiapine. Many suggest that the metabolic burden of olanzapine limits its long-term use. The wide uptake of these drugs may have been due to marketing and expectations of clozapine-type results rather than to true clinical advantages.

Although clozapine heralded a new era in the pharmacotherapy of psychosis, particularly with neuroleptic-resistant patients and other subpopulations (e.g., patients with Parkinson's disease), the risk of agranulocytosis complicated the use of this agent. The efficacy of clozapine for both positive and negative symptoms in acute and chronic schizophrenia is an additional feature of this compound and demonstrated that the effective treatment of psychoses was not inexorably linked with EPS. This observation prompted the search for similar compounds without the hematologic side effect.

All of the compounds approved as antipsychotic drugs in the United States are efficacious. Clozapine is more effective than the others in the treatment of schizophrenia. The second-generation antipsychotic drugs differ only in their potency (the dosage needed to produce the desired effect) and side effects. Among the older antipsychotics, drugs that are most potent tend to produce more EPS and those

1 haloperidol 2 mg → 100 CPZ

that are less potent produce more sedation, postural hypotension, and anticholinergic effects (Table 2.2). For example, 8 mg of haloperidol and 400 mg of chlorpromazine are equivalent regarding antipsychotic efficacy; however, the patient receiving haloperidol would be more likely to develop EPS, and the patient taking chlorpromazine would be more likely to feel sedated and to develop postural hypotension. The first-generation compounds are more likely to induce EPS than the second-generation compounds, though all of the second-generation drugs, particularly risperidone and aripiprazole, can cause EPS. In addition, they **all can cause sedation and postural hypotension** and, except possibly ziprasidone and aripiprazole, can cause weight gain (particularly clozapine and olanzapine). Among the newer agents, risperidone and paliperidone are especially likely to elevate plasma prolactin, whereas the other second-generation agents are rarely associated with prolactinemia. Aripiprazole can even lower prolactin levels. With the exception of clozapine in treatment-refractory schizophrenia, because there is no established difference in the therapeutic effectiveness of these drugs, side-effect profiles are a central consideration when starting a patient on antipsychotic treatment.

A patient who has responded well to a particular psychotropic drug in the past is likely to do well on the same drug again. On the other hand, even if a patient has no history of severe EPS or other troublesome side effects with a particular **first generation** antipsychotic, the physician should consider initiating therapy with a newer compound that would have considerably less or no EPS or risk of TD over the long term. In considering the acute advantages offered by more sedating agents (e.g., for the young patient with severe insomnia), the clinician could also consider the acute use of a less sedating compound combined with temporary use of a benzodiazepine (e.g., lorazepam or clonazepam) to achieve sedation so that when the acute episode passes, the sedation can be dissected from the treatment by stopping the hypnotic medication if desired. For example, although olanzapine may allow for greater sedation in acute treatment than ziprasidone or aripiprazole, long-term use of olanzapine may lead to daytime sedation and weight gain, whereas ziprasidone or aripiprazole may be better tolerated over the long term.

For certain groups of patients, **toxic effects determine drugs to avoid.** Common examples are as follows: (a) patients with cardiac conduction problems should avoid pimozide; (b) patients with Parkinson's disease should avoid high-potency antipsychotics; (c) patients with diabetes should generally avoid clozapine or olanzapine; and (d) clozapine should be administered only to patients who are adequately compliant so that they will comply with frequent blood drawing.

Use of Antipsychotic Drugs
Because antipsychotic drugs can produce striking changes in the thinking, language, and behavior (including motor behavior) of the patients who receive them, a **thorough examination of physical and mental status** should be performed before initiating therapy. In psychotic disorders, the mental status may fluctuate markedly; thus, on occasion a brief initial period of drug-free observation may be helpful for the hospitalized patient when the diagnosis is unclear. A reliable history must always supplement the mental status examination. In all cases, but especially when the diagnosis is unclear, it is important to objectively rate target symptoms that can be monitored throughout the treatment with antipsychotic drugs. The physician must have a clear notion of the symptoms that are likely to respond specifically to antipsychotic drugs and the symptoms (e.g., anxiety) that may be better treated by other classes of drugs.

The latency of response of psychotic symptoms such as delusions, hallucinations, and bizarre behavior is usually several days, with nonspecific sedation occurring more rapidly. The full benefit in antipsychotic-responsive disorders usually takes at least 2 to 6 weeks. Unfortunately, physicians are often impatient in treating psychoses given the level of patient and family distress and the pressure of disruptive behavior on the inpatient unit. **Thus, premature dosage increases occur,** and when symptoms finally remit, the time course of improvement is often mistaken for a requirement for high doses of antipsychotic drugs. Aripiprazole has a half-life of 3 days, and dose adjustments during a brief hospitalization would not even be apparent until after hospital discharge. If dangerous behavior must be rapidly controlled, the physician may choose to increase the antipsychotic drug dosage temporarily to exploit its nonspecific sedative properties or perhaps more wisely choose to use an adjunctive benzodiazepine as needed. Valproate can be added to reduce agitation in acute psychosis, although it has no benefit in the long run for patients with schizophrenia. In either case, once the acute symptoms subside, extra medications administered for sedation should be tapered and an optimal antipsychotic drug dosage established.

Switching Antipsychotic Drugs

Many patients switch antipsychotics, whether from lack of efficacy or side-effect problems. The debate as to whether to switch stable patients on older antipsychotics to newer agents is unfortunately not yet informed by data as to which populations will benefit most from changing their medication. Studies conflict over the relative benefits or tolerability of second-generation compared with first-generation antipsychotics. A recent nationwide practical clinical trial [Clinical Antipsychotic Trials of Intervention Effectiveness (CATIE) study] found that few patients persisted on antipsychotics over an 18-month period, and perphenazine, when combined with an anticholinergic agent, was tolerated by patients as well as second-generation antipsychotics. In the cost-sensitive environment of managed health care, the significantly higher (sometimes 10-fold) cost of a regimen of second-generation drugs versus traditional compounds raises questions about the cost effectiveness of switching. **Some fundamental points can be made presently regarding the question of switching a patient's regimen.**

In the outpatient setting, the clinician should consider a switch if the patient is not doing well on an older antipsychotic medication and is able to comply with oral medication (accepts illness and can recognize symptomatic worsening) and if there is family support for such a change. Before switching, the clinician should be certain that the patient is taking the drug. Learning from family or the patient that the patient is not taking the drug allows a more reasoned decision. The switch should generally be made slowly, tapering the previous drug while titrating the first. In our experience, some patients may have a relapse if the change happens too abruptly. However, most switches can be accomplished in about 1 month to avoid the phenomenon of "stalled taper." A switch should not be executed to an oral second-generation antipsychotic if compliance dictates use of a long-acting preparation. Patients who are not compliant with oral medication may be switched to depot haloperidol or depot fluphenazine if either of those parent drugs was known to be well tolerated and effective when taken. On the other hand, nonadherent patients known to respond to risperidone or not tolerate first-generation antipsychotics are candidates for a trial of long-acting risperidone. Switching between second-generation antipsychotics happens frequently. Changes often happen because of side effects, but sometimes patients' symptoms are poorly maintained on an individual drug. If medication adherence is clear, then a switch may help patients who are not doing well. A common scenario finds that patients improve from acute use with olanzapine, but following significant weight gain or persisting sedation, they require a switch to another agent.

In the inpatient setting, a history of nonresponse or partial response on traditional antipsychotics and a clear history of compliance with oral medication are factors that should encourage a switch to a second-generation compound. If the patient has a history of excellent response to a traditional drug, may not comply with an oral regimen, or requires a depot preparation, or if the side-effect profile of the second-generation drug is more challenging (e.g., an angina patient unable to tolerate hypotensive effects), a switch to newer medication could be less advantageous. Generally, patients with chronic schizophrenia who are doing well, without TD or EPS, and are stable on a traditional medication most probably can remain on their regimen. Patients who are not doing well on a traditional compound, are relatively unstable on traditional treatment, are having difficulty with EPS, and are able to comply with oral medicines should be given a trial course of newer drugs. Keep in mind that the newer drugs may not have as much EPS, but they may contribute new problems of sedation, weight gain, dyslipidemia, or insulin resistance.

Specific Clinical Situations

In the treatment of any psychotic disorder, certain paradigmatic situations arise, each requiring a distinct approach to the use of antipsychotic drugs. These include (a) acute psychoses in which the symptoms may constitute a medical emergency, (b) long-term treatment aimed at minimizing residual symptoms or prophylaxis of recurrent psychosis, and (c) use of antipsychotics on an as-needed basis.

Acute Psychosis

When a patient with known or suspected schizophrenia develops an exacerbation of psychotic symptoms, it is important to **consider all possible causes.** These include worsening course of illness (despite medication), noncompliance with medication, a superimposed medical disorder, a superimposed mood disorder, drug abuse, psychosocial crises, or toxic effects of the antipsychotic drugs (especially akathisia or neuroleptic-induced catatonia). If the exacerbation involves florid psychotic symptoms, the treatment is the same as that for acute psychosis. Identification of the cause for the exacerbation is helpful in the treatment of acute relapse and is necessary for long-term planning. If **noncompliance** is the problem, it is often helpful for the physician to explore with the patient the reasons for avoiding medication. If the physician and patient agree that compliance could be improved with injectable drug preparations, the use of long-acting depot preparations may be indicated. If drug abuse or an intercurrent medical or psychiatric illness (e.g., depression) is to blame, disorder-specific treatment is necessary. Failure to address psychosocial factors in relapse (e.g., family problems or lack of an adequate living situation) will predispose the patient to further difficulties.

Acute psychosis is a clinical syndrome that may be caused by a wide variety of disorders (Table 2.4), and it typically presents in patients with a rapid onset (days to weeks) of psychotic symptoms (e.g., hallucinations, delusions, ideas of reference), agitation, insomnia, and often hostility or combativeness. It is important to rule out acute medical illness by obtaining as much history as possible, monitoring vital signs, performing a physical examination, and ordering necessary laboratory work.

During an acute presentation (having excluded a medical disorder), it may still be difficult to make a definitive psychiatric diagnosis. Because a diagnosis cannot be made from mental status alone and because acutely psychotic patients often have difficulties relating their story, a definitive diagnosis may be difficult to establish immediately. To make a diagnosis, the following factors need to be considered:

1. Clinical presentation
2. Medical history, including any prescription or other drug use
3. Physical examination and any relevant laboratory tests
4. Psychiatric history

TABLE 2.4	Causes of Acute Psychotic Syndromes
Major psychiatric disorders	Acute exacerbation of schizophrenia Atypical psychoses (e.g., schizophreniform) Depression with psychotic features Mania
Drug abuse and withdrawal	Alcohol withdrawal Amphetamines and cocaine Phencyclidine and hallucinogens Sedative-hypnotic withdrawal
Prescription drugs	Anticholinergic agents Digitalis toxicity Glucocorticoids and adrenocorticotropic hormone Isoniazid L-Dopa and other dopamine agonists Nonsteroidal antiinflammatory agents Withdrawal from monoamine oxidase inhibitors
Other toxic agents	Carbon disulfide Heavy metals
Neurologic causes	AIDS encephalopathy Brain tumor Complex partial seizures Early Alzheimer's or Pick's disease Huntington's disease Hypoxic encephalopathy Infectious viral encephalitis Lupus cerebritis Neurosyphilis Stroke Wilson's disease
Metabolic causes	Acute intermittent porphyria Cushing's syndrome Early hepatic encephalopathy Hypo- and hypercalcemia Hypoglycemia Hypo- and hyperthyroidism Paraneoplastic syndromes
Nutritional causes	Niacin deficiency (pellagra) Thiamine deficiency (Wernicke–Korsakoff syndrome) Vitamin B_{12} deficiency

5. Mental status examination
6. Baseline of premorbid functioning
7. Time course of onset of symptoms and overall duration of illness
8. History of prior treatment response, especially to traditional antipsychotics, antidepressants, lithium, or electroconvulsive therapy
9. Family history of psychiatric or neurologic disorders

When patients are extremely agitated, combative, or hyperactive, it may be necessary to **begin treatment before a definitive diagnosis can be made.** Fortunately, most acute primary psychotic disorders, and many psychoses secondary to medical and neurologic disorders, respond to antipsychotic drug treatment regardless of the specific disorder. Optimal long-term treatment requires that a correct diagnosis be made. In addition, it is important to identify conditions that might be worsened by some or all of the antipsychotic agents (e.g., low-potency antipsychotic drugs may worsen symptoms of phencyclidine toxicity or anticholinergic delirium; catatonic states may be caused by neuroleptic toxicity in some patients).

Because acutely psychotic patients are potentially dangerous to themselves and others, even if not immediately agitated or threatening, rapid treatment is an important goal. For the clinician, the question is which antipsychotic and what dose should be used?

The second-generation antipsychotics, despite sobering nonpharmaceutical sponsored prospective studies that question their clear superiority over the older drugs, remain the most commonly selected treatments for a variety of psychoses. Any one of the newer antipsychotics is a reasonable first-line treatment of new-onset psychosis, whether schizophrenia or concomitant symptoms of another illness (i.e., bipolar disorder, acute psychotic disorder). It would also be reasonable to use an older drug in combination with an anticholinergic agent, particularly if there are cost issues or a past known response to an older agent. Their efficacy in well-controlled trials over 4 to 20 weeks is well established; the latency to full antipsychotic effect in the 75% of patients who respond remains approximately 2 to 4 weeks. If there is **insufficient control of agitated behavior,** it is recommended that additional dosing with a benzodiazepine (e.g., lorazepam, usually as needed 1 to 2 mg per 4 to 6 hours) be used over the course of the first week. The addition of a high-potency conventional antipsychotic (e.g., haloperidol) should be reserved for patients whose symptoms are not controlled with these two medications. Haloperidol is often used as adjunctive treatment with the second-generation drugs for patients who are particularly agitated or have a history of responding to a specific antipsychotic. Acute, sometimes life-threatening syndromes such as **NMS or acute dystonic reactions are far less likely with the newer compounds.** Evidence to date suggests a low likelihood of TD. Following the acute phase of either a first episode of psychotic illness or exacerbation of a chronic disorder, the goal is eventual monotherapy with a single drug.

Optimal dosing of the older agents in schizophrenia and schizoaffective disorder has been addressed in several studies. In one study, patients were treated with fixed doses of haloperidol (5, 10, or 20 mg per day) for 4 weeks. The 20-mg dose was superior to the 5-mg dose throughout the trial and was marginally superior to the 10-mg dose after the first 2 weeks of treatment. By the second week, however, the group given 20 mg per day experienced symptomatic worsening with respect to blunted affect, motor retardation, and emotional withdrawal. In addition, a significantly higher percentage of patients on the 20-mg dose left the hospital against medical advice than those on lower doses, suggesting that, at high doses, toxicity of typical antipsychotics outweighs benefits. Some studies show efficacy of haloperidol as low as 2.5 mg per day. In general, haloperidol has been used at excessive doses, and it often works well at low doses although large interindividual variability makes haloperidol dosing difficult. In addition, many comparison studies with second-generation antipsychotics employed high doses of haloperidol, often without anticholinergic agents, thereby establishing a tolerability imbalance. If a high-potency traditional antipsychotic drug is used, an anticholinergic drug should be added as prophylaxis against EPS and dystonia; benztropine mesylate, 2 mg twice a day (b.i.d.), may be used. Evidence from various studies has demonstrated that such a regimen decreases the incidence of acute dystonia, which is a problem particularly in individuals younger than 40 years. If anticholinergic side effects become a problem, the dosage can be decreased to benztropine 1 mg b.i.d.

Treatment studies with all newer antipsychotic drugs have shown that their efficacy for acute psychosis is at least equivalent to that of traditional compounds, with 4 to 6 mg per day of risperidone, 6 mg per day of paliperidone, 10 to 20 mg per day of olanzapine, 600 mg per day of quetiapine, 160 mg per day of ziprasidone, or 15 mg per day of aripiprazole being reasonable doses to target.

It should be recognized that a substantial number of patients with schizophrenia will not benefit from first-line antipsychotic drugs. For these patients, very high doses are more likely to produce more side effects than therapeutic benefit. Schizophrenic patients who have been unresponsive to two or more adequate trials (8 to 12 weeks on therapeutic doses) of antipsychotic drugs should be considered for a trial of clozapine. Approaches to refractory mania are discussed in Chapter 4.

At the recommended doses of antipsychotic drugs, many patients will remain agitated in the short term. Therefore, in acute psychoses, in addition to effective doses of an antipsychotic drug, short-term use of benzodiazepines may be required. Lorazepam, which has a relatively short half-life, has no active metabolites, is well absorbed intramuscularly, and is a good choice. Other clinicians prefer the longer-acting benzodiazepine clonazepam, which has the disadvantage of lacking a parenteral form. Lorazepam, 1 to 2 mg orally or i.m., or clonazepam, 0.5 to 1.0 mg orally, could be given every 2 hours as needed to calm an agitated patient. Benzodiazepines appear to be relatively free of dangerous side effects if used carefully in the short term but should be avoided with clozapine. The physician should monitor the course of psychotic symptoms over the first 2 weeks of treatment, being alert to the fact that as the acute psychosis improves, the requirement of adjunctive benzodiazepine is likely to decrease. **It is recommended that the sedative drug be tapered as agitation subsides.**

Long-Term Use

Because most patients for whom antipsychotic drugs are effective have chronic or relapsing illnesses, long-term use of these drugs is usually indicated. Because with first-generation antipsychotic drugs the danger of producing TD is significant, the clinician should continually monitor the duration of treatment and consider alternative treatments whenever possible. Because a number of the second-generation antipsychotics are associated with weight gain, dyslipidemias, and diabetes, the clinician must carefully monitor for these metabolic side effects. See Table 2.5 for suggested monitoring.

Long-Acting Preparations. When patients with schizophrenia or other chronic psychoses relapse because of noncompliance, consideration should be given to the use of long-acting antipsychotic preparations. Of course, in some patients, non-

TABLE 2.5	Metabolic Monitoring for Second-Generation Antipsychotics
Measure	**Frequency**
Weight	Each visit
Blood pressure	Baseline + quarterly
Lipids	Baseline, 3 months, annually
Glucose (A1c or fasting)	Baseline, 3 months, annually

compliance may respond to psychosocial measures, obviating the need for depot antipsychotic drugs, and some might prefer long-acting preparations to pills.

The first generation antipsychotic depot preparations are available in the United States at the time of this writing are fluphenazine decanoate and haloperidol decanoate. Long-acting injectable risperidone (Consta) is only second generation antipsychotic available in long acting form. Controlled studies of fluphenazine decanoate have covered a 100-fold range in dosage (1.25 to 125 mg every 2 weeks). High doses (25 mg every 2 weeks) appear to be associated with an inferior outcome. Although these studies may have been skewed by assignment of sicker patients to higher dosages, the general impression is that the dosages used in current clinical practice are often too high. Long-acting risperidone studies show efficacy in doses of 25 to 50 mg every 2 weeks. Stable patients on oral risperidone switched to long-acting form tend to improve modestly. Many of the more ill patients switched to risperidone generally need doses in the higher range, 37.5 to 50 mg every 2 weeks. Although some patients can tolerate longer durations between injections, most patients require the 2-week frequency.

There are no ideal conversion ratios from oral dosages to long-acting preparations. For fluphenazine, one reasonable estimate is that 0.5 mL of fluphenazine decanoate (12.5 mg) given every 2 weeks is equivalent to 10.0 mg per day of fluphenazine hydrochloride. For haloperidol decanoate, the ratio of decanoate to oral dose is about 10:1 to 15:1, so that 150 mg of the decanoate given every 4 weeks is equivalent to 10 mg per day of oral haloperidol. For risperidone, 25 mg long-acting preparation is equivalent to about 2 to 3 mg oral risperidone. Because these conversions are only approximate, individual dosage adjustments will have to be made. For haloperidol, the best outcomes are associated with doses between 150 and 200 mg every 4 weeks. Fluphenazine and risperidone injections are best given every 2 weeks, though longer periods between injections may be tolerated by some.

Because these are long-acting preparations, patients should be exposed to the oral form of the drug prior to their first injection to minimize the possibility of a long-lasting idiosyncratic reaction. It is safest to start long-acting agents at low dosages and then carefully adjust them to maximize the safety of therapy and minimize side effects. For fluphenazine and haloperidol, extrapyramidal side effects are to be expected. With long-acting risperidone, EPS is uncommon.

The **long-acting risperidone** preparation is different from the oil-based decanoate preparations. Long-acting **risperidone is a water-based suspension** of the risperidone encapsulated in a carbohydrate polymer. The polymer is similar to the compound used in dissolvable sutures. The injected suspension allows for gradual absorption that escapes first-pass metabolism by the liver.

The preparation comes as a powder that requires refrigeration before it is mixed with a wetting solution to make the injectable suspension. Once mixed, the preparation must be used within 6 hours and must be shaken just before injection. Unlike the decanoate preparations, the long-acting risperidone preparation is not viscous and causes little, if any, swelling or pain at the injection site.

Absorption of the injectable risperidone is gradual, **taking more than 3 weeks to reach peak concentration.** Therefore, regular dose of oral medication needs to continue for at least 3 weeks after the first injection. The effective dose of injectable risperidone appears to be between 25 and 50 mg every 2 weeks. Lower dosing may be reasonable for geriatric patients with dementia and psychosis if this approach is used. Some patients need oral supplementation in addition to long-acting risperidone (the highest available injection strength, 50 mg of injectable risperidone, given every 2 weeks corresponds to only about 4 to 6 mg per day of oral risperidone). In general, patients stable on relatively low doses of antipsychotics (e.g., 4 mg risperidone, 5 mg haloperidol, 10 mg olanzapine) can be switched to 25 mg of injectable risperidone, and patients taking higher doses will likely need 50 mg every 2 weeks. Patients being switched from fluphenazine or haloperidol decanoate to long-acting risperidone should receive overlapping treatment for approximately 1 month after starting the injectable risperidone.

The following recommendations apply for the long-acting preparations:

1. Ensure that the patient has had a test of the drug orally to make certain that it is tolerated.
2. Start injections at low doses, for example, 5.0 to 12.5 mg (0.2 to 0.5 mL) of fluphenazine decanoate, 50 to 100 mg (1 to 2 mL) of haloperidol decanoate, or 25 mg of risperidone. Give fluphenazine decanoate and long-acting risperidone every 2 weeks and haloperidol decanoate every 4 weeks. At the start of treatment, haloperidol decanoate and fluphenazine decanoate may be given weekly for 2 to 3 weeks to reach steady state more quickly.
3. With the low initial doses, oral supplementation may be necessary temporarily. Do not increase doses of the depot preparation too rapidly because steady state is reached only after four to five dosing intervals.
4. Average effective maintenance dosages are in the range of 12.5 mg (0.5 mL) every 2 weeks for fluphenazine, 25 to 50 mg every 2 weeks for risperidone, and 150 to 200 mg (1.5 to 2 mL) every 4 weeks for haloperidol decanoate.
5. For haloperidol- and fluphenazine-treated patients, observe for akinesia, depression-like symptoms, or increasing withdrawal. Because these symptoms may be drug induced, it may be necessary to lower the dosage. Parkinsonism and akathisia are also common and may require treatment with benztropine or propranolol.
6. Recall that worsening of psychotic symptoms with dosage reduction may not become evident for several weeks; hence, the clinician must monitor patients for an extended period before assuming that the reduction has been successful.

As-Needed Use

Antipsychotic drugs are often prescribed in the hospital on an as-needed basis for the acute treatment of psychotic symptoms or agitation. Although not an uncommon practice, the use of antipsychotics on an as-needed basis likely reflects the absence of a clear diagnosis or treatment strategy. The time course of improvement for psychotic disorders in response to antipsychotic drugs is such that intermittent dosing is unlikely to help and may confuse the physician as to the amount of antipsychotic drug the patient is receiving daily. **Patients receiving only intermittent antipsychotic drug doses for psychotic symptoms are more likely to do poorly;** this would be much like using an antidepressant on an as-needed basis. In addition, clinicians sometimes combine second-generation antipsychotics, using one drug as the base drug and then adding a second as-needed for agitation or insomnia. This practice makes little sense, particularly when a side effect of a drug (e.g., sedation from quetiapine) is being used, whereas the patient may need more time or a drug such as benzodiazepine that targets the acute anxiety or insomnia need. A second-generation antipsychotic like quetiapine used for insomnia increases the side-effect burden and exposes patients to unnecessary potential metabolic risks (i.e., weight gain, diabetes, and dyslipidemia).

Frequent examinations by a physician are preferable to long-standing as-needed orders for antipsychotic drugs that may mask or exacerbate side effects or undiagnosed medical illness. For example, patients with akathisia on older antipsychotics have been given extra (as-needed) doses of an antipsychotic drug because their symptoms were misinterpreted as agitation. If more medication is needed to provide sedation for an acutely disturbed patient, benzodiazepines (e.g., lorazepam) may be preferred to antipsychotic drugs because they are reliable and limit the side effects with higher doses of antipsychotics (e.g., >6 mg per day of risperidone) (see Chapter 5). It should be recalled that even hallucinations may worsen with anxiety, fear, and agitation and are likely to respond to adequate anxiolysis without additional antipsychotic drugs.

Clozapine

In well-designed clinical trials, albeit most of them short-term, and in clinical experience, clozapine has proven to be more effective in reducing symptoms of schizophrenia and in preventing relapses than first-generation antipsychotic drugs. The CATIE trial had a treatment arm that included clozapine, which showed that clozapine is superior to second-generation antipsychotics as well. Moreover, there are studies comparing clozapine and olanzapine, which show that clozapine is superior to olanzapine in preventing suicide attempts in schizophrenic patients with a history of suicide attempts or suicidal thinking at study entry. Indeed, the FDA has approved clozapine to reduce the risk of suicidal behavior in schizophrenia or schizoaffective disorder.

There is evidence that clozapine also may have advantages in schizoaffective disorders and in some treatment-refractory bipolar patients as well. Clozapine is also effective at lower doses in the treatment of L-Dopa–induced psychotic symptoms in patients with Parkinson's disease, a patient group that cannot tolerate first-generation antipsychotic drugs. Although clozapine was the first tolerable treatment of psychosis in Parkinson's disease or Lewy body disease, today most patients are treated with quetiapine. Clozapine has the significant advantage of being almost free of EPS and of not causing TD. Thus, it has not only produced improvement in previously refractory patients, but it has also been used effectively in some patients with severe EPS, including akathisia, who could not tolerate typical antipsychotic drugs. It has also been reported that clozapine may improve existing TD, but further data are needed to support this contention.

Unfortunately, clozapine has a rather severe side effect burden in its own right, which limits its general utility. Clozapine was first tested in the 1960s but was withdrawn from general use when several deaths from agranulocytosis occurred in Europe. It was introduced in the United States in 1990, bundled by its manufacturer with a mandatory program of weekly blood counts. Although the programs available for blood count determinations have since been broadened, weekly determination of granulocyte counts remains necessary with clozapine for the first 6 months of therapy, after which biweekly measures suffice. The rate of agranulocytosis with clozapine has been approximately 1%, although it has been greater in some trials. Despite appropriate monitoring, there have been fatalities due to agranulocytosis in the United States. More than 95% of cases of agranulocytosis occur within the first 6 months of treatment, with the period of highest risk between weeks 4 and 18. The risk also appears to increase with age and may be higher in women. The mechanism of agranulocytosis is not known. **It is imperative to monitor WBC counts and the absolute neutrophil count before starting the treatment and then weekly for the first 6 months.** If the WBC count is stable, counts can be taken biweekly for 6 months, and if no significant drop in WBC counts occurs, then blood counts can be checked monthly. WBC counts should also be monitored for several weeks after discontinuation. Treatment should not be started unless the WBC count is more than 3,500 cells/mm³ and the absolute neutrophil count is more than 2,000 cells/mm³. If there is a 50% decrease in the WBC count, a WBC count of less than 3,000 cells/mm³, or an absolute neutrophil count of less than 1,500 cells/mm³, immediately discontinue treatment. Following discontinuation, the WBC count should be monitored twice weekly until the WBC count normalizes. Gradual clozapine reintroduction can then be considered on a case-by-case basis after the WBC count returns to normal. All patients treated with clozapine must be registered with one of the manufacturers, either the original manufacturer, Novartis, or one of the generic makers. Each company records the laboratory results from the blood count and reports to the original manufacturer. Detailed information from the original manufacturer can be found at www.clozaril.com

As previously described, clozapine has a relatively low affinity for D_2 dopamine receptors compared with typical antipsychotic drugs and a higher affinity for D_4 versus D_2 dopamine receptors than older antipsychotic drugs. However, the role of D_4 dopamine receptors in treatment, if any, remains unclear. Its relatively low affinity for D_2 dopamine receptors and high affinity for 5-HT$_{2A}$ serotonin receptors likely explains much of its low liability for causing EPS. It also interacts with D_1 and D_3 dopamine receptors, serotonin 5-HT$_6$ and 5-HT$_7$ receptors, α_1-adrenergic receptors, histamine H_1 receptors, and muscarinic cholinergic receptors. The mechanism of its unique efficacy remains unknown.

To minimize side effects and orthostatic hypotension, begin clozapine with a single 12.5- or 25-mg daily dose, increase to 25 mg b.i.d., and then increase by not more than 25 mg per day to a dosage of 300 to 450 mg per day over a period of 2 to 3 weeks. Dosage should subsequently be increased no more rapidly than weekly in increments no greater than 100 mg. During the initial titration, it may be useful to administer another antipsychotic, either a lower dose of the drug it is replacing or a low dose of nonsedating drugs, such as haloperidol. This overlapping drug will limit the psychotic exacerbation that may accompany the gradual titration of clozapine. Adjunctive benzodiazepines are best avoided because they may combine with clozapine to cause profound sedation, though some clinicians use benzodiazepines judiciously at the start of treatment. The manufacturer recommends against combining benzodiazepines with clozapine. At the start of clozapine treatment, we have successfully used adjunctive low-dose trazodone for insomnia. Careful monitoring for significant tachycardia and postural hypotension is important in the first month of treatment. Should these occur, the dosage may be temporarily decreased and then increased again more slowly. Most clozapine-responsive patients are effectively treated at dosages between 300 and 600 mg per day in divided doses, with most of the total given at bedtime. Some patients have been treated with doses as high as 900 mg per day in divided doses, but at doses of 600 mg and above, the risk of seizures increases significantly (from 1%–2% to 3%–5%). For patients who require high doses and develop seizures, the addition of therapeutic doses of valproate is often quite helpful. The optimal duration of a trial to identify clozapine-responsive patients remains unknown. Patients should be treated for at least 12 weeks, and some clinicians would recommend considerably longer (e.g., 6 months) trials of clozapine before declaring the treatment ineffective.

In addition to agranulocytosis, seizures, and postural hypotension, other problematic side effects include sedation (which may be marked), sialorrhea, tachycardia (which may be persistent), constipation, transient hyperthermia, and weight gain (which can be substantial; 20% to 30% increase over baseline weight). Eosinophilia without serious consequences has also rarely been reported. There have also been a number of cases of myocarditis and heart failure associated with clozapine. The reason is not clear, though a chest x-ray is currently advised before starting clozapine. Because of clozapine's potential for cardiovascular adverse effects, other baseline measurements should include an ECG, weight, and fasting glucose and lipids. These parameters should be monitored regularly, particularly at the start of treatment. Some patients may develop new-onset diabetes or worsening of existing diabetes. For patients who develop diabetes, the risks of treatment must be carefully weighed against the benefits. In cases of diabetes associated with ketoacidosis, clozapine should be stopped. In less severe cases, the degree of improvement will guide the decision whether to treat the diabetes or change drugs. Because weight gain is so problematic, patients must be educated and trained regarding diet and exercise. Smoking cessation may also be helpful to reduce cardiovascular risk, though if patients stop smoking during clozapine treatment, clozapine levels may rise considerably. This is because during clozapine use cytochrome 1A2 enzymes are induced. Following smoking cessation, the primary enzyme that metabolizes clozapine (1A2) returns to normal levels and clozapine concentrations rise. Some patients who discontinued clozapine when starting another antipsychotic drug, such as risperidone, have experienced marked agitation and even rebound psychotic symptoms. The mechanism is unknown but likely represents, in part, a cholinergic withdrawal syndrome. Slow tapering of clozapine rather than abrupt termination is recommended, even when switching to another antipsychotic drug.

Plasma concentrations of clozapine may be increased by drugs that inhibit the 1A2 cytochrome P450 hepatic enzymes, such as ciprofloxacin and fluvoxamine. In addition, clozapine moderately inhibits the 2D6 cytochrome enzyme, and this may result in higher concentrations than normal for concomitant drugs primarily metabolized by this enzyme, including haloperidol, risperidone, and tricyclic antidepressants (Table 2.6).

Risperidone/Paliperidone

Risperidone (Risperdal) combines high affinity for D_2 dopamine receptors with high affinity for $5-HT_{2A}$ receptors. Risperidone's high D_2 affinity is similar to that of haloperidol (rather than clozapine), whereas its high $5-HT_{2A}$ affinity is similar to that of clozapine. Risperidone also has high affinity for α_1-adrenergic receptors

TABLE 2.6	Clinically Significant Cytochrome P450 Drug Interactions of Second-Generation Antipsychotics		
Drug	**Major Substrate**	**Inducers of Substrate Enzyme**	**Inhibitors of Substrate Enzyme**
Olanzapine	1A2	Smoking, barbiturates (e.g., phenobarbital)	Fluvoxamine, ciprofloxacin, carbamazepine, norfloxacin, ofloxacin, rifampin, ketoconazole
Clozapine[a]	1A2		
Risperidone	2D6	Carbamazepine, rifampin, quinidine	Fluoxetine, paroxetine, duloxetine, bupropion, protease inhibitors (e.g., ritonavir), ropinirole, terbinafine, ranitidine, cimetidine
Aripiprazole[b]	2D6		
Ziprasidone	3A4	Barbiturates (e.g., phenobarbital), carbamazepine, modafinil, phenytoin, pioglitazone	Erythromycin, azithromycin, cimetidine, fluvoxamine, protease inhibitors (indinavir), St. John's wort, ketoconazole, itraconazole, nefazodone, verapamil
Quetiapine	3A4		
Aripiprazole[b]	3A4		

Enzyme inducers—reduce expected plasma concentration of antipsychotic.
Enzyme inhibitors—raise expected plasma concentration of antipsychotic.
[a]Clozapine also inhibits cytochrome 2D6, which can lead to increased concentrations of drugs metabolized by 2D6 including haloperidol, risperidone, tricyclic antidepressants, paroxetine, duloxetine, venlafaxine, and β-blockers.
[b]Aripiprazole is a major substrate of two cytochrome enzymes.

and α_2-adrenergic receptors but low affinity for muscarinic cholinergic receptors, making it devoid of anticholinergic effects. Based on the studies to date and early clinical experience, risperidone is as effective as haloperidol and in some specific cases may be more effective, particularly in preventing relapse. It is certainly better tolerated when used at the lower end of its dose range. It may still cause EPS, however, and regularly does so at higher doses. It also appears to lack the degree of enhanced efficacy exhibited by clozapine. Overall, given its efficacy and tolerability, it is justifiably a widely used first-line drug. Of the second-generation antipsychotics, it behaves most like the older antipsychotics.

Since its introduction, the average doses of risperidone have decreased and the rate of titration has slowed. Patients may be started on 1 mg per day or b.i.d. (0.5 mg b.i.d. for elderly patients or for those with impaired hepatic function). Although the dosage can be increased over several days to the target dose of 4 to 6 mg per day range, most patients require dose escalation over several weeks. The average dosage in use in the United States for schizophrenia is now just over 4 mg per day. Dosage increases should be slow in elderly patients and in those who experience postural hypotension with initial dosing. Elderly schizophrenic patients benefit from doses ranging from 0.5 to 2 mg per day. Optimal antipsychotic effects for most schizophrenic patients are seen at 6 mg per day or less in divided doses. If response is poor, upward adjustments may be made, but dosages above 8 mg per day do not appear to offer added benefit, whereas EPS becomes more prominent. The incidence of EPS appears to be dose related; at dosages of 10 mg per day or greater, the incidence of EPS is similar to that with haloperidol.

In addition to postural hypotension (and reflex tachycardia), risperidone may produce sedation, insomnia, and difficulty concentrating. Dizziness, galactorrhea, sexual dysfunction, and weight gain are also common.

Like other D_2 receptor antagonists, risperidone may eventually reveal the potential to cause TD, and cases of NMS have been reported with this drug, although these risks at this point are decidedly less than those for the older agents. The combination of D_2 antagonism and high 5-HT$_{2A}$ affinity likely explains risperidone's propensity to cause prolactin elevation, which accounts for the occasional report of galactorrhea and menstrual irregularities in women. The long-term implications of elevated prolactin levels, if any, particularly in the absence of side effects or menstrual irregularities is unclear, though there are some studies associating elevated prolactin levels with decreased bone mineral density.

Risperidone is primarily metabolized by cytochrome P450 2D6. When used in combination with inhibitors of the 2D6 enzyme, such as fluoxetine, duloxetine, or paroxetine, patients may have significant rises in risperidone concentrations and more side effects than usual. Lower dose of risperidone are often needed in combination with these agents.

The primary metabolite of risperidone, 9-hyroxyrisperidone, has been marketed under the name paliperidone **(Invega)**. It has much the same properties and adverse effects as risperidone and appears to be generally well tolerated. Increases in prolactin are reportedly less in manufacturer-conducted studies, though this metabolite of risperidone is thought to be the primary cause for the rise in prolactin levels. It is formulated as a slow release preparation and studies find it effective as a once daily dose. The effective dose is generally between 6 and 9 mg per day. It is available in 3-, 6-, and 9-mg extended release tablets that allow for once daily dosing. The coated tablet has microscopic holes through which the drug is released via osmotic pressure into the intestines over 24 hours. The time-release system allows for a narrow range between peak and trough concentrations. The finished tablet is excreted in the feces. As with risperidone, the propensity for weight gain, lipid rises, or insulin resistance is relatively low, though still present. Despite its relative advantages compared with olanzapine, the drug use still requires metabolic monitoring.

Olanzapine

Olanzapine **(Zyprexa)** (2-methyl-4-(4-methyl-1-piperazinyl)-10H-thieno-[2,3-b] [1,5] benzodiazepine) is a thienobenzodiazepine compound related to clozapine. Like clozapine, it has a complex pharmacology, interacting with D_1 and D_2 family dopamine receptors, multiple serotonin receptors (5-HT_{2A}, 5-HT_{2C}, and 5-HT_6), histamine H_1 receptors, and muscarinic cholinergic receptors (Table 2.1). In clinical trials, olanzapine is at least as effective as haloperidol and better tolerated. Some data indicate that it may be more effective than haloperidol for negative symptoms of schizophrenia, but this has been difficult to establish with certainty.

Olanzapine treatment of schizophrenia is typically begun with a single dose of 10 mg, although some patients who are particularly sensitive to sedation do best starting at 5 mg. The recommended maximum dose is 20 mg daily, but higher doses have been well tolerated, and in one study of 148 patients with acute schizophrenia, patients tolerated 40 mg per day for 2 days before the dose was gradually reduced. The drug is generally well tolerated because patients report improved sleep and anxiety. It is best given all at bedtime. The average prescribed dosage is 10 to 20 mg per day, though some patients require higher maintenance doses. The drug reaches peak plasma levels in 5 to 8 hours and has a half-life of about 35 hours; drug–drug interactions are unlikely to influence olanzapine levels. Abnormalities of the QTc on electrocardiogram (ECG) are unlikely to occur, so there is no need for a baseline ECG. The most common side effects are mild to moderate sedation, dizziness, and weight gain, but the latter, in a subgroup of patients, can be substantial and a primary reason for drug discontinuation. About 40% of patients in clinical trials gain weight, with reported anecdotes of significant weight gain associated with new onset of diabetes. Although new-onset diabetes is relatively rare, the drug clearly leads to increased insulin resistance and, sometimes, worsened preexisting diabetes. Olanzapine also frequently leads to rises in triglycerides and, to a lesser degree, cholesterol elevation. Patients receiving olanzapine need careful monitoring for weight, lipids, and fasting glucose. There are few established methods to reduce weight gain, though one controlled trial found that the addition of topiramate (100 to 200 mg per day) led to modest weight loss. Metformin has shown promise as an adjunctive agent to prevent or blunt the metabolic abnormalities associated with antipsychotics, but metformin is not a benign treatment either. The H_2 blockers nizatidine and famotidine have also been studied as antidotes to olanzapine-induced weight gain. Findings have been mixed for nizatidine and negative for famotidine. EPS has not been observed at higher rates than placebo in dosages of up to 20 mg per day, though some patients develop akathisia or parkinsonism. TD appears uncommonly from olanzapine alone.

Olanzapine is available in tablets of various strengths as well as in a rapidly dissolvable tablet for patients who have difficulty swallowing or "cheeking" medication. For use in the emergency setting, an injectable, rapidly effective i.m. formulation is also available in a 10-mg/mL dose. A long-acting form, which unfortunately has potential for severe somnolence, is under review by the FDA.

Quetiapine

Quetiapine (Seroquel) is a dibenzothiazepine compound with relatively low affinity for 5-HT_{1A} and 5-HT_{2A} receptors; moderate to high affinity for α_1, α_2, and H_1 receptors; and weaker activity at D_1, D_2, D_3, D_4, and D_5 dopamine receptors. Interestingly, one of its metabolites, N-desalkyl quetiapine, moderately blocks the reuptake of norepinephrine, and this property may underlie its antidepressant properties. It is available in tablets and in an extended release formulation that allows for somewhat more rapid titration. Some initial concerns among clinicians about the efficacy of quetiapine appear to have reflected inadequate dosing.

Although the drug is more effective than placebo in the dosage range of 150 to 800 mg per day, 400 to 800 mg per day is the usual effective range of dosing. More severely ill patients may require even higher doses. It has a relatively mild side-effect profile with respect to EPS (no worse than placebo), with initial sedation being the main reason; the drug should be started at low doses and titrated upward. Sedation tends to resolve over several weeks. However, weight gain and orthostatic hypotension can occur, as can other effects such as insomnia, headache, and dry mouth. Some patients report restless legs at bedtime after starting quetiapine, though the mechanism is uncertain. It does not elevate prolactin.

Because it has a short half-life, b.i.d. or three times a day (t.i.d.) dosing was initially recommended, though most clinicians dose it once daily after reaching the final dose. Although the original dosing schedule was quite modest, with more experience, inpatient clinicians generally start at 100 or 200 mg at bedtime. The recently introduced extended-release preparation makes this rapid titration easier. In acutely ill patients, dosing can then be gradually increased as tolerated, generally by no more than 100 to 200 mg per day until reaching a dose of 500 to 800 mg per day. Weight gain is intermediate compared with the other second-generation antipsychotics. We have seen, however, some patients gain tremendous amounts of weight while others gain little. As with olanzapine, weight, lipid level, and glucose level should be monitored on a regular basis. The emergence of cataracts in toxicology studies of dogs has unclear, if any, implications for human use; although the manufacturer suggests twice-yearly slit lamp examinations for cataracts, most clinicians do not follow this. A large prospective study in humans comparing quetiapine with risperidone is under way to determine if there is any reason for cataract concern. Ophthalmology studies conclude that eye examinations are unnecessary for patients taking quetiapine.

Quetiapine is not common among the antipsychotics because it is popular among patients with drug addiction, despite its lack of usual reinforcing properties associated with addiction. Some stimulant abusers use it to counter the anxiety-producing effects of cocaine or amphetamine. It is known as "quell" for this street use. It has also been used in prison populations, where it is known as "Suzie-Q," because it produces an altered state when injected or snorted.

Ziprasidone

Ziprasidone (Geodon) is a 3-benzisothiazolyl-piperazine derivative with high 5-HT_{2A} and moderate D_2 antagonism with antagonism at 5-HT_{1D} and 5-HT_{2C} receptors and antagonism at 5-HT_{1A} and 5-HT_{1C} receptors. Like other second-generation antipsychotics, it is a moderately potent α_1 and H_1 histamine receptor blocker. Although the FDA made note of the propensity of ziprasidone to prolong the QTc this effect is modest and rarely of clinical significance. An ECG is not required but should be considered for patients with a family history of sudden death or known heart disease or for patients taking drugs known to prolong the QTc such as the quinolones. The available clinical trial data indicate that ziprasidone is efficacious, although not superior to other antipsychotics. Ziprasidone has a favorable profile with respect to weight gain, lipids and glucose metabolism, and effects on prolactin. Sedation may be the most common side effect but emerged in fewer than 20% of subjects in clinical trials. It is much less sedating than olanzapine, risperidone, and quetiapine, and some patients may require a benzodiazepine to help with sleep. Of note, it may be activating at low doses, and the original low dosing has since been dropped and replaced with a more vigorous starting dose and titration schedule. Dosing should be started at 40 to 60 mg twice daily and increased over several days as tolerated to 160 mg per day in divided doses or as a single dose with the evening meal. Ziprasidone has a short half-life of 4 to 5 hours, and blood levels are increased with food; thus, dosing should initially be b.i.d. with meals, although many patients do well with once daily dosing. The drug absorption is greatly affected by taking it with food; taking it on an empty stomach results in a 50% reduction in the plasma concentration compared with taking it with a meal. The effective dose range is usually between 120 and 160 mg per day. Some patients may require doses above 160 mg per day, but the benefit of higher doses has not been established in clinical trials. EPS was rare at the 40-mg dose but was reported in 9% of subjects on 80 mg per day, with akathisia noted in 15%. A short-acting injectable preparation is available for emergency use. The injectable-preparation dose is 10 to 20 mg and has been shown to be effective for agitated psychotic patients within 15 to 30 minutes of administration. At this dose range, ziprasidone is not associated with EPS or excessive sedation.

Monitoring for weight, lipids, and glucose appears less important for ziprasidone than for most of the other antipsychotics. Because this patient group is at risk for the metabolic syndrome, regular monitoring remains a useful measure.

Aripiprazole

Aripiprazole (**Abilify**) is a quinolinone derivative unrelated to other antipsychotics that shows moderate to high antagonism at the dopamine D_2 receptor and shows partial D_2 agonist effects in vivo. Although the property of antagonizing D_2 receptors in the presence of high dopamine concentrations and activating D_2 receptors in the absence of dopamine is of theoretical interest, the clinical benefits of this unique D_2 property are still not known. Aripiprazole also shows high affinity for $5HT_{2A}$ and $5HT_{1A}$ receptors. Aripiprazole has no affinity for muscarinic receptors and very mild effects on α_1 and H_1 histamine receptors, thus providing a favorable side-effect profile for long-term use. Although α_1 and H_1 blockade is mild, some patients may still suffer orthostasis or sedation, although these effects are uncommon. In the treatment of acute psychosis, the lack of sedating qualities may limit its ability to rapidly quell agitation or insomnia. Some patients may require added benzodiazepines for insomnia or anxiety associated with psychosis. Adverse effects are otherwise minimal, although some patients may experience nausea when they initiate treatment. EPS is relatively uncommon, though akathisia is possible, and at higher doses, patients may develop parkinsonism. Aripiprazole generally does not elevate prolactin levels (it might even decrease prolactin levels), and in one study adjunctive aripiprazole reversed haloperidol-induced prolactinemia. Although some patients may gain weight, on average, the drug is weight neutral. The drug is generally benign with respect to lipids and glucose metabolism, though diabetic ketoacidosis remains a rare possibility for all of these antipsychotics. Patients should still be monitored for weight, lipids, and glucose, though surveillance need not be as close as with some others. There are no significant effects on the QTc.

Aripiprazole has a half-life of 75 hours allowing for once daily dosing. Absorption is not affected by food. Dosing can usually be started at 10 to 15 mg per day and there is no controlled evidence that higher doses are more effective than 15 mg per day, though 30 mg is the commonly used dose. Elderly patients can be started at lower doses (e.g., 2 to 5 mg per day). Patients treated with inhibitors of cytochrome P450 isoenzyme 3A4 (e.g., ketoconazole) or 2D6 (paroxetine or fluoxetine) can be treated with lower doses. Patients treated with inducers of the P450 isoenzyme 3A4 (e.g., carbamazepine) should be treated with higher doses (20 to 30 mg per day).

Aripiprazole is best started in the morning with the first meal. Most patients can be started at a dosage of 10 to 15 mg daily. Because it takes about 2 weeks to reach steady state, dose adjustments are often made too quickly. Increasing the dose rapidly to 30 or 45 mg may lead to mild sedation and delayed parkinsonism or akathisia. About 1 in 10 patients experience agitation, which spontaneously resolves in about half or which is managed with a benzodiazepine or β-blocker.

Switching Among the Second-Generation Antipsychotics

Although, on average, the second-generation drugs are equally effective, for the individual patient there may be differences, and no drug is completely satisfactory. **Most patients have switched drugs,** and patients rarely stay on one drug indefinitely for a variety of reasons. Indeed, in the much discussed nationwide study, the CATIE, only 25% of patients stayed on the drug they began with over an 18-month period. This study employed an unusual measure of effectiveness, using time to discontinuation of drug for any cause, rather than a symptom measure as its primary outcome measure. Although changing drugs for any reason is a clinically useful measure of effectiveness, in the study patients and clinicians knew there were several phases of the study, and this may have led to premature switches to enroll in the next, possibly better treatment. Other criticisms of the study were that the olanzapine dose was better optimized compared to the other antipsychotics, the exclusion of patients with TD in some treatment arms, and the differences in prestudy treatments.

Many of these patients had taken several antipsychotics before they started the trial, and few found the new blind treatment more effective than the past treatment. Although there were minor treatment adherence advantages held by olanzapine compared to the others, the problematic side effects of weight gain and dyslipidemia make this advantage marginal. Interestingly, the advantages found with olanzapine were attenuated when the data were analyzed to compare how patients did if they were assigned to the drug they were taking before the study started. That is, patients taking risperidone before the study continued longer on the drug if they continued on risperidone rather than if they were switched to another medication at the start of the study. Even so, if patients continued on their original drug, more than half discontinued the drug before the study ended.

A drug change is reasonable if a patient has unsatisfactory clinical response or if side effects are problematic. What is to be gained by switching? What is to be lost by switching? Resolving side effects and improving tolerance and function without losing benefit is the best outcome, though some switches lead to loss of clinical stability. Hence, we recommend that switches be taken cautiously when patients are stable, and with the involvement of patients' families. Simple titration schedules, over a short time, are best used to prevent confusion. For example, reducing the first drug by half while starting the second drug at half its projected dose, and then completing the switch within a week is generally manageable. A common area of potential improvement is to switch from a sedating drug to one that is less sedating. If dose reduction does not improve daytime sedation, then a switch from olanzapine, risperidone, or quetiapine to ziprasidone or aripiprazole often leads to greater daytime alertness. Unfortunately, this switch may lead to insomnia, necessitating the addition of bedtime trazodone or a benzodiazepine. Metabolic side effects are common with several of the drugs, and switches may help here. Weight gain is often problematic with olanzapine and sometimes with quetiapine; a switch to ziprasidone or aripiprazole frequently helps. Glucose intolerance or dyslipidemia associated with olanzapine is best treated with a switch to ziprasidone or aripiprazole.

Parkinsonism or elevated prolactin levels are most common with risperidone; if dose reduction does not suffice, these signs are best reversed by switching to olanzapine or quetiapine. Akathisia, though also potential with any of the second-generation drugs, is most common with aripiprazole and ziprasidone. If this cannot be reversed by the addition of propranolol or a benzodiazepine, it usually resolves by switching to olanzapine or quetiapine. For patients who experience insomnia that is not resolved by the addition of a hypnotic, a switch to olanzapine or

	Approximate Dose Equivalent (mg)	Sedative Effect	Hypotensive Effect	Appetite Effect	Lipid Effect	Extrapyramidal Effect
Drug						
Haloperidol	5	Low	Low	Low	Low	High
Clozapine	200	High	High	High	High	Low
Olanzapine	10	High	Medium	High	High	Low
Quetiapine	250	High	Medium	Medium	Low	Low
Risperidone	2	Medium	Medium	Medium	Low	Medium
Ziprasidone	80	Low	Low/medium	Low	Low	Low
Aripiprazole	15	Low	Low	Low	Low	Low/medium

TABLE 2.7 Second-Generation Antipsychotic Drugs: Relative Potencies and Side-Effect Profiles

quetiapine may be best. Orthostasis may be problematic with quetiapine and risperidone, and typically least problematic with ziprasidone and aripiprazole (Table 2.7). The advantages and disadvantages of switching among the second-generation drugs are summarized below.

Advantages of Switching

Olanzapine/quetiapine—improved sleep, well tolerated, low parkinsonism, low prolactin.

Risperidone—moderate sedation, improved sleep, moderate appetite, well tolerated.

Aripiprazole/ziprasidone—more daytime alertness, reduced appetite, lipids and glucose neutral, limited effects on blood pressure, low prolactin.

Disadvantages of Switching

Olanzapine—significant appetite and weight gain, rise in lipids, glucose intolerance, sedation.

Quetiapine—sedation, moderate weight gain, hypotension.

Risperidone—elevated prolactin, parkinsonism at higher doses, hypotension.

Aripiprazole/ziprasidone—insomnia, akathisia with aripiprazole.

USE OF ANTIPSYCHOTIC DRUGS IN PREGNANCY AND NURSING

Antipsychotic medications, capable as they are of crossing the blood–brain barrier, are also **generally able to cross the maternal–placental barrier** and be present in the fetus and amniotic fluid. A preliminary study of the second-generation antipsychotics found that olanzapine, risperidone, and quetiapine all passed through the placenta, and olanzapine had the highest placental passage ratio. The limited prospective data regarding the second-generation antipsychotics suggest that they are not associated with fetal malformation or pregnancy loss. The effects of chlorpromazine have been most carefully studied in pregnancy, although other agents also have been investigated regarding teratogenicity. No clear patterns of teratogenicity have emerged. Given the relative paucity of safety data, it is best, if possible, to avoid antipsychotic agents in pregnancy, especially in the first trimester. Nonetheless, there are many situations in which failure to treat the mother creates a graver risk to the fetus than any established risk of antipsychotic drugs. Reasonable efforts should be made to avoid antipsychotic exposure during pregnancy, most particularly in the first trimester. As with other psychotropics, these drugs should be used only if the benefits outweigh the risks.

There are well-documented problems with the use of antipsychotics in late pregnancy. Chlorpromazine has been associated with an increased risk of neonatal jaundice. In addition, there are reports that mothers treated with antipsychotics, including some of the second-generation antipsychotics, have given birth to infants with EPS. The washout time for these drugs in the fetus is at least 7 to 10 days. Therefore, to avoid EPS in the newborn, it has been recommended that the antipsychotic be discontinued 2 weeks before the due date. If the discontinuance predisposes the expectant mother to severe psychotic symptoms, the clinician must carefully weigh the risks of the psychotic disorder against the potential for neuroleptic toxicity in the child.

Antipsychotics are secreted in breast milk, although likely at very low levels. A nursing infant of a mother treated with antipsychotics is therefore at some risk for the development of EPS. Because the effect of antipsychotic drugs on development is unknown, mothers who must take antipsychotic agents should strongly consider alternatives to breast-feeding.

USE OF ANTIPSYCHOTIC DRUGS IN ELDERLY PATIENTS

Elderly persons have a slower hepatic metabolism of antipsychotic drugs (pharmacokinetic effects) and an **increased sensitivity of the brain** to dopamine antagonism and anticholinergic effects (pharmacodynamic effects). Thus, lower dosages should be used, and longer waiting periods should be respected before increasing doses. When older antipsychotics are being used, recall that high-potency antipsychotic drugs (e.g., haloperidol) are less likely than low-potency drugs to cause anticholinergic symptoms such as constipation, urinary retention, tachycardia, sedation, and confusion or to cause postural hypotension. Unfortunately, in elderly patients, high-potency antipsychotic drugs have a higher likelihood of causing drug-induced parkinsonism and a higher risk of causing TD; with clozapine, there may be a higher risk of drug-induced agranulocytosis in elderly populations. Low dosages should therefore be the rule; dosages in the range of 0.5 to 2.0 mg per day of haloperidol are often adequate in elderly persons. **The second-generation agents are generally the treatment of first choice for initial therapy in the elderly.** For those who are doing well on older agents or who have failed using second-generation antipsychotics, the older drugs may be reasonable. The newer drugs, especially risperidone and quetiapine, however, often cause orthostasis and starting doses should be very low. The FDA placed warnings on the second-generation antipsychotics because in a pooled analysis of elderly dementia patients treated with these agents there were more deaths on drug than placebo-treated patients (4.5% vs 2.5%). Causes of death were not necessarily attributable to the drugs, though this warning serves as a reminder that these drugs should be used cautiously, carefully weighing the possible benefits with the risks. They are best used for psychosis and delirium rather than for nonspecific agitation or insomnia.

USE OF ANTIPSYCHOTICS IN DELIRIUM

Delirium, acute confusional states, and toxic and metabolic encephalopathy are among the many terms that have been used to describe a clinical syndrome that consists of acute global depression of cerebral function generally accompanied by abnormalities in arousal. Delirium is always the result of at least one medical condition, which can constitute a medical emergency. The cornerstone of treatment of delirium is supportive care while specific therapy for the underlying medical disorder is provided. Because delirious patients are unpredictable and may either harm themselves by falling or by pulling out necessary lines and tubes in a hospital setting or harm others, restraints or constant observation is generally indicated. Pending the results of specific therapy for an underlying disorder or while waiting for an offending drug to be metabolized and excreted, symptomatic use of psychotropics is often necessary, although use should be minimized, if possible, especially when the diagnosis is unclear. The choice of agent will be dictated by the cause of the delirium and the patient's medical status.

Delirium due to ethanol, benzodiazepine, or barbiturate withdrawal is best treated with a cross-reactive agent, generally a benzodiazepine (see Chapter 5). Antipsychotic drugs are not effective sole treatment for ethanol withdrawal. When delirium is caused by anticholinergic drugs, it is also wise to avoid antipsychotics because of the risk of increasing anticholinergic toxicity. For many other causes of delirium, especially in medically fragile patients, an antipsychotic, but particularly the high-potency typical agent haloperidol, has long been the acute agent of choice because it has little effect on the cardiovascular system, little effect on respiratory drive, and very low anticholinergic potency and because tablet, liquid, and rapidly acting parenteral formulations are available. Low-potency first-generation antipsychotic drugs lower the seizure threshold, increase the risk of postural hypotension, and may be strongly anticholinergic; thus, they should be avoided. In older patients, doses of haloperidol as low as 0.5 mg b.i.d. may be effective in symptomatic treatment of delirium. In younger patients, higher doses may be used at least initially (doses of 2 to 5 mg may be given parenterally every 30 to 60 minutes as needed). The major liability of haloperidol in older patients is the emergence of parkinsonian symptoms (although younger men are most at risk for acute dystonias). When elderly patients are given older antipsychotics, however, they should be monitored frequently for cogwheel rigidity, changes in gait, and the development of masked facies. Late reemergence of agitation while a patient is on haloperidol should raise the suspicion of akathisia. If antipsychotic treatment beyond the acute intervention is required, the second-generation agents are the treatments of choice. The availability of short-acting injectable second-generation drugs (e.g., ziprasidone) permits greater flexibility of administration of medication and increased use of newer agents for delirium.

SIDE EFFECTS AND TOXICITY

Neurologic Side Effects

Acute Dystonia

Clinical Presentation. Acute dystonia is most likely to occur within the first week of treatment with high-potency first-generation antipsychotics (e.g., haloperidol or fluphenazine). Despite the expected rarity of the event with the newer agents, the continued acute use of parenteral first-generation antipsychotics in emergency settings indicates that clinicians need to be familiar with the recognition and treatment of acute dystonia. There is a higher incidence in patients younger than 40 years, in males, and in patients on high-potency first-generation antipsychotic drugs. Patients may develop acute muscular rigidity and cramping, usually in the musculature of the neck, tongue, face, and back. Occasionally, patients report the subacute onset (3 to 6 hours) of tongue "thickness" or difficulty in swallowing. Opisthotonos and oculogyric crises also may occur. Acute dystonia can be very uncomfortable and frightening to patients, and occasionally it has serious sequelae; muscular cramps can be severe enough to cause joint dislocation, and, most dangerously, laryngeal dystonia can occur with compromise of the airway.

Treatment. Anticholinergic drugs (Table 2.8), such as benztropine, 2 mg i.m. or i.v., or diphenhydramine, 50 mg i.m. or i.v., usually bring rapid relief. Benztropine may be preferred because it lacks the antihistaminic effects of diphenhydramine. If there is no effect in 20 minutes, a repeat injection is indicated. If the dystonia is still unresponsive after two injections, a benzodiazepine, such as lorazepam 1 mg

TABLE 2.8	Commonly Used Antiparkinsonian Drugs
Drug	**Usual Dosage Range**
Anticholinergic drugs	
Benztropine (Cogentin)	1–2 mg b.i.d.
Biperiden (Akineton)	1–3 mg b.i.d.
Trihexyphenidyl (Artane)	1–3 mg t.i.d.
Anticholinergic antihistamine	
Diphenhydramine (Benadryl)	25 mg b.i.d. to q.i.d.; 50 mg b.i.d.
Dopamine-releasing agent	
Amantadine (Symmetrel)	100 mg b.i.d. to t.i.d.

b.i.d., twice a day; q.i.d., four times a day; t.i.d., three times a day.

i.m. or i.v., may be tried. In cases of laryngeal dystonia with airway compromise, repeat dosing should occur at shorter intervals unless the dystonia resolves. The patient should receive 4 mg of benztropine i.v. within 10 minutes and then 1 to 2 mg of lorazepam i.v. slowly if needed.

With reversal of dystonia, if the antipsychotic medication is to be continued, standing doses of an anticholinergic drug (e.g., benztropine, 2 mg b.i.d) should be prescribed for 2 weeks (Table 2.8). Even if the antipsychotic is discontinued, an anticholinergic should be taken for 2 to 3 days to prevent a recurrence of the dystonic reaction. There is evidence that the prophylactic use of benztropine, 2 mg b.i.d, begun at the same time as the antipsychotic drug, significantly reduces the incidence of dystonia. Dystonias are much less likely with low-potency older drugs (e.g., chlorpromazine) or second-generation antipsychotics compared with **high-potency** first-generation drugs.

Antipsychotic Drug–Induced Parkinsonism

Clinical Presentation. Symptoms include bradykinesia, rigidity, cogwheeling, tremor, masked facies, stooped posture, festinating gait, and drooling. When these side effects are severe, akinesia, which can be indistinguishable from catatonia, may develop. Onset is usually after several weeks of therapy and is more common in elderly patients and with high-potency drugs. These symptoms rarely limit therapy with the newer antipsychotics except for risperidone at doses of 8 mg and higher and are rare with olanzapine, ziprasidone, aripiprazole, or quetiapine. They are virtually absent with clozapine.

Switching treatment for a stable, psychotic patient from a typical agent to an atypical compound is certainly reasonable when that patient suffers drug-induced parkinsonism. If the clinician does choose to switch to a newer antipsychotic, response must be closely examined to ensure comparable efficacy, in addition to reduced parkinsonian side effects.

Treatment. If the antipsychotic is to be unchanged, a fixed dose of an antiparkinson drug should be prescribed, and the antipsychotic drug dosage should be decreased to the lowest that is effective for the patient. In elderly patients, lower doses of antiparkinson drugs should be used (e.g., benztropine, 1 mg b.i.d.). A switch to a newer agent is preferable. Because there is some evidence that long-term use of anticholinergics may increase the risk of TD, periodic attempts should be made to wean these drugs during maintenance therapy, assuming there remains a clinical rationale for use of the older compound.

Akathisia

Clinical Presentation. Akathisia is experienced subjectively as an intensely unpleasant sensation of restlessness and the need to move, especially the legs. Patients often appear restless, with symptoms of anxiety, agitation, or both. It can be difficult to distinguish akathisia from anxiety related to the psychotic disorder. Increased restlessness following the institution of typical antipsychotics should always raise the question of akathisia. Recent evidence suggests that akathisia may be more prevalent in patients treated with these drugs than previously thought. Akathisia is a leading cause of noncompliance and treatment refusal. The inescapable distress associated with akathisia may amplify the hopelessness of the patient and may be a factor in suicidal ideation. As with parkinsonism, akathisia is unlikely with risperidone at low doses, rare with olanzapine and quetiapine, and virtually absent with clozapine. Anxiety and agitation occur with ziprasidone and aripiprazole, typically a state of activation that resembles akathisia, but can resolve spontaneously over time.

Treatment. First-generation antipsychotic drugs should always be prescribed at the minimum effective dose. Low-potency antipsychotics, especially thioridazine, have a significantly lower incidence of akathisia than high-potency agents do. A variety of compounds have been reported effective for the treatment of akathisia including β-adrenergic blockers as first-line remedies, anticholinergic drugs, and benzodiazepines. There have also been reports on the use of clonidine for akathisia, but the evidence in its favor is scant, and clonidine has the additional problem of causing hypotension. Recently, mirtazapine has been shown to be an effective intervention for antipsychotic-induced akathisia and could be tried if first-line approaches prove ineffective.

In the treatment of akathisia, various situations that call for differing approaches can arise. We recommend the following:

A. When the patient is treated with an antipsychotic drug and does not have other EPS (e.g., haloperidol or aripiprazole)
1. First choice: a β-adrenergic blocker, such as propranolol, 10 to 30 mg t.i.d. (nadolol also can be used) (see Chapter 6).
2. Second choice: an anticholinergic, such as benztropine, 1 to 2 mg b.i.d.
3. Third choice: a benzodiazepine, such as lorazepam, 1 mg t.i.d., or clonazepam, 0.5 mg b.i.d.

B. When the patient is treated with a low-potency older antipsychotic drug (e.g., chlorpromazine) or an antipsychotic and a cyclic antidepressant and does not have other EPS
1. First choice: propranolol, 10 to 30 mg t.i.d.
2. Second choice: lorazepam, 1 mg t.i.d., or clonazepam, 0.5 mg b.i.d.
3. Third choice: benztropine, 1 mg b.i.d. (additive anticholinergic toxicity)

C. When the patient is treated with an antipsychotic and manifests other EPS (dystonias or parkinsonism)
1. First choice: benztropine, 1 to 2 mg b.i.d.
2. Second choice: benztropine with propranolol, 10 to 30 mg t.i.d.
3. Third choice: benztropine with lorazepam, 1 mg t.i.d., or clonazepam, 0.5 mg b.i.d.

D. When other EPS are present and akathisia is unresponsive to an anticholinergic alone
1. First choice: benztropine, 1 to 2 mg b.i.d., with propranolol, 10 to 30 mg t.i.d.
2. Second choice: benztropine, 1 to 2 mg b.i.d., with lorazepam, 1 mg t.i.d., or clonazepam, 0.5 mg b.i.d.

    E. When EPS or akathisia is present, the clinician should review again the possibility of switching to a second-generation antipsychotic with low propensity for EPS, such as quetiapine or olanzapine, recognizing that when interchanging agents, comparable efficacy on a different drug is not certain.

Neuroleptic Malignant Syndrome

Clinical Presentation. NMS is an extremely serious idiosyncratic reaction to neuroleptic drugs. The major symptoms of NMS are **rigidity, fever, autonomic instability, and delirium.** Symptoms usually develop over a period of several hours to several days, with rigidity typically preceding fever and autonomic instability. Fever may be high, with temperatures of 41°C or higher commonly reported. Lead pipe rigidity is typical, with increased muscle tone leading to myonecrosis in some cases. When patients are also dehydrated, the resulting myoglobinuria may be severe enough to cause renal failure. Autonomic symptoms include instability of blood pressure, often including both hypertension and hypotension, tachycardia, diaphoresis, and pallor. Cardiac arrhythmias may occur. In addition to rigidity, motor abnormalities including akinesia, tremor (which may fluctuate in severity), and involuntary movements have been reported. The patients are usually confused and often mute. There may be fluctuations in level of consciousness from agitation to stupor. Seizures or coma also may occur.

    NMS is a clinical diagnosis with a relatively wide continuum of severity. Because there are no clear criteria for making a diagnosis, especially in milder cases, it is difficult to state mortality rates. Although there are no specific laboratory findings, creatinine phosphokinase is usually elevated. For unknown reasons, liver function test results also may be abnormal, including elevations of transaminases and lactic dehydrogenase. The WBC count also may be slightly elevated.

    Risk factors for development of NMS include dehydration, poor nutrition, external heat load, and possible intercurrent medical illness. Although all antipsychotics have been associated with NMS, there is evidence to suggest that high doses of older high-potency antipsychotics (e.g., haloperidol or fluphenazine) increase the risk. Although NMS is extremely rare with newer drugs, a number of cases have been reported with all of the second-generation antipsychotics, including clozapine.

    In severely psychotic patients, the following question often arises: Can the patient receive antipsychotics again after having had NMS? In fact, it appears that not all patients who have had NMS suffer a recurrence, even with the same drug that had previously caused the syndrome. Nonetheless, case reports accumulating in the literature suggest that a substantial percentage of patients who have developed NMS once have a recurrence. Given the serious morbidity and possible lethality of this syndrome, it is prudent to withhold older antipsychotics from patients who have had NMS unless there are compelling indications to resume this treatment and no alternative can be found. We suggest that all patients with a high likelihood for a recurrence should receive a trial of quetiapine or clozapine. If for whatever reason this is not possible, the other alternative is to use the lowest possible doses of olanzapine or another low-potency drug, such as thioridazine. Ideally, treatment will not be resumed for at least 4 weeks after full resolution of NMS symptoms. Lorazepam 1 to 2 mg b.i.d. can be used in the interim for agitation or sleep disturbance. The risks and benefits of such a decision should be fully discussed with the patient and, if appropriate, with his or her family.

    Treatment. Meticulous supportive care is critical, including adequate hydration, use of cooling blankets for high fever, turning of patients to avoid decubitus ulcers, cardiac monitoring, and monitoring of urine output and renal function. Should renal failure occur, dialysis may be necessary, but dialysis cannot be expected to remove antipsychotics because they are highly bound to plasma proteins and peripheral tissues. Dantrolene, a direct-acting muscle relaxant, may decrease rigidity, secondary hyperthermia, and tachycardia. Response usually occurs rapidly. Dosages for this indication are not well established, but dosages in the range of 0.8 to 10.0 mg per kilogram per day have been advocated. In general, dosages of 1 to 3 mg per kilogram per day orally or i.v., divided into a four times a day regimen, seem to be effective. Dosages above 10 mg per kilogram per day have been associated with hepatotoxicity. The dopamine agonist bromocriptine is thought to act centrally to decrease some of the symptoms of NMS. There are conflicting opinions on whether bromocriptine hastens recovery. Full response is said to require several days of treatment. Treatment with bromocriptine usually begins at 2.5 mg orally t.i.d. and is increased as tolerated to 5 to 10 mg orally t.i.d. Dantrolene and bromocriptine can be administered together. The duration of therapy with either drug is not well established, but it is prudent to continue the drugs for a week after symptoms of NMS have passed. In cases of rigidity and life-threatening hyperthermia, general anesthesia and paralysis may be life saving.

Tardive Dyskinesia

TD is a syndrome of long-standing or permanent abnormal involuntary movements that is most commonly caused by the long-term use of first-generation antipsychotic drugs. At least 20% of patients who are treated with first-generation antipsychotics long-term develop TD. It presents clinically as **involuntary athetoid movements of the tongue, facial and neck muscles, upper and lower extremities, truncal musculature**, or occasionally muscle groups that subserve breathing and swallowing. Buccolingual–masticatory movements are usually seen early in the course of the disorder and are characterized by tongue thrusting (often visible to the observer as the tongue pushing against the cheeks or lips), tongue protrusions, lip smacking, puckering of the lips, chewing movements, and cheek puffing. Excessive unnecessary facial movements, including grimacing, blinking, and rapid tic-like movements of the face or periorbital musculature, also can be seen in the early phases of TD. Although the movements may occasionally be difficult to distinguish from stereotyped posturing that may occur spontaneously in chronically psychotic individuals, TD generally appears less voluntary and usually has a more choreoathetoid quality. TD rarely develops in patients who have had less than 3 to 6 months of antipsychotic drug exposure, though elderly patients may develop dyskinesias after shorter exposure. The only firmly established risk factor for TD besides first-generation antipsychotic drug exposure is **being older than 50 years**, although there is some evidence that women may be at greater risk than men. There is inconsistent evidence that patients with mood disorders may be at greater risk for developing TD and that intermittent dosing (particularly among patients with mood disorders) may increase the risk of TD. None of the older antipsychotic drugs is known to be more or less likely to cause TD than another. Some evidence supports that the presence of EPS during antipsychotic treatment predicts the development of TD. There is also some suggestion that chronic use of anticholinergic compounds may increase the risk of TD; thus, their use should be minimized if possible. With the advent of newer antipsychotics, the clinician is compelled to consider a variety of factors in deciding the course of treatment for patients on older antipsychotics at risk for TD. The choice may vary with the clinical situation, ranging from the patient doing very well on typical antipsychotics with no TD, to well-controlled psychotic patients with minimal TD, to well-controlled patients with moderate to severe TD, to poorly controlled patients with minimal TD, to poorly controlled patients with severe TD. Except for the well-controlled patient with no symptoms of TD, any evidence that TD is present compels the clinician to justify withholding a trial of newer antipsychotics. Initial treatment of all patients, especially high-risk patients such as elderly patients or those with a history of TD, should be with second-generation antipsychotics. TD often emerges while the patient is still on medication. However, antipsychotic drugs can mask the symptoms of TD, and the abnormal involuntary movements may become apparent only on discontinuation or lowering of the drug dosage. When TD-like movements occur after a decrease in drug dosage or discontinuation and then regress over several days or weeks, they are defined as withdrawal dyskinesia. If relatively permanent, they are defined as TD. Although there is no solid evidence to suggest that withdrawal dyskinesia portends TD if antipsychotics are resumed, it would be judicious to discontinue treatment with first-generation antipsychotic drugs if clinically possible. Treatment with a newer antipsychotic should be considered in this situation.

Several long-term naturalistic studies have shown that **TD is generally mild and fluctuates over time.** Many patients' symptoms remit over time, although TD often returns after antipsychotic treatment resumes. Limited longitudinal study suggests that the rate of TD is approximately five times less with the newer agents than with the older agents. Pending additional research, the clinician must make a judgment for patients with serious psychotic disorders responsive to first-generation drugs who are unable to take clozapine or other atypical drugs. It currently appears that if the psychotic disorder has been serious, it may cause less morbidity to continue treatment, even with an older antipsychotic drug, than to make TD the sole focus of the treatment. Clearly, this clinical judgment requires a full discussion with the patient and family.

Tardive dystonia, a syndrome of late-onset refractory dystonias, follows less commonly in patients treated chronically with first-generation antipsychotic drugs. There may be considerable overlap with TD. Dystonias may respond to benztropine 1 to 2 mg b.i.d. The natural history and risk factors are not well understood.

Prevention. There is no reliable treatment of TD. Thus, the optimal approach is to prevent it by limiting use of older antipsychotics to situations in which they are truly indicated. In general, patients with mood, anxiety, or personality disorders should not be treated with first-generation antipsychotic drugs for protracted periods unless there is some compelling clinical evidence to show that the benefits outweigh the potential risks of developing TD. It is also judicious to avoid long-term use of first-generation antipsychotics whenever possible in the treatment of **mental retardation, dementia, traumatic brain injury, substance abuse, or in elderly patients, because these patients may be at particular risk for TD.**

The clinician should examine all patients prior to initiating antipsychotic drug treatment. Optimally, a standardized scale for abnormal movements should be used, such as the Abnormal Involuntary Movement Scale (AIMS), published by the National Institute of Mental Health. These examinations should be repeated no less than every 6 months while the patient is on antipsychotic drugs. If treatment with an antipsychotic is required for 1 year, the clinician should attempt to taper or discontinue the drug and perform the evaluation at a lowered dosage of antipsychotic or while the patient is off the drug. If evidence of TD is noted, the clinician should discuss the implications with the patient and family so that an informed decision can be made regarding continuing the antipsychotic drug or switching to an atypical antipsychotic.

Differential Diagnosis. A variety of primary neurologic disorders are similar to TD (Table 2.9).

Drugs. Although many treatments, including lithium, lecithin, physostigmine, and benzodiazepines, have been tried, there is no consistently successful treatment of TD. Initial reports suggested that prophylaxis with the antioxidant vitamin E

TABLE 2.9	Differential Diagnosis of Tardive Dyskinesia
Neurologic disorders	Wilson's disease Huntington's disease Brain neoplasms Fahr's syndrome Idiopathic dystonias (including blepharospasm, mandibular dystonia, facial tics) Meige's syndrome (spontaneous oral dyskinesias) Torsion dystonia (familial disorder without psychiatric symptoms) Postanoxic or postencephalitic extrapyramidal symptoms
Drugs and other toxicities	Antidepressants Lithium Anticholinergics Phenytoin L-Dopa and dopamine agonists Amphetamines and related stimulants Magnesium and other heavy metals

might prevent development or worsening of TD, but subsequent larger studies have shown no benefit compared with placebo. There is some evidence that TD improves when patients are switched to clozapine or other second-generation antipsychotics.

Cardiac Toxicity
Pimozide and a number of first-generation antipsychotics may slow cardiac conduction. Thus, they are mildly antiarrhythmic but can cause problems including heart block and prolongation of the QTc with risk of torsades de pointes ventricular tachycardia. Intravenous haloperidol, particularly in high doses, has been recently highlighted for these cardiac conduction abnormalities by the FDA. Although the toxicity of these drugs is most likely to be evident in overdose, it may occur in therapeutic doses as well. Patients with known cardiac disease should therefore be treated with newer agents. The newer agents typically have modest and clinically unimportant effects on the Q-T interval. Risperidone has been associated with QTc prolongation in some cases, and although ziprasidone has been singled out by the FDA because of mild prolongation of the QTc available clinical and research data do not reveal significant ECG abnormalities. In patients with known elevated QTc, follow-up ECGs should be considered when these agents are used.

Clozapine is known to cause tachycardia independent of postural hypotension, which can be severe at times and may limit its use. The ECG in patients on the older drugs, particularly the low-potency agents, may show an increase in the Q-T and P-R intervals, ST-segment depression, and increased heart rate, which may be of little clinical consequence, except in patients who have underlying cardiac disease or preexisting heart block. QT prolongation should prompt the physician to change to a high-potency antipsychotic (e.g., haloperidol) or a newer drug.

Postural Hypotension
Postural hypotension most commonly develops with the use of the lower potency antipsychotic drugs, especially chlorpromazine, thioridazine, and clozapine. However, the newer antipsychotic drugs, especially risperidone, olanzapine, and

quetiapine, may also produce postural hypotension. This side effect is due to α-adrenergic receptor blockade by these compounds and may be associated with reflex tachycardia. Postural hypotension may be severe enough to cause syncope. Hypotension usually improves when the patient is supine; patients should be warned to get up from recumbency slowly.

Weight Gain

Both first- and second-generation antipsychotic drugs may cause weight gain. The only first-generation antipsychotic drug that is thought to be free of this side effect is molindone. Haloperidol is also generally weight neutral in studies comparing it with second-generation antipsychotics. Of the second-generation antipsychotic drugs, the greatest weight gain has been associated with clozapine and the closely related compound olanzapine. In short-term studies, weight gain is approximately 15lb, though extreme weight gains of 50 to 70 lb over a year with either of these drugs are possible. Quetiapine and risperidone also have been associated with weight gain, although to a lesser extent than olanzapine and clozapine. Ziprasidone and aripiprazole, on average, induce minimal, if any, weight gain. Given the long-term nature of antipsychotic drug use, this is more than a cosmetic issue. First, it may affect compliance. In addition, it puts patients at risk of obesity with associated risk of heart disease, hypertension, and diabetes. Cases of treatment-emergent diabetes have been observed with all of the second-generation antipsychotics, though more commonly with olanzapine and clozapine. Because the clinician cannot readily predict in advance which patient on clozapine, olanzapine, or other agents will be among the subgroup (a minority, but up to 40% on olanzapine in some studies) to develop significant weight gain, patients should be informed of the risk, and exercise and diet counseling should be offered to minimize the likelihood of being surprised or overwhelmed by dramatic weight change. If weight gain occurs, a change to ziprasidone or aripiprazole can be instituted. See Table 2.5 for suggested metabolic monitoring.

Ocular Side Effects

Blurred Vision

Because the low-potency agents such as chlorpromazine, thioridazine, and clozapine are relatively anticholinergic, they may cause cycloplegia (the inability to accommodate). Patients may complain of blurred vision, usually with the greatest difficulty in reading. The medium-potency first-generation drugs (e.g., perphenazine) occasionally cause this effect as well. In addition, blurred vision can be caused by anticholinergic compounds given to treat EPS. Often, reading glasses can address the problem. Ocular problems are generally not an issue with the second-generation antipsychotics, and although olanzapine has relatively high anticholinergic properties in pharmacologic studies, blurred vision is rare.

Glaucoma

Any anticholinergic drug may precipitate an attack of narrow-angle glaucoma; therefore, a history of glaucoma should prompt the use of a high-potency first-generation antipsychotic agent (i.e., haloperidol), avoidance of antiparkinson drugs, and an ophthalmologic follow-up. Narrow-angle glaucoma is a medical emergency. Patients with open-angle glaucoma can be managed on neuroleptics if their glaucoma is concomitantly treated by an ophthalmologist.

Ocular Pigmentation

This side effect can be divided into two categories. Pigmentation of the lens, cornea, conjunctiva, and retina (often associated with skin pigmentation) is one category. This occurs mostly with the use of low-potency antipsychotics and is un-likely to interfere with vision except in extremely severe cases. The second cate-gory is pigmentary retinopathy, which is associated with the use of thioridazine above dosages of 800 mg per day and which leads to irreversible degenerative changes with visual impairment. Thioridazine should never be used at dosages above 800 mg per day for this reason. Patients on thioridazine with visual com-plaints should be examined by an ophthalmologist.

Cataracts

Although quetiapine induces cataracts in beagles, and the product label suggests slit-lamp examinations before and regularly after starting the drug, this toxicity does not appear pertinent to humans. Ophthalmologic studies find no evidence supporting regular eye examinations. Because patients with schizophrenia have other risk factors for cataracts, however, a referral to an ophthalmologist for an eye examination can be part of routine medical care.

Cutaneous Side Effects

As with any class of drugs in medicine, the antipsychotics can cause allergic rashes, usually within the first 2 months of treatment. These are most commonly maculopapular erythematous rashes that affect the upper trunk, face, neck, and extremities. Although rashes are usually mild, exfoliative dermatitis has been re-ported. Discontinuation of the drug is followed by a remission of these symptoms. The physician should choose a compound from another chemical class if antipsy-chotic treatment is to be resumed. Low-potency typical antipsychotics can act as photosensitizers, leading to severe sunburn. In addition, there are rare reports of blue-gray discoloration of the patient's skin, usually associated with ocular pig-mentary changes. Although cosmetically undesirable, this effect has not been shown to predispose patients to further cutaneous pathology.

Hypothalamic and Pituitary Side Effects

The major pituitary effect of risperidone and its metabolite, paliperidone, shared with many of the older antipsychotic compounds, is hyperprolactinemia; the nor-mal tonic dopaminergic inhibition of prolactin in the pituitary is blocked by these antipsychotics but not by clozapine and other newer agents. In women, this can result in galactorrhea (also seen rarely in men), amenorrhea, or both. In men, hy-perprolactinemia may cause impotence. Because of their low affinity for D_2 dopamine receptors, clozapine and quetiapine have little or no effect on prolactin levels. Similarly, despite being reasonably potent D_2 blockers, ziprasidone, olanzapine, and aripiprazole have little effect on prolactin levels, and aripiprazole can even lower prolactin levels. **Risperidone and paliperidone, however, frequently elevates prolactin levels** and may cause galactorrhea and amenorrhea in women and galactorrhea and erectile dysfunction in men. Both libido and arousal are frequently affected as well. High-potency older drugs such as haloperidol and fluphenazine are highly prone toward causing erectile failure. The second-generation antipsychotics also frequently cause sexual dysfunction, and it is not clear that any of the newer drugs is superior to another in this regard. For erectile dysfunction associated with second-generation antipsychotics, preliminary placebo-controlled studies find that sildenafil, 50 to 100 mg, improves this side effect. Finally, antipsychotics with prominent α-1 blockade may rarely induce priapism. This requires prompt treatment with intracavernous injection of sympathomimetics or blood drainage.

Although the effects are poorly understood, antipsychotics are known to pre-dispose certain patients to hyperthermia or to marked weight gain, possibly by a hypothalamic mechanism. Severe antipsychotic-induced obesity may lead to drug refusal. There are several reports that molindone causes less obesity than do the other older antipsychotics, and among the newer agents, ziprasidone and aripiprazole have the most favorable profiles for weight gain.

Endocrine Side Effects

Clozapine and olanzapine are nearly free of neurologic side effects, but they frequently cause prominent **lipid and insulin abnormalities.** In rare cases, patients experience acute diabetes with ketoacidosis, but more often patients experience increased appetite, weight gain, and insulin resistance, sometimes leading to new-onset diabetes or worsening of existing diabetes. The exact mechanism by which olanzapine or clozapine affect insulin resistance remains unknown, though there is preliminary evidence that the drugs may directly affect the pancreatic β-cells. Risperidone and quetiapine are less likely to cause weight gain or insulin resistance, though they are not problem-free in this regard. Aripiprazole and **ziprasidone generally do not cause glucose abnormalities. All patients with** schizophrenia treated with second-generation antipsychotics should be monitored for glucose abnormalities and lipid profile, at baseline and then at least twice yearly. See Table 2.5 for suggested metabolic monitoring.

Olanzapine and clozapine often lead to significantly elevated triglyceride levels. The mechanism by which this occurs is unknown. This triglyceride increase occurs much less often with quetiapine or risperidone and rarely occurs with ziprasidone or aripiprazole. Patients changed from risperidone or olanzapine to ziprasidone experience significant reductions in triglyceride levels. Cholesterol levels are affected to a lesser degree by the newer antipsychotics, though they may sometimes be elevated by olanzapine and clozapine treatment.

Hepatic Side Effects

Antipsychotics, especially chlorpromazine, have been associated with cholestatic jaundice, probably secondary to a hypersensitivity reaction in certain predisposed individuals. This presents typically within the first 2 months of treatment and includes nausea, malaise, fever, pruritus, abdominal pain, and jaundice. Elevations of alkaline phosphatase and bilirubin accompanied by minor elevations of the transaminase are seen. Hepatitis should prompt discontinuation of the drug. The syndrome usually remits within 2 to 4 weeks after discontinuation. If further antipsychotic therapy is indicated, a different chemical class should be chosen. Jaundice or transaminase elevations do not appear problematic with the newer agents.

Hematologic Side Effects

Agranulocytosis is a potentially life-threatening hematologic side effect seen most commonly with clozapine and very rarely with aliphatic (e.g., chlorpromazine) and piperidine (e.g., fluphenazine) phenothiazine antipsychotics. The incidence with clozapine may be 1% to 3%. Because of the frequency of agranulocytosis with clozapine, regular monitoring is required indefinitely. The details are listed in the section covering clozapine. **Neutropenia or thrombocytopenia** has been rarely reported with all of the second-generation antipsychotics. Patients on antipsychotics should be counseled to report signs of infection (e.g., sore throats) rather than to monitor blood counts. Symptomatic agranulocytosis requires immediate discontinuation of the medication. When agranulocytosis is associated with an antipsychotic drug in a particular patient, that drug should never be resumed.

OVERDOSAGE

Although the antipsychotic drugs have many toxicities that interfere with their therapeutic use, they have little potential for causing death if taken in overdose. Generally, the most serious complications of overdose are coma and hypotension, both of which should respond to volume expansion. Rarely, lethal cardiac arrhythmias may occur, probably most commonly with pimozide, thioridazine, and mesoridazine. These drugs may prolong the Q-T interval and precipitate heart block or torsades de pointes ventricular tachycardia.

The more common manifestations of overdose may differ between high- and low-potency antipsychotics. Low-potency drugs such as chlorpromazine and thioridazine generally produce CNS depression. Coma may result after administration of 3 to 4 g of chlorpromazine. Low-potency drugs also may lower the seizure threshold markedly when taken in overdose, and thioridazine has potent anticholinergic effects. In addition, these drugs have potent anti–α-adrenergic effects and may cause significant hypotension. Like all antipsychotics, these drugs may produce hypothermia or hyperthermia. Cardiac manifestations occur infrequently but may include Q-T prolongation and ventricular tachyarrhythmias, especially with thioridazine. The second-generation antipsychotics appear safer than the first-generation antipsychotics in overdose, although there have been reports of death from cardiovascular complications. Seizures and status epilepticus may occur. There is one report of a lethal overdose with olanzapine in which the patient developed coma and persistent choreoathetosis, with basal ganglia damage on autopsy. For the newer agents there are reports of massive overdose without serious complication, but some patients have died following a single drug overdose. Higher-potency older antipsychotic drugs can produce either CNS depression or CNS excitation with agitation, delirium, and severe extrapyramidal effects, such as muscular rigidity, tremor, or catatonic symptoms. Thermoregulation also may be impaired. Cardiac arrhythmias are rare but have been reported.

With serious overdoses, the basis of treatment is meticulous supportive care. CNS excitation can be treated with low doses of lorazepam. Hypotension that does not respond to volume expansion will respond to vasopressors such as norepinephrine or phenylephrine. β-Adrenergic agonists should be avoided because they may worsen vasodilation. Hypothermia should be treated with slow warming. Hyperthermia should be treated with antipyretics and, if necessary, cooling blankets. Severe extrapyramidal effects should be treated with diphenhydramine, 50 mg i.m. or i.v., or benztropine, 2 mg i.m. or i.v. Because cardiac arrhythmias may occur, cardiac monitoring is necessary.

Ventricular tachyarrhythmias may be treated with lidocaine. Direct current cardioversion is the treatment of life-threatening tachyarrhythmias. Torsades de pointes ventricular tachycardia, which may occur with pimozide, thioridazine, or mesoridazine, is best managed with isoproterenol or overdrive pacing.

If an ingestion was recent, induction of emesis (which may be difficult because of the antiemetic properties of the drug) or evacuation of the gastric contents through a nasogastric tube is indicated. After emesis is complete, administration of activated charcoal with a cathartic is helpful in adsorbing any remaining drug. Forced diuresis or dialysis is not helpful in removing antipsychotic drugs.

ANTIPSYCHOTICS IN DEVELOPMENT

Several antipsychotics in development are similar (blocking D_2 and $5HT_2$ receptors) to the existing second-generation antipsychotics, and one appears truly novel. All of these have preliminary studies showing superiority to placebo. Iloperidone, asenapine, bifeprunox, and GSK 773812 appear to have relatively mild side-effect profiles, behaving more like aripiprazole or ziprasidone than olanzapine in their side-effect profile. That is, these agents are not associated with lipid or glucose metabolism problems and do not seem to increase appetite. Dosing is not yet established for these drugs, and their efficacy and role vis-à-vis existing second-generation antipsychotics remain unknown. Asenapine and Iloperidone are closest to FDA to approval, though as of this writing they are not yet approved.

A drug manufactured by Eli Lilly, LY 404039, is distinctly different from the others in development. Instead of blocking D_2 receptors and $5HT_2$ receptors, it is a selective agonist for metabotropic glutamate type 2 and 3 receptors. These receptors are found throughout the brain, both on neurons and glia, and are thought to be modulators of dopamine and glutamate transmission. The drug does not directly affect N-methyl-D-aspartate or kainate glutamate receptors, though it does reverse phencyclidine-induced locomotor effect in mice. Hence, its exact mechanism of action remains unknown. In the only published study, in an inpatient phase II clinical trial, LY 404039 was compared with placebo and olanzapine, 15 mg. Two hundred patients were studied for 4 weeks. The drug was clearly superior to placebo (though interestingly there was no improvement among placebo-treated patients) but not as effective as olanzapine [mean Positive and Negative Syndrome Scale (PANSS) change: LY404039 −13; placebo +8; olanzapine −19). The drug did not have any significant laboratory or ECG effects and did not induce parkinsonism. These preliminary results are promising but await replication and dose determination. Although it is tantalizing that drugs could be developed with a mechanism of action that avoids blocking dopamine directly, it is unclear how satisfactory these drugs would treat schizophrenia. Indeed, the drug was less effective than a relatively low dose of a standard drug, so it may only be the start of a new area of inquiry. Mild symptom reduction is far from providing an effective treatment of debilitating schizophrenia.

VALPROATE OR LITHIUM IN THE TREATMENT OF SCHIZOPHRENIA

Valproate and lithium have modest roles in the treatment of schizophrenia. Limited study suggests that lithium is beneficial as an adjunct in schizoaffective disorder for improving both manic and depressive symptoms. Studies have been conducted with haloperidol and clozapine, though the findings likely hold for other antipsychotics. Used in combination with antipsychotics, lithium modestly improves anxiety and mood symptoms in schizophrenia but not core psychotic symptoms. Lithium is likely more effective in patients with schizoaffective disorder than in patients with schizophrenia. In fact, some studies show no benefit of lithium in schizophrenia. Adjunctive lithium is generally used at the therapeutic doses used in bipolar disorder. Although there have been reports about the neurotoxicity of lithium combined with antipsychotics, in these cases lithium concentrations were high, patients were old, and antipsychotic doses were higher than currently employed. We find that lithium may readily be combined with antipsychotics, though patients may experience usual neurologic side effects associated with lithium. Dosing increase should be gradual; the target plasma concentration should be 0.5 to 1.0 mEq/L.

Valproate may be useful for schizoaffective disorder, though it is **better for the manic than the depressive features.** It may also be effective for treating aggression in schizophrenia or schizoaffective disorder. Systematic study is limited, and some studies find little or no benefit for valproate in schizophrenia. One placebo-controlled study in schizophrenia found that usual therapeutic doses of valproate added to risperidone or olanzapine improved hostility more than placebo during the first week, but the difference was minimal after the first week. Presumably, valproate's benefits accrue earlier than the antipsychotic's effects. Thus, although valproate may be helpful in the short-term for agitation or hostility in schizophrenia, caution should be exercised before undertaking long-term use, particularly because side effects such as sedation and weight gain may persist. Long-term treatment with valproate in schizophrenia or schizoaffective disorder has not been established, even if it is common practice. In our clinical experience, psychosis may worsen following valproate withdrawal, though in other cases patients improve because they are less sedated. If valproate is used in conjunction with antipsychotics for acute schizophrenia to control aggression or manic symptoms, it should be dosed much the same as in acute mania, starting at 10 to 20 mg per kilogram per day with the aim of a plasma concentration of 50 to 100 ng/mL. Consideration should be given to remove the valproate after the acute behavior problem resolves.

ANTIDEPRESSANTS IN SCHIZOPRENIA

Depression commonly occurs in schizophrenia. In some cases, depression is relatively clear-cut, as when it follows a psychotic exacerbation (postpsychotic depression). In many cases, depression is insidious and difficult to distinguish from negative symptoms intrinsic to the disorder. In these cases, neurovegetative symptoms of depression and new-onset suicidal thoughts may help distinguish depression from negative symptoms. A number of antidepressants, including the tricyclic antidepressants, selective serotonin reuptake inhibitors (SSRIs), and bupropion may be helpful for treating depression in schizophrenia. We have found that some patients do not tolerate antidepressants and experience worsening of their psychosis, though in general they are well tolerated. The overall benefit from SSRIs, though commonly prescribed to patients with schizophrenia and depression, appears modest. Negative symptoms in stable schizophrenia may show modest improvement with antidepressant use, though some studies find no change.

Hostility and aggression may be centerpiece behaviors for some paranoid patients, and though the antipsychotics are frequently helpful for these behaviors, sometimes they are insufficient. We have found the addition of mood stabilizers such as valproate or lithium helpful for aggression, though the adjunctive use of these agents may lead to problematic weight gain. On the other hand, the SSRIs offer a less complex alternative and these may prove quite helpful in some patients with schizophrenia. In a small placebo-controlled, crossover study, violent inpatients ($N = 15$) with schizophrenia who were stable on antipsychotics were given adjunctive citalopram (20 to 60 mg daily). Over the course of the 48 weeks, there were significant reductions in aggressive behaviors in patients taking citalopram. These findings require replication, but they are consistent with the general finding that the SSRIs treat hostility and aggression.

Although the SSRIs have not been systematically studied for treating anxiety disorders such as panic disorder or obsessive compulsive disorder, we have found these drugs to be somewhat helpful, though more helpful for comorbid panic than for obsessive-compulsive disorder. Sexual side effects, which may already be problematic with the antipsychotics, however, are compounded by the SSRIs and may limit the combination's tolerability.

Care should be taken when adding paroxetine, bupropion, or fluoxetine to risperidone or haloperidol because these antidepressants inhibit the antipsychotic's metabolism (via cytochrome 2D6) and may lead to worsened antipsychotic side effects. Usual antidepressant doses have been used when combining them with antipsychotics.

Although we have seen clinical benefit using bupropion for depression in schizophrenia or for treating sedation associated with antipsychotics, controlled study has been primarily conducted for smoking cessation in schizophrenia. In these trials, bupropion dosed between 150 and 300 mg per day has been safely used in combination with antipsychotics. Bupropion generally does not worsen positive symptoms of schizophrenia in these studies, though it leads to only modest benefit on reducing smoking, even when combined with cognitive behavioral therapy or nicotine replacement therapy. Clinical trials have generally been short-term, and as in other patient groups, benefits decay following short-term trials. Compared to the general population, patients with schizophrenia might require longer treatment with bupropion, nicotine replacement, or the newer smoking cessation aid varenicline to prevent smoking relapse.

BENZODIAZEPINES

Anxiety is common among patients with schizophrenia, whether as a component of an acute psychotic exacerbation or with common co-occurring disorders such as obsessive-compulsive disorder or panic disorder. The pharmacology of the benzo-diazepines is extensively covered in Chapter 5. Lorazepam is frequently helpful in acute psychosis, whether given orally or parenterally. Patients with acute exacerbations of schizophrenia are frequently very agitated and cannot sleep. Lorazepam 2 to 8 mg per day may help improve sleep and prevent behavioral escalation during the early phases of antipsychotic use. Other benzodiazepines may also be helpful, though versatility of lorazepam makes it a good choice. Unlike in acute mania, in schizophrenia treatment the benzodiazepines rarely lead to behavioral dyscontrol or a drunk-like state. Treating anxiety and agitation with benzodiazepines may reduce the need for seclusion and restraint as well as treat some psychotic symptoms. Although we frequently think of the benzodiazepines as primarily helping anxiety symptoms, one 4-week study ($N = 53$) found that diazepam was as helpful as fluphenazine and superior to placebo in treating early signs and symptoms of psychotic exacerbation in schizophrenia. Hence, in addition to treating florid agitation, the benzodiazepines may also be useful during mild psychotic symptom worsening.

Bibliography

Mechanism of Action

Agid O, Kapur S, Arenovich T, et al. Delayed-onset hypothesis of antipsychotic action: a hypothesis tested and rejected. *Arch Gen Psychiatry* 2003;60:1228–1235.

Clinton S, Meador-Woodruff J. Thalamic dysfunction in schizophrenia: neurochemical, neuropathological, and in vivo imaging abnormalities. *Schizophr Res* 2004;69:237.

Costa E, Davis JM, et al. GABAergic cortical deficit dominates schizophrenia pathophysiology. *Crit Rev Neurobiol* 2004;16:1.

Frost DO, Tamminga CA, Medoff DR, et al. Neuroplasticity and schizophrenia. *Biol Psychiatry* 2004;56:540.

Hyman SE, Nestler EJ. *Molecular foundations of psychiatry*. Washington, DC: American Psychiatric Press, 1993.

Jensen NH, Rodriguiz RM, Caron MG, et al. N-desalkylquetiapine, a potent norepinephrine reuptake inhibitor and partial 5-HT(1A) agonist, as a putative mediator of quetiapine's antidepressant activity. *Neuropsychopharmacology* 2008;33:2303–2312.

Moghaddam B. Targeting metabotropic glutamate receptors for treatment of the cognitive symptoms of schizophrenia. *Psychopharmacology* 2004;174:39.

Nyberg S, Eriksson B, Oxenstierna G, et al. Suggested minimal effective dose of risperidone based on PET-measured D_2 and 5-HT_{2A} receptor occupancy in schizophrenic patients. *Am J Psychiatry* 1999;156:869.

Schizophrenia and Other Schizoaffective Disorders

American Psychiatric Association. Practice guidelines for the treatment of patients with schizophrenia. *Am J Psychiatry* 1997;154(4 suppl):1.

Breier A, Buchanan RW, Kirkpatrick B, et al. Effects of clozapine on positive and negative symptoms in outpatients with schizophrenia. *Am J Psychiatry* 1994;151:20.

Carlsson A, Waters N, Carlsson ML. Neurotransmitter interactions in schizophrenia—therapeutic implications. *Biol Psychiatry* 1999;46:1388.

Davis JM, Chen N. Dose response and dose equivalence of antipsychotics. *J Clin Psychopharmacol* 2004;24:192.

Kane JM. Pharmacologic treatment of schizophrenia. *Biol Psychiatry* 1999;46:1396.

Mueser KT, McGurk SR. Schizophrenia. *Lancet* 2004;363(9426):2063.

Robinson DG, Woerner MG, Alvir JM, et al. Predictors of treatment response from a first episode of schizophrenia or schizoaffective disorder. *Am J Psychiatry* 1999;156:544.

Small JG, Hirsch SR, Arvanitis LA, et al. Quetiapine in patients with schizophrenia: a high- and low-dose double-blind comparison with placebo. *Arch Gen Psychiatry* 1997;54:549.

Tollefson GD, Beasley CM, Tran PV, et al. Olanzapine versus haloperidol in the treatment of schizophrenia and schizoaffective and schizophreniform disorders: results of an international collaborative trial. *Am J Psychiatry* 1997;154:457.

Van Putten T, Marder SR, Mintz J. A controlled dose comparison of haloperidol in newly admitted schizophrenic patients. *Arch Gen Psychiatry* 1990;47:754.

Viguera AC, Baldessarini RJ, Hegarty JM, et al. Clinical risk following abrupt and gradual withdrawal of maintenance neuroleptic treatment. *Arch Gen Psychiatry* 1997;54:49.

Second-Generation Antipsychotic Drugs

Awad AG, Voruganti LN. New antipsychotics, compliance, quality of life, and subjective tolerability—are patients better off? *Can J Psychiatry* 2004;49:297.

Brier AF, Malhotra AK, Su T-P, et al. Clozapine and risperidone in chronic schizophrenia: effects on symptoms, parkinsonian side effects, and neuroendocrine response. *Am J Psychiatry* 1999;156:294.

Copolov DL, Link CG, Kowalcyk B. A multicentre, double-blind, randomized comparison of quetiapine (ICI 204,636, "Seroquel") and haloperidol in schizophrenia. *Psychol Med* 2000;30:95.

Csernansky JG, Mahmoud R, Brenner R, et al. A comparison of risperidone and haloperidol for the prevention of relapse in patients with schizophrenia. *N Engl J Med* 2002;346:16–22.

Jackson CT, Covell NH, Essock SM. Differential effectiveness of clozapine for patients nonresponsive to or intolerant of first generation antipsychotic medications. *Schizophr Bull* 2004;30:219.

Jones PB, Barnes TR, Davies L, et al. Randomized controlled trial of the effect on Quality of Life of second- vs first-generation antipsychotic drugs in schizophrenia: Cost Utility of the Latest Antipsychotic Drugs in Schizophrenia Study (CUtLASS 1). *Arch Gen Psychiatry* 2006;63(10):1079–1087.

Kane J, Honigfeld G, Singer J, et al. Clozapine for the treatment-refractory schizophrenic: a double-blind comparison with chlorprozamine. *Arch Gen Psychiatry* 1988;45:789.

Khan AY, Preskorn SH. Examining concentration-dependent toxicity of clozapine: role of therapeutic drug monitoring. *J Psychiatr Pract* 2005;11:289–301.

Kramer M, Simpson G, Maciulis V. Paliperidone extended-release tablets for prevention of symptom recurrence in patients with schizophrenia: a randomized, double-blind, placebo-controlled study. *J Clin Psychopharmacol* 2007;27(1):6–14.

McEvoy JP, Lieberman JA, Stroup TS, et al. Effectiveness of clozapine versus olanzapine, quetiapine, and risperidone in patients with chronic schizophrenia who did not respond to prior atypical antipsychotic treatment. *Am J Psychiatry* 2006;163:600–610.

Potkin SG, Saha AR, Kujawa MJ, et al. Aripiprazole, an antipsychotic with a novel mechanism of action, and risperidone vs placebo in patients with schizophrenia and schizoaffective disorder. *Arch Gen Psychiatry* 2003;60:681.

Rosenheck RA, Leslie DL, Sindelar J, et al. Cost-effectiveness of second-generation antipsychotics and perphenazine in a randomized trial of treatment for chronic schizophrenia. *Am J Psychiatry* 2006;163:2080–2089.

Rosenheck R, Perlick D, Bingham S, et al. Effectiveness and cost of olanzapine and haloperidol in the treatment of schizophrenia: a randomized controlled trial. *JAMA* 2003;290:2693.

Swartz MS, Perkins DO, Stroup TS. Effects of antipsychotic medications on psychosocial functioning in patients with chronic schizophrenia: findings from the NIMH CATIE study. *Arch Gen Psychiatry* 2006;63:1079–1087.

Wahlbeck K, Cheine M, Essali A, et al. Evidence of clozapine's effectiveness in schizophrenia: a systematic review and meta-analysis of randomized trials. *Am J Psychiatry* 1999;156:990.

Wirshing DA, Marshall BD, Green MF, et al. Risperidone in treatment-refractory schizophrenia. *Am J Psychiatry* 1999;156:1374.

Depot Antipsychotic Drugs

Carpenter WT Jr, Buchanan RW, Kirkpatrick B, et al. Comparative effectiveness of fluphenazine decanoate injections every 2 weeks versus every 6 weeks. *Am J Psychiatry* 1999;156:412.

Kane JM, Davis JM, Schooler N, et al. A multidose study of haloperidol decanoate in the maintenance treatment of schizophrenia. *Am J Psychiatry* 2002;159:554.

Kane JM, Eerdekens M, Lindenmayer JP, et al. Long-acting injectable risperidone: efficacy and safety of the first long-acting atypical antipsychotic. *Am J Psychiatry* 2003;160:1125.

Parellada E. Long-acting injectable risperidone in the treatment of schizophrenia in special patient populations. *Psychopharmacol Bull* 2007;40:82–100.

Side Effects and Toxicity

Allison DB, Mentore JL, Heo M, et al. Antipsychotic-induced weight gain: a comprehensive research synthesis. *Am J Psychiatry* 1999;156:1686.

Bhanushali MJ, Tuite PJ. The evaluation and management of patients with neuroleptic malignant syndrome. *Neurol Clin* 2004;22:389.

Casey DE. Side effect profiles of new antipsychotic agents. *J Clin Psychiatry* 1996;57(suppl 11):40.

Correll CU, Leucht S, Kane JM. Lower risk for tardive dyskinesia associated with second-generation antipsychotics: a systematic review of 1-year studies. *Am J Psychiatry* 2004;161:414.

Davis LE, Becher MW, Tlomak W, et al. Persistent choreoathetosis in a fatal olanzapine overdose: drug kinetics, neuroimaging, and neuropathology. *Am J Psychiatry* 2005;162:28.

Gardos G, Casey DE, Cole JO, et al. Ten-year outcome of tardive dyskinesia. *Am J Psychiatry* 1994;151:836.

Gareri P, De Fazio P, De Fazio S, Marigliano N, et al. Adverse effects of atypical antipsychotics in the elderly: a review. *Drugs Aging* 2006;23:937–956.

Goff DC, Cather C, Evins AE, et al. Medical morbidity and mortality in schizophrenia: guidelines for psychiatrists. *J Clin Psychiatry* 2005;66:183–194.

Henderson DC. Weight gain with atypical antipsychotics: evidence and insights. *J Clin Psychiatry* 2007;68(suppl 12):18–26.

Meyer JM, Koro CE. The effects of antipsychotic therapy on serum lipids: a comprehensive review. *Schizophr Res* 2004;70:1.

Nasrallah HA. Metabolic findings from the CATIE trial and their relation to tolerability. *CNS Spectr* 2006;11(7 suppl 7):32–39.

Sussman N. The implications of weight changes with antipsychotic treatment. *J Clin Psychopharmacol* 2003;23(3 suppl 1):S21.

Tamminga C, Woerner M. Clinical course of cellular pathology of tardive dyskinesia. In: Davis K, Charney D, Coyle J, Nemeroff C, eds. *Neuropsychopharmacology—the fifth generation of progress*. Philadelphia: Lippincott Williams & Wilkins, 2003:1831–1841.

Tarsy D, Baldessarini RJ, Tarazi FI. Effects of newer antipsychotics on extrapyramidal function. *CNS Drugs* 2002;16:23.

Trenton A, Currier G, Zwemer F. Fatalities associated with therapeutic use and overdose of atypical antipsychotics. *CNS Drugs* 2003;17:307.

VanderZwaag C, McGee M, McEvoy JP, et al. Response of patients with treatment-refractory schizophrenia to clozapine within three serum level ranges. *Am J Psychiatry* 1996;153:1579–1584.

Drug Interactions

Conley RR, Kelly DL. Drug-drug interactions associated with second-generation antipsychotics: considerations for clinicians and patients. *Psychopharmacol Bull* 2007;40(1):77–97.

Prior TI, Baker GB. Interactions between the cytochrome P450 system and the second-generation antipsychotics. *J Psychiatry Neurosci* 2003;28:99.

Antipsychotic Drugs in Elderly Patients

Aupperle P. Management of aggression, agitation, and psychosis in dementia: focus on atypical antipsychotics. *Am J Alzheimers Dis Other Demen.* 2006;21:101–108.

Jeste DV. Tardive dyskinesia rates with atypical antipsychotics in older adults. *J Clin Psychiatry* 2004;65(suppl 9):21.

Jeste DV, Lacro JP, Bailey A, et al. Lower incidence of tardive dyskinesia with risperidone compared with haloperidol in older patients. *J Am Geriatr Soc* 1999;47:716.

Lee PE, Gill SS, Freedman M, et al. Atypical antipsychotic drugs in the treatment of behavioural and psychological symptoms of dementia: systematic review. *BMJ* 2004;329(7457):75.

Antipsychotic Drugs in Pregnancy

Gentile S. Clinical utilization of atypical antipsychotics in pregnancy and lactation. *Ann Pharmacother* 2004;38:1265.

McKenna K, Koren G, Tetelbaum M, et al. Pregnancy outcome of women using atypical antipsychotic drugs: a prospective comparative study. *J Clin Psychiatry* 2005;66:444–449.

Newport DJ, Calamaras MR, DeVane CL, et al. Atypical antipsychotic administration during late pregnancy: placental passage and obstetrical outcomes. *Am J Psychiatry* 2007; 164(8):1214–1220.

Patton SW, Misri S, Corral MR, et al. Antipsychotic medication during pregnancy and lactation in women with schizophrenia: evaluating the risk. *Can J Psychiatry* 2002;47:959.

Other Drugs Used in Schizophrenia

Carpenter WT Jr, Buchanan RW, Kirkpatrick B, et al. Diazepam treatment of early signs of exacerbation in schizophrenia. *Am J Psychiatry* 1999;156:299–303.

Citrome L, Casey DE, Daniel DG, et al. Adjunctive divalproex and hostility among patients with schizophrenia receiving olanzapine or risperidone. *Psychiatr Serv* 2004;55(3): 290–294.

Patil ST, Zhang L, Martenyi F, et al. Activation of mGlu2/3 receptors as a new approach to treat schizophrenia: a randomized phase 2 clinical trial. *Nat Med* 2007;13(9):1102–1107.

Vartiainen H, Tiihonen J, Putkonen A, et al. Citalopram, a selective serotonin reuptake inhibitor, in the treatment of aggression in schizophrenia. *Acta Psychiatr Scand* 1995; 91(5):348–351.

3 Drugs for the Treatment of Depression

Depressive disorders are debilitating medical conditions that are associated with significant distress, impairment of social and occupational functioning, and elevated risks for cardiovascular and other medical disorders and mortality. Major depressive disorder (MDD) and related unipolar depressive disorders, which include dysthymic disorder and minor depressive disorder, are among the leading causes of disability in the United States.

MAJOR DEPRESSIVE DISORDER

MDD typically presents with a complex set of overlapping symptoms in varying degrees of severity. These symptoms can be classified as **psychological, behavioral, and physical.** According to the *Diagnostic and Statistical Manual of Mental Disorders,* 4th edition (*DSM-IV*), two of the essential features of MDD are depressed mood and loss of interest or pleasure in nearly all activities for a period of at least 2 weeks. Emotional, psychological, and cognitive symptoms of MDD may also include anxiety, irritability, reduced concentration and motivation, feelings of hopelessness and helplessness, excessive guilt, thoughts of suicide, hypersensitivity to criticism, low self-esteem and feelings of worthlessness, and indecisiveness. Common behavioral symptoms include psychomotor retardation or agitation, crying spells, anger attacks and interpersonal confrontation, social withdrawal, reduced productivity, compulsive or ritualistic behaviors, substance abuse, and self-injury. Physical symptoms of MDD comprise a third and equally important set of manifestations. These include sleep disturbances, changes in appetite and weight, fatigue, overall aches and pains, gastrointestinal disturbances, backaches and headaches, and sexual dysfunction. Some of these symptoms, of course, overlap with those of a variety of medical conditions, complicating the differential diagnosis. However, for many patients with MDD, these physical symptoms are an important part of their initial presentation. Given the comorbidity of MDD and various medical conditions, a diagnosis of a coexisting medical condition does not exclude a diagnosis of MDD. The *DSM-IV* diagnostic criteria for MDD, in addition to depressed mood, are captured by the mnemonic SIGECAPS (S for Sleep disturbances; I for Interest, diminished; G for Guilt, excessive or feelings of worthlessness; E for Energy, diminished; C for Concentration, diminished or indecisiveness; A for Appetite disturbances; P for Psychomotor retardation or agitation; and S for Suicidal thoughts or behaviors). MDD is heterogeneous clinically and likely heterogeneous in etiology.

The lifetime risk of MDD ranges from 7% to 12% in men and from 20% to 25% in women. Medical and psychiatric comorbidities are very common in MDD. It has been estimated that only 20% to 25% of the patients with MDD in the community receive adequate treatment. For patients who meet the *DSM-IV* criteria for MDD, it can be expected that approximately 30% to 40% will achieve remission with a single adequate trial (i.e., adequate dose for at least 6 weeks) of any effective antidepressant. Of the remainder, the majority will show some improvement, but 15% to 30% will not improve. The most common reasons for failure of drug treatment are **inadequate drug dosage, intolerance to the pharmacological treatment, and inadequate duration of drug trial.** For those who respond inadequately to initial treatment, there are dozens of alternatives when one considers the various permutations of switching agents, as well as augmenting and combining treatments. Most patients who fail adequate trials of drug therapy for moderate to severe depression could respond to electroconvulsive therapy (ECT) if the treatment were available and acceptable to the patient. However, for most of these patients, a continuation and maintenance treatment would still be required, a need that usually calls for continued efforts to find an effective pharmacologic regimen. Recent studies have suggested that some forms of short-term psychotherapy [cognitive-behavioral therapy (CBT) and interpersonal therapy (IPT)] may be as effective as pharmacotherapy in MDD and that the combination of an antidepressant with cognitive therapy can be more efficacious than either treatment alone. Some researchers have argued that the more serious the depression, the clearer the advantage of drug therapy over psychotherapies in terms of efficacy. In fact, there are no published, adequately powered, comparative studies between CBT or IPT and pharmacotherapy in severe and melancholic depression. Nonetheless, many clinicians would argue that given the effectiveness of medications there would need to be compelling evidence before using CBT or IPT as a single initial therapy for melancholic and/or severely ill depressed patients. For residual depressive symptoms that persist despite pharmacotherapy, CBT and its variants may prove to be particularly useful and the improvement in residual symptoms may remove one of the common risk factors (negative cognitions) for recurrence of depression. The combination of pharmacotherapy and IPT has also been shown to reduce the risk of recurrences more effectively than pharmacotherapy alone, at least in a large sample of geriatric depressed patients.

MINOR DEPRESSION
Minor depression is characterized by the presence of depressed mood and/or reduced interest and pleasure (present most of the time for at least 2 weeks) accompanied by fewer of the symptoms of MDD. There is some evidence from twin studies that minor depression is very closely related to MDD and that in reality these disorders ought to be understood on a continuum rather than as different illnesses. Although milder in severity of symptoms than MDD, this disorder is associated with significant disability.

DYSTHYMIC DISORDER
Dysthymic disorder is characterized by the presence of chronically depressed mood (present, at least intermittently, much of the time for at least 2 years) accompanied by fewer symptoms than would be required to reach the threshold for MDD. Dysthymic disorder is heterogeneous clinically and likely heterogeneous in etiology, although clearly related to MDD. More than 70% of the patients with dysthymic disorder will go on to develop MDD and to have recurrent major depressive episodes superimposed on the dysthymic disorder (double depression). As in the case of MDD, most dysthymic patients have comorbid medical or psychiatric disorders. Although milder than MDD, this disorder may have profound consequences for quality of life and for effective functioning in multiple life roles; this degree of morbidity is reflective of the duration of dysthymic disorder rather than the number of symptoms. It was once thought that dysthymic patients would not respond to antidepressants, an opinion that may have reflected the mistaken idea that patients with milder symptoms should require only low doses of antidepressants, leading to inadequate dosing or duration of treatment for dysthymic patients. More recent studies of dysthymic disorder treatment with various classes of antidepressants indicate that this is a drug treatment—responsive condition; moreover, the benefit of treatment is maintained with continued therapy as in MDD. Because psychotherapies such as IPT and CBT for depression have proven efficacious in patients with depressions of milder severity and in patients with

chronic depressions, these strategies should be considered as alternatives or adjuncts to antidepressant treatment.

SUBTYPES OF DEPRESSIVE DISORDERS

The *DSM-IV* criteria for depression are very useful for clinical practice and research but likely include heterogeneous subgroups based on genetic and other risks and on pathophysiology. Attempts to identify more homogenous groups of depressive disorders are currently ongoing. In the meantime, it has been possible to identify groups of patients with specific clinical features that may predict differential treatment responses.

Melancholic Depression

The *DSM-IV* uses the term melancholic depression to describe severely depressed patients who are unable to experience pleasure (anhedonia) and who lose normal emotional responsiveness to life experiences. These patients also exhibit early morning awakenings, excessive guilt, reduced appetite and weight loss, and psychomotor retardation and agitation. In this population, serotonin-norepinephrine reuptake inhibitors (SNRIs) and those tricyclic antidepressants (TCAs) that act on both the neurotransmitters have shown fairly consistently a modest but significant superiority over selective serotonin reuptake inhibitors (SSRIs).

Anxious Depression

The term anxious depression historically has been used to refer to depressed patients with prominent anxiety symptoms. Many of these patients suffer from comorbid anxiety disorders, whose onset may have either preceded or followed the onset of MDD. Patients with anxious depression are also significantly more likely than patients with nonanxious MDD to be unemployed, to have less education, to be more severely depressed, and to report more melancholic/endogenous features, even after adjustment for severity of depression. Patients with anxious depression have been shown to be less likely to respond to antidepressant treatment than do patients with nonanxious depression, but there is no clear evidence yet of differential antidepressant treatment responsiveness, despite the common belief that certain antidepressants or antidepressant classes may be more anxiolytic than others. However, there is some preliminary evidence that SNRIs may be relatively more efficacious than SSRIs in this subtype. In addition, given the relative modest efficacy of antidepressant monotherapy with these patients, clinicians often augment antidepressants with antianxiety, anticonvulsant, and antipsychotic drugs, despite the limited evidence for their efficacy.

Atypical Depression

In the *DSM-IV*, atypical depression refers to a subtype of depression characterized by mood reactivity, accompanied by symptoms such as hypersensitivity to rejection or criticism, hypersomnia, hyperphagia (often related to carbohydrate craving), and prominent physical fatigue (leaden paralysis; e.g., feelings of heaviness in arms and legs as if they were full of lead). These patients respond better to monoamine oxidase inhibitors (MAOIs; phenelzine is best studied) than to TCAs, although TCAs are superior to placebo. The only adequately powered study in the literature comparing SSRIs with TCAs and placebo has shown comparable efficacy for TCAs and SSRIs, although both drugs were superior to placebo. One of the theories concerning the superior efficacy of MAOIs over TCAs is that the effect of MAOIs on dopamine neurotransmission may play a key role in this patient population. Given safety and tolerability concerns about MAOIs, some clinicians thereby favor antidepressants with norepinephrine and dopamine mechanisms such as bupropion or antidepressant augmentation with psychostimulants, modafinil, and dopamine D_2 and D_2 receptor agonists such as pramipexole or ropinirole. Despite the lack of evidence for superiority of SSRIs over TCAs, SSRIs are often used as first-line treatment of atypical depression, and the switch to bupropion or the augmentation with dopaminergic agents is typically pursued only if the patient fails to respond to an SSRI.

Depression with Anger Attacks

Past attempts to classify subtypes of MDD yielded a possible hostile depressive subtype. Recent work indicates that a significant proportion (30% to 40%) of outpatients with MDD are predominantly irritable when depressed and manifest intermittent outbursts of anger or rage, which have been termed *anger attacks*. Anger attacks emerge abruptly with minimal interpersonal provocation and are associated with a paroxysm of autonomic arousal reminiscent of panic attacks but feature explosive verbal or physical anger, usually directed at close companions or family members. Both anecdotal and systematically ascertained data suggest an important therapeutic role for antidepressants, especially SSRIs, in these patients. In fact, anger attacks cease in the majority of patients with MDD treated with antidepressants. Interestingly, these patients also appear to have decreased central serotonergic activity compared with patients without anger attacks. The depression in irritable patients with anger attacks responds to antidepressants as well as it does in patients without anger attacks.

Secondary Mood Disorders

A large number of medical illnesses and drugs can produce secondary depressive syndromes (Table 3.1). When the depression is due to a treatable disorder or medication, it may remit with appropriate medical care or discontinuation of the offending drug. If, however, the depression is severe or does not remit after treatment of the medical condition, it is reasonable to initiate antidepressant therapy. For example, certain neurologic disorders (e.g., stroke, Parkinson's disease, Huntington's disease) are commonly associated with MDD. Dominant hemisphere stroke patients, in particular, develop MDD with an incidence greater than would be predicted by the degree of disability. Aggressive treatment of the depression may improve the patient's quality of life and his or her ability to participate in rehabilitation. For patients with depression secondary to an untreatable medical or

 TABLE 3.1 Conditions Associated with Secondary Depression

Drug-induced: reserpine, interferon, β-blockers, α-methyldopa, levodopa, estrogens, corticosteroids, cholinergic drugs, benzodiazepines, barbiturates and similarly acting drugs, ranitidine, calcium channel blockers

Related to drug abuse: alcohol abuse, sedative/hypnotic abuse, cocaine and other psychostimulant withdrawal

Metabolic and endocrine disorders: hyperthyroidism (especially in elderly patients), hypothyroidism, Cushing's syndrome, Addison's disease, hypercalcemia, hyponatremia, diabetes mellitus

Neurologic disorders: stroke, subdural hematoma, multiple sclerosis, brain tumors (especially frontal), Parkinson's disease, Huntington's disease, uncontrolled epilepsy, syphilis, dementias, closed head injuries

Nutritional disorders: vitamin B_{12} or folate deficiency, pellagra

Other: pancreatic carcinoma, viral infections (especially mononucleosis and influenza)

neurologic illness, the duration of therapy is undetermined. However, many patients with brain injuries or neurodegenerative disorders (e.g., Alzheimer's disease) manifest elevated susceptibility to the side effects of psychotropic medications, especially typical antipsychotics, any compounds with anticholinergic activity, and sedative-hypnotics including benzodiazepines. Thus, medications must be prescribed with care.

Grief, Bereavement, and Loss

Following bereavement, loss of a job, or a life event leading to significant loss of self-esteem, individuals may experience symptoms of depression. It is important to distinguish depressive illness from normal grief or sadness. Although normally grieving individuals commonly sleep poorly and have decreased appetite, poor concentration, and other apparent neurovegetative symptoms immediately following the loss, these symptoms improve spontaneously over several weeks' or months' time in most cases. If depressive symptoms are particularly severe, persistent, or pervasive; are accompanied by serious suicidal thoughts or behavior; or are protracted beyond what might be reasonably expected for the precipitating stressor, treatment is indicated.

In many cases, the preferred treatment modality is psychotherapy aimed at helping the patient develop adequate coping skills to deal with the loss and associated problems. However, if the depressive symptoms are severe and unremitting, antidepressant therapy should be considered. Indeed, patients are thought to be better able to engage in psychotherapy if severe depressive symptoms are alleviated. Dosages are the same as for the treatment of MDD occurring outside the setting of loss.

Depression with Psychotic Features

MDD accompanied by psychotic symptoms (e.g., delusions or hallucinations) responds poorly to treatment with antidepressants alone. Controlled studies demonstrate that depression with psychotic features is more effectively treated with the combination of an antidepressant and an antipsychotic drug (70% to 80% exhibiting significant improvement) than if treated with either class of drugs alone (30% to 50% response rate). Although some reports describe the efficacy of monotherapy with SSRIs in psychotic depression, the accuracy of diagnosis in these studies has been questioned. ECT is at least as effective as the combined antidepressant–antipsychotic regimen and is the treatment of choice if this combination fails.

The recommended dosage of antipsychotic medication for depression with psychotic features has not been clearly established, but it appears that slightly lower dosages of conventional and second-generation antipsychotic drugs than those used in schizophrenia may be adequate, in addition to full doses of an antidepressant. Individual dosage adjustments are then made as needed. Although exhibiting fewer of the anticholinergic, sedative, and hypotensive side effects of tricyclics, SSRIs may exacerbate the extrapyramidal side effects of both typical and second-generation antipsychotic drugs. Moreover, because of their relatively greater potential to inhibit the hepatic metabolism of drugs metabolized by the P450 2D6 isoenzyme, fluoxetine and paroxetine are more likely than sertraline, citalopram, or escitalopram to produce increases in typical antipsychotic drug levels and thus side effects or toxicity. In contrast to the SSRIs, the anticholinergic effects of TCAs offer some levels of prophylaxis against extrapyramidal symptoms; thus, additional anticholinergics should not initially be prescribed when tricyclics are used in combination with a typical antipsychotic drug. Tricyclics should not generally be combined with low-potency typical antipsychotic drugs (e.g., thioridazine, mesoridazine, or chlorpromazine) because of additive anticholinergic toxicity and postural hypotension. If multiple anticholinergic medications prove necessary for extrapyramidal symptoms, careful monitoring for anticholinergic toxicity is important. Fixed combinations (e.g., perphenazine/amitriptyline, fluoxetine/olanzapine) are available to treat depression with psychotic features but limit the flexibility of the clinician to adjust medications individually as needed. Amoxapine, a cyclic antidepressant with metabolites possessing some antipsychotic potential, is used rarely as monotherapy to treat psychotic depression; there are scant supporting data for this approach.

It should be recalled that antipsychotic drugs, particularly the first generation ones, may cause apathy, akinesia, and blunting of affect, which can be confused with depressive symptoms; thus, other target symptoms, such as sleep, guilt, or psychotic symptoms, may be better indicators of improvement when patients are on combined antipsychotic–antidepressant regimens.

Increasingly, the second-generation antipsychotics (e.g., olanzapine, risperidone, quetiapine, ziprasidone, aripiprazole, and paliperidone) have replaced the first generation antipsychotics for use in mood-disordered patients with psychotic features given the relative lack of extrapyramidal adverse effects and the reduced risk for tardive dyskinesia for which mood-disordered patients appear to be more vulnerable. These drugs also appear to offer some antidepressant potential. Whether they might be used alone, without antidepressants, for psychotic depression remains to be demonstrated. A recent study has yielded fairly low response rates to monotherapy treatment with second-generation antipsychotic agents in psychotic depression, suggesting that the old principle of combining antidepressants and antipsychotics in this population may still be valid even in the era of second-generation antipsychotic agents.

Given the serious morbidity and high suicide risk in depression with psychotic features, **maintenance treatment is recommended.** However, there are few data to guide the decision of whether to continue with combined treatment or either agent alone. For a patient who continues to do well, usual clinical practice involves the gradual (over 3 or 4 months) discontinuation of the antipsychotic drug first, while maintaining the antidepressant treatment for the longer term. In some cases, however, even the gradual discontinuation of the antipsychotic drug may precipitate the emergence of significant symptoms and patients may be kept on the combination therapy for the longer term.

Depression Comorbid with Other Psychiatric Disorders

More than 50% of patients with MDD suffer comorbid psychiatric disorders, in particular, anxiety disorders, substance use disorders, and personality disorders. Relatively higher rates of comorbidity are observed among individuals with early-onset MDD, suggesting that comorbid conditions may in fact be risk factors for the development of MDD.

Depression with Comorbid Anxiety Disorders

Anxiety disorders commonly accompany MDD and generally respond to antidepressant treatment along with the symptoms of the depressive episode. Because SSRIs and SNRIs are antidepressants with Food and Drug Administration (FDA) approval for certain anxiety disorders, such as obsessive-compulsive disorder (OCD), generalized anxiety disorder, panic disorder, and social anxiety disorder, many clinicians use SSRIs and SNRIs as the first-line treatment of MDD with comorbid anxiety disorders. As in the case of anxious depression, many clinicians also administer adjunctive benzodiazepines, second-generation antipsychotics, or anticonvulsants to target comorbid anxiety disorder symptoms. Adjunctive benzodiazepines offer initial relief of anxiety symptoms prior to onset of antidepressant efficacy. They also may be useful for residual symptoms that do not improve with the antidepressant. Because of its delayed onset of efficacy, the antianxiety drug buspirone is not used to provide initial relief but may be used to help with co-morbid generalized anxiety. It is important to recognize that antidepressants are the essential therapeutic agents in these cases and that full antidepressant doses are needed whether or not a benzodiazepine produces initial improvements in anxiety and insomnia. Combining high-potency benzodiazepines with SSRIs for initiation of antidepressant treatment has been reported to enhance treatment compliance and improve early response but can be followed by tapering off the benzodiazepine as the antidepressant response emerges.

Depression with Comorbid Personality Disorders

Personality disorders often co-occur with MDD. That said, it is treacherous to make a new personality disorder diagnosis during a depressive episode; some studies have shown that patients diagnosed with a personality disorder prior to treatment for their mood disorder no longer met criteria for a personality disorder after treatment. Although initial reports suggested that the presence of comorbid personality disorders, particularly borderline personality disorder, was associated with relatively poorer treatment outcome in MDD, subsequent reports using monotherapy with SS-RIs have failed to support this view. SSRIs are often used in patients with borderline personality disorder and other cluster B personality disorders to (a) treat intercurrent MDD; (b) reduce chronic depressive symptoms that do not meet criteria for MDD; (c) modulate anger, hostility, and irritability; (d) diminish impulsivity; and (e) improve other comorbid conditions such as bulimia nervosa or panic disorder. Because personality disorder patients with MDD are often impulsive, angry, and self-destructive, **SSRIs also make good first-choice medications** because they are less dangerous and lethal in overdose than TCAs or MAOIs. Moreover, in one report, the TCAs amitriptyline and desipramine produced worsening in some such patients—both in self-destructive episodes and in global ratings.

Depression Comorbid with Substance Use Disorders

A substantial proportion of patients with MDD have either current or lifetime history of substance use disorders. In some cases, the substance abuse emerges in the context of already existing MDD, whereas in others, MDD may occur in the context of alcohol abuse and abuse of other central nervous system (CNS) depressants (e.g., barbiturates). In the latter case, often the depressive symptoms are presumed to be due to effects of the alcohol or the other substance of abuse; ideally, therefore, the primary treatment should be detoxification. Given the possibilities of drug interactions with alcohol or barbiturates (including altered pharmacokinetics and possible additive CNS depression), prescription of the older antidepressants to actively drinking alcoholics should be avoided if possible, and the newer antidepressants, safer in overdose, should be preferred. Generally, antidepressants are indicated only if depressive symptoms persist for 4 weeks or more after successful detoxification or if the history indicates that mood disorder may be primary and not secondary to substance abuse. There is some support for the potential of SSRIs to reduce drinking for some patients unrelated to an antidepressant effect and for antidepressant treatment to increase the likelihood of abstinence in depressed alcoholics. There also has been interest in the possibility that antidepressants may help maintain abstinence from cocaine based on early reports with desipramine and later anecdotes involving fluoxetine or other SSRIs, but the evidence for the usefulness of antidepressants in nondepressed cocaine abusers is not compelling.

ANTIDEPRESSANTS

A large number of compounds were initially developed to treat depression. Typically, these compounds are called antidepressants, even though most of these drugs are also effective in the treatment of several disorders such as panic and

TABLE 3.2	Indications for Antidepressants
Effective	Major depressive disorder and other unipolar depressive disorders
	Bipolar depression
	Panic disorder
	Social anxiety disorder
	Generalized anxiety disorder
	Posttraumatic stress disorder
	Obsessive-compulsive disorder (e.g., clomipramine and SSRIs)
	Depression with psychotic features in combination with an antipsychotic drug
	Bulimia nervosa
	Fibromyalgia and neuropathic pain (tricyclic drugs and SNRIs)
	Insomnia (e.g., trazodone, amitriptyline)
	Enuresis (imipramine best studied)
	Atypical depression (e.g., monoamine oxidase inhibitors)
	Smoking cessation (e.g., bupropion)
	Attention deficit disorder with hyperactivity (e.g., desipramine, bupropion)
Probably effective	Narcolepsy
	Organic mood disorders
	Pseudobulbar affect (pathologic laughing and weeping)
Possibly effective	Personality disorders

SSRIs, selective serotonin reuptake inhibitors; SNRIs, serotonin-norepinephrine reuptake inhibitors.

other anxiety disorders, and some are effective in the treatment of OCD and a variety of other conditions (Table 3.2). The antidepressant drugs are a heterogeneous group of compounds that have been traditionally subdivided into major groups according to their chemical structure or, more commonly, according to their effects on monoamine neurotransmitter systems: (a) SSRIs, (b) SNRIs, (c) TCAs and the related cyclic antidepressants (i.e., amoxapine and maprotiline), (d) MAOIs, (e) norepinephrine reuptake inhibitors (NRIs), (f) norepinephrine-dopamine reuptake inhibitors (NDRIs), (g) serotonin receptor antagonists and agonists, and (h) α_2-adrenergic receptor antagonists. Because they overlap, the mechanisms of action and indications for use for the antidepressants are discussed together, but separate sections are provided for the method of administration and side effects.

MECHANISM OF ACTION

The precise mechanisms by which the antidepressant drugs exert their therapeutic effects remain unknown, although much is known about their initial actions within the nervous system. All of the currently marketed antidepressants interact with the monoamine neurotransmitter systems in the brain, particularly the norepinephrine and serotonin systems and to a lesser extent the dopamine system. Essentially all currently marketed antidepressants have as their molecular targets components of monoamine synapses, including the reuptake transporters (that terminate the action of norepinephrine, serotonin, or dopamine in synapses), monoamine receptors, or enzymes that serve to metabolize monoamines. What remains unknown is how these initial interactions produce a therapeutic response often after a latency of weeks. The search for the molecular events that convert altered monoamine neurotransmitter function into the lifting of depressive symptoms is currently a matter of intense research.

The architecture of monoamine neurotransmitter systems in the brain is based on the synthesis of the neurotransmitter within a restricted number of nuclei within the brainstem with neurons projecting widely throughout the brain and, for norepinephrine and serotonin, the spinal cord as well. Norepinephrine is synthesized within a series of nuclei in the medulla and pons, of which the largest is the nucleus locus ceruleus. Serotonin is synthesized in the brainstem raphe nuclei. Dopamine is synthesized in the substantia nigra and the ventral tegmental area of the midbrain. Through extensive projection networks, these neurotransmitters influence a large number of target neurons in the cerebral cortex, basal forebrain, striatum, limbic system, and brainstem where they interact with multiple receptor types to regulate arousal, vigilance, attention, sensory processing, emotion, and cognition (including memory).

One of the classic animal models of depression uses the drug reserpine, which depletes neurons of monoamine neurotransmitters, including norepinephrine, serotonin, and dopamine, and causes hypomotility. Similarly, reserpine was believed to induce depression in some humans (although this is a matter of some dispute), which may be clinically indistinguishable from major depressive illness. In animal models, the cyclic antidepressants are partly able to reverse the hypomotility induced by reserpine and other amine-depleting agents, such as tetrabenazine.

Norepinephrine, serotonin, and dopamine are removed from synapses after release by reuptake, mostly into presynaptic neurons. This mechanism of terminating neurotransmitter action is mediated by specific norepinephrine, serotonin, and dopamine reuptake transporter proteins. After reuptake, norepinephrine, serotonin, and dopamine are either reloaded into vesicles for subsequent release or broken down by the enzyme monoamine oxidase (MAO). MAO is present in two forms (MAOA and MAOB), which differ in their substrate preferences, inhibitor specificities, tissue expression, and cell distribution. MAOA preferentially oxidizes serotonin and is irreversibly inactivated by low concentrations of the acetylenic inhibitor clorgyline. MAOB preferentially oxidizes phenylethylamine and benzylamine and is irreversibly inactivated by low concentrations of pargyline and deprenyl. Dopamine, tyramine, and tryptamine are substrates for both forms of MAO. Catecholamines are also broken down by catechol-O-methyltransferase, an enzyme that acts extracellularly. Two common alleles of catechol-O-methyltransferase have been identified, resulting in high and low enzyme activity. There is now research attempting to determine whether these alleles contribute to risk of mental disorders or to interindividual responses to drugs.

The TCAs and other cyclic antidepressants, as well as the SNRIs, block the reuptake of norepinephrine and serotonin in varying ratios, thus potentiating their action (Fig. 3.1). The TCAs doxepin, amitriptyline, and nortriptyline also inhibit glycine uptake by equally blocking the glycine transporters 1b (GLYT1b) and 2a (GLYT2a). The cyclic antidepressant amoxapine is a selective inhibitor of GLYT2a. Whether these properties are relevant to antidepressant action is unclear. Amoxapine is also a dopamine D_2 receptor antagonist *in vivo*, although, interestingly, *in vitro* data suggest that trimipramine and clomipramine have comparable affinity for the dopamine D_2 receptor. There is concern that amoxapine, therefore, could exhibit neuroleptic-like side effects. TCAs, to varying degrees, are also fairly potent blockers of histamine H_1 receptors, serotonin 5-HT$_2$ receptors, muscarinic acetylcholine receptors, and α_1-adrenergic receptors. All the available SNRIs (venlafaxine, duloxetine, and milnacipran) share the property of being relatively potent inhibitors of serotonin and norepinephrine uptake with minimal

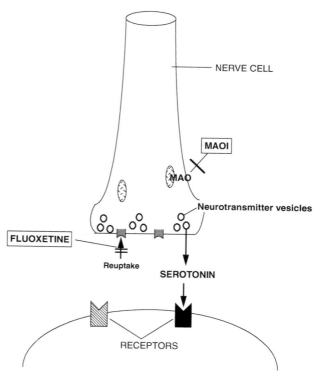

FIGURE 3.1 Fluoxetine blocks reuptake of serotonin into presynaptic serotonin neurons by blocking the reuptake transporter protein. The action of monoamine neurotransmitters in the synapse is terminated by reuptake via specific reuptake transporters. The selective serotonin reuptake inhibitors (SSRIs), such as fluoxetine, specifically block the serotonin transporter; the tricyclics and serotonin-norepinephrine reuptake inhibitors (SNRIs) block both the norepinephrine and serotonin transporters. The resulting increase in synaptic neurotransmitters initiates slow adaptive responses that produce clinical improvement. MAOI, monoamine oxidase inhibitor.

affinity for postsynaptic receptors, with the exception of venlafaxine, which acts as a mild antagonist of nicotinic cholinergic receptors.

At therapeutically relevant doses, the SSRIs exhibit significant effects primarily on serotonin reuptake in the human brain. The SSRIs also appear to have effects at other monoamine transporters that vary from agent to agent, with sertraline demonstrating modest dopamine reuptake inhibition and paroxetine demonstrating modest norepinephrine reuptake inhibition. In addition, fluoxetine, particularly the R-isomer, has mild 5-HT$_{2A}$ and 5-HT$_{2C}$ antagonist activity, as well as weak noradrenergic reuptake inhibition. SSRIs have minimal or no affinity for muscarinic cholinergic receptors with the exception of **paroxetine, which is a weak cholinergic receptor antagonist;** SSRIs also have negligible effects on histaminergic and adrenergic receptors. The lack of significant action on these receptors contributes the mild side-effect profile of SSRIs compared with TCAs.

At therapeutically relevant doses, the NRIs have significant effects primarily on norepinephrine reuptake, although the NRI atomoxetine is also a weak inhibitor of serotonin uptake. The NRI reboxetine appears to have antagonist properties at nicotinic cholinergic receptors.

MAOIs potentiate the action of biogenic amines by inhibiting MAO activity, thus blocking the intracellular catabolism of monoamines. The MAOIs available in the United States are all irreversible inhibitors of MAOA and MAOB activity. Newer MAOIs, such as brofaromine and moclobemide, reversibly inhibit MAOA activity. More recently, additional pharmacologic properties for the MAOIs have been revealed. MAOIs, for instance, also appear to inhibit the binding of [3H] quinpirole, a dopamine agonist with high affinity for D_2 and D_3 dopamine receptors. To complicate the pharmacology of MAOIs, two of the MAOIs, **selegiline and tranylcypromine, have methamphetamine and amphetamine as metabolites;** phenelzine and its yet unidentified metabolite also elevate brain gamma-aminobutyric acid levels. $R(-)$-selegiline but not $S(+)$-selegiline also appears to induce dopamine release by directly modulating ATP-sensitive potassium channels, and the $(-)$ enantiomer of tranylcypromine also appears to inhibit catecholamine uptake.

Serotonin receptor agonists and antagonists primarily bind to serotonin 5-HT_2 receptors. The serotonin receptor antagonists (nefazodone and trazodone) primarily block serotonin 5-HT_{2A} receptors (in some cases, demonstrating partial agonist properties) and share a rather complex pharmacology. Findings from *in vitro* and *in vivo* studies support the hypothesis that *m*-chlorophenylpiperazine (*m*-CPP), an active metabolite of both trazodone and nefazodone, releases neuronal 5-HT via a nonexocytotic carrier-mediated exchange mechanism involving 5-HT transporters. In addition, both trazodone and nefazodone are relatively weak inhibitors of serotonin and norepinephrine uptake, and trazodone appears to stimulate μ-opioid receptors and is a potent agonist of the serotonin 5-HT_{2C} receptors, which are able, when activated, to inhibit the *N*-methyl-D-aspartate-induced cyclic guanosine monophosphate elevation. Both trazodone and, to a lesser degree, nefazodone block α_1-adrenergic receptors. Buspirone and gepirone act as full agonists at the serotonin 5-HT_{1A} autoreceptors and are generally, although not exclusively, partial agonists at postsynaptic serotonin 5-HT_{1A} receptors. Both compounds also have weak affinity for the α_1-adrenoceptors and have mild dopamine D_2 antagonism. Buspirone also has α_2-adrenoceptor antagonist properties via its principal metabolite, 1-(2-pyrimidinyl)-piperazine.

The NDRIs primarily block the reuptake of dopamine and norepinephrine and have minimal or no affinity for postsynaptic receptors. Although bupropion has been recently characterized by some researchers as an NDRI, both bupropion and its metabolite S,S-hydroxybupropion display only weak affinity for the dopamine transporter, and only S,S-hydroxybupropion appears to possess measurable affinity at the norepinephrine transporter level. In addition, other researchers have argued that the NDRI bupropion's effect on norepinephrine is primarily through an increase in presynaptic release. Therefore, one may argue that bupropion's effects on both norepinephrine and dopamine neurotransmission may be due to mechanisms other than those of pure NDRIs. It also appears that bupropion is able to antagonize $\alpha_3\beta_2$ and $\alpha_3\beta_4$ nicotinic cholinergic receptors.

The α_2-adrenergic receptor antagonists (e.g., mirtazapine, mianserin) appear to enhance the release of both serotonin and norepinephrine by blocking auto- and hetero-α_2-receptors. Because mirtazapine appears to be a blocker of serotonin 5-HT_2 and 5-HT_3 receptors as well, it is thought to enhance the release of norepinephrine and enhance 5-HT_{1A}-mediated serotonergic transmission. **Mirtazapine is also a potent histaminergic H_1-receptor antagonist** and is more sedating than the SSRIs. Mianserin is also a 5-HT_2 antagonist.

Because TCAs and MAOIs were the first antidepressants to be introduced in the market, this was initially interpreted as suggesting that antidepressants work by significantly increasing noradrenergic or serotonergic neurotransmission, thus compensating for a postulated state of relative deficiency. However, this simple theory could not and cannot fully explain the action of antidepressant drugs for a number of reasons. The most important of these includes the lack of convincing evidence that depression is characterized by a state of inadequate monoamine neurotransmission. In fact, the results of studies testing the monoamine depletion hypothesis in depression have yielded inconsistent results. Moreover, blockade of reuptake by the cyclic antidepressants and SSRIs and inhibition of MAO by MAOIs occur rapidly (within hours) after drug administration, but antidepressants are rarely clinically effective prior to 2 weeks and may require 6 weeks or more.

These considerations have led to the idea that inhibition of monoamine reuptake or inhibition of MAO by antidepressants represents an initiating event. The actual therapeutic actions of antidepressants, however, result from slower adaptive responses within neurons to these initial biochemical perturbations. Research investigating slow-onset changes in neurons that might better reflect the time course of antidepressant action is ongoing. It has been found, for example, that chronic (2 weeks) treatment of rats with cyclic antidepressants or MAOIs is associated with a reduction in number (downregulation) of β_1-adrenergic receptors, accompanied by a decreased activation of adenyl cyclase by norepinephrine. Many antidepressants also downregulate α_2-adrenergic receptors and have variable effects on 5-HT$_2$ serotonin receptors. Changes in receptor number are currently seen as correlates of long-term administration (established largely in normal rat brain), not a likely therapeutic mechanism. Slow-onset changes in the nervous system that may be related convincingly to the mechanism of action of antidepressants are actively being sought. It is now well established that antidepressants, like other drugs that affect neurotransmitters, **alter the expression of a large number of genes** in the brain. The question is which genes are relevant and what is the effect of increasing or decreasing the levels of the proteins that they encode. For example, increased neurogenesis in areas of the brain, such as the hippocampus, is considered one of the possible downstream effects of antidepressants.

Although research to understand the therapeutic actions of antidepressants has been challenging, receptor studies have been useful in understanding some of their side effects. For example, the rank order of binding affinities of cyclic antidepressants at muscarinic cholinergic receptors generally parallels the potency of their clinical anticholinergic effects. Similarly, high affinities for histamine H_1 receptors may partially explain their strong sedative effects and their ability to increase appetite, while high affinities for α_1-adrenergic receptors may be related to the risk of orthostatic hypotension. Such information is very useful for clinicians to understand and treat side effects and to those attempting to develop new antidepressants.

Given that antidepressants that act via monoamine systems have similar efficacy for MDD, attempts have been made to find antidepressant compounds that act independently of monoamines. For example, attempts are being made to develop corticotropin-releasing factor 1 receptor antagonists and drugs that block the neurokinin 1 receptors (NK-1 antagonists) to treat depression.

CLINICAL USES

As one would expect, the newer antidepressants (SSRIs, SNRIs, NRIs, NDRIs, and serotonin receptor antagonists) all have safety and side-effect advantages over the TCAs and MAOIs. Since the introduction of fluoxetine, the SSRIs and SNRIs have become the most often prescribed initial treatment for MDD. The success of the SSRIs and SNRIs in displacing tricyclic drugs as first-choice agents is not based on established differences in efficacy but rather on a generally more favorable side-effect profile such as lack of anticholinergic and cardiac side effects and a high therapeutic index (ratio of lethal dose to therapeutic dose), combined with ease of administration. Furthermore, with certain comorbidities of depression, such as OCD, SSRIs offer advantages in efficacy over the tricyclics. Some of the meta-analytic studies of the efficacy of SSRIs and TCAs have even concluded that some of the tertiary amine tricyclics may be slightly more efficacious than SSRIs in more severe, melancholic depression. Because of their toxicity and risk, MAOIs are a class of drugs reserved for patients for whom other treatments have failed.

Suicide Risk

The tricyclic and related cyclic antidepressants (maprotiline and amoxapine) and the MAOIs are potentially lethal in overdose, unlike the SSRIs, the SNRIs, and the other newer antidepressants. Thus, a careful evaluation of impulsiveness and suicide risk influences not only the decision as to the need for hospitalizing a person with depression but also the choice of an antidepressant. For potentially suicidal or highly impulsive patients, the SSRIs, the SNRIs, and the other newer agents would be a better initial choice than a cyclic compound or an MAOI. Patients at elevated suicide risk who cannot tolerate these safer compounds or who do not respond to them should not receive large quantities or refillable prescriptions for TCAs or MAOIs. Generally, patients who are new to treatment or those at more than minimal risk for suicide whose therapeutic relationship is unstable should receive a limited supply of any medication.

Evaluation for suicide risk must continue even after the initiation of treatment. Although suicidal thoughts are often among the first symptoms to improve with antidepressant treatment, they may also be slow to respond to treatment, and patients may become demoralized before therapeutic efficacy is evident. Side effects such as agitation and restlessness and, most important, intercurrent life events may exacerbate suicidal thoughts prior to a full therapeutic response. Thus, rarely, for a variety of reasons, patients may temporarily become more suicidal following the initiation of treatment. Should such worsening occur, appropriate interventions may include management of side effects, more frequent monitoring, discontinuation of the initial treatment, or hospitalization. The FDA has asked manufacturers of almost all the antidepressant drugs to include in their labeling a warning statement that recommends close observation of adult and pediatric patients treated with these drugs for worsening depression or the emergence of suicidality. This warning was based on the analyses of clinical trials data comparing the relative risk of emergence of suicidal ideation in patients on these drugs and placebo following initiation of treatment. The difference was small (less than twofold) but statistically significant. This finding underscores the need for good practice, which includes education of patients (and families if the patient is a child) about side effects of drugs (including the possible emergence of suicidal thoughts and behaviors), close monitoring (especially early in treatment), and the availability of a clinician in case suicidality emerges or worsens. Further analyses from the FDA on the relative risk of treatment-emergent suicidal ideation with the SSRIs have demonstrated that a very small increase in risk is observed only in adolescents and young adults. A consensus remains, however, that the **risks associated with withholding antidepressant treatment** from patients, including pediatric patients, with serious depression outweighs the risks associated with the drugs.

Treatment-Resistant Depression

A large number of patients respond **partially or not at all to an initial antidepressant trial.** When evaluating possible causes for antidepressant nonresponse, it is important to ensure that the initial diagnosis is correct and that there is no unsuspected comorbid psychiatric or medical condition (e.g., alcoholism or thyroid disease) negatively affecting treatment response. There are three general strategies for treating resistant depression that can be used in an orderly fashion (these strategies are discussed in detail for each specific class of drug):

1. **Optimization/dose increase**—ensuring adequate drug doses for the individual, which may be higher than initial doses (e.g., fluoxetine, 40 to 80 mg; desipramine, 200 to 300 mg) and adequate duration of treatment (8 to 12 weeks or longer). In addition, the possibility of failure of the patient to adhere to the regimen, which occurs more commonly than most practitioners appreciate, should be considered. Dose increases above the FDA-recommended dose range may occur in clinical practice when patients have partial or nonresponse in the absence of side effects. In some cases, obtaining blood levels of the antidepressant (typically 24 hours after the last dose) may help and guide this decision.

2. **Augmentation or combination**—addition of drugs (to the ongoing treatment) that are not antidepressant agents themselves is termed *augmentation therapy*; well-studied augmentation strategies included, for example, adjunctive second-generation antipsychotic agents, lithium, or L-triiodothyronine (T_3). Other less well-studied augmentation strategies include the use of buspirone, modafinil, psychostimulants, methylfolate, and S-adenosyl-methionine (SAMe). Combination treatment generally refers to the prescribing of more than one antidepressant. Examples of this approach include adding antidepressants such as bupropion or mirtazapine to SSRIs or SNRIs. The array of putative augmentation and combination strategies has dramatically increased with the newer antidepressant agents. Although there are many commonly used augmentation and combination strategies, few have been well studied and supported by clinical research.

3. **Switching**—change in the primary drug. If lack of efficacy was the problem, a switch to an agent from a different drug class is reasonable, particularly when the first drug is poorly tolerated; for example, if the first drug was an SSRI, switch to bupropion or to an SNRI. If, however, the first drug failed because of side effects, a drug within the initial class may be effective if it is tolerated. For reasons that are unclear but likely reflect the minor pharmacological differences between SSRIs, a switch within the class is clinically helpful for primary efficacy failures sufficiently often to warrant a second SSRI trial for some patients before switching out of class. If the patient remains seriously depressed despite additions or changes in medication, consideration should be given to the relative risks of additional trials (based on severity of symptoms and concern about time delay) versus the use of ECT.

Continuation and Maintenance Treatment

Originally based on studies with TCAs, patients with unipolar depressive disorders were observed to be at high risk for relapse when treatment was discontinued within the first 16 weeks of therapy. Therefore, in treatment responders, most experts favor a continuation of antidepressant therapy for a minimum period of 6 months following the achievement of remission. The value of continuation therapy for several months to prevent relapse into the original episode has also been established for virtually all the newer agents. Risk of recurrence after this 6- to 8-month continuation period, that is, the development of a new episode after recovery from the index episode, is particularly elevated in patients with a chronic course before recovery, residual symptoms, and multiple prior episodes (three or more). For these individuals, the **optimal duration of maintenance treatment is unknown but is often measured in years.** Based on research to date, prophylactic efficacy of an antidepressant has been observed for as long as 5 years with clear benefit. In contrast to the initial expectation that maintenance therapy would be effective at dosages lower than that required for acute treatment, the current consensus is that full-dose therapy is required for effective prophylaxis. In some cases, adequate maintenance may actually require doses of antidepressants higher than those that were acutely effective and therefore some dose flexibility.

Two of the main issues in the use of antidepressants for continuation and maintenance treatment are the persistence of troublesome side effects emerging during the acute phase of treatment and the emergence of side effects during the continuation and maintenance phases. For example, continuation and maintenance therapy with TCAs is often difficult because of early-onset, persisting side effects such as weight gain, dry mouth, and constipation. With the newer drugs, in particular the SSRIs, the main issue is often the emergence of certain side effects during the continuation and maintenance therapy such as **apathy, cognitive side effects, sexual dysfunction, weight gain, fatigue, and sleepiness.**

About 20% to 30% of patients who are treated with each of the classes of antidepressants will experience a return of depressive symptoms despite continued treatment. In such patients, a dose increase of the antidepressant is typically the first-line approach, although the same considerations and strategies described for treating resistant depression are also of potential value.

Except for amoxapine, which possesses some antipsychotic drug properties and has been implicated in tardive dyskinesia, there are no known severe adverse effects specifically due to long-term antidepressant treatment, except that the risk of a discontinuation syndrome with TCAs, MAOIs, SSRIs, and SNRIs is more likely after abrupt interruption of chronic treatment especially with shorter half-life agents. Discontinuation syndromes are typically characterized by the emergence of transient, short-lived physical (e.g., dizziness, headache, nausea, flulike symptoms) and psychological (e.g., dysphoria, irritability, anxiety) symptoms that abate rapidly on reintroducing the antidepressant agent. To minimize the risk for discontinuation reactions, it is always advisable to gradually taper and discontinue antidepressants after chronic exposure.

CHOICE OF ANTIDEPRESSANT

A large number of antidepressants are available (Table 3.3), including SSRIs, SNRIs, tricyclic and related compounds, MAOIs, NRIs, NDRIs, serotonin receptor antagonists and agonists (e.g., nefazodone and trazodone), and the α_2-adrenergic receptor antagonists. Successful use of antidepressants requires the following:

1. Good patient selection as determined by a thorough and comprehensive diagnostic evaluation. In particular, attention should be paid to comorbid psychiatric and medical disorders.
2. Choice of a drug with an acceptable side-effect profile for the given patient.
3. Adequate dosage. In the absence of side effects and response, dose escalations within the recommended range should be pursued aggressively.
4. Drug trial of at least 6 to 12 weeks for MDD and other unipolar depressive disorders.

Many patients with potentially treatable depression fail to improve because of inadequate dosing or duration of treatment or both. Every physician does not need to be thoroughly familiar with every antidepressant on the market, but it is useful for the clinician to be comfortable prescribing several drugs that differ in mechanism and side-effect profile. The most important considerations in choosing among these drugs are efficacy for the condition being treated and side effects. The

TABLE 3.3 — Available Preparations of Antidepressants

Drug	Dose Forms	Usual Daily Dose (mg)	Extreme Daily Dosage (mg)	Therapeutic Plasma Levels (ng/mL)
Selective serotonin reuptake inhibitors (SSRIs)				
Fluoxetine (Prozac and generics)	C: 10, 20, 40 mg LC: 20 mg/5 mL Weekly: 90 mg	20–40	5–80	
Fluvoxamine (Luvox and generics) (not indicated for depression in the United States)	T: 50, 100 mg CR: 100, 150 mg	50–150	50–300	
Paroxetine (Paxil and generics)	T: 10, 20, 30, 40 mg LC: 10 mg/5 mL CR: 12.5, 25, 37.5 mg	20–40 25–37.5	10–50 12.5–50	
Sertraline (Zoloft and generics)	T: 25, 50, 100 mg LC: 20 mg/mL	50–150	25–300	
Citalopram (Celexa and generics)	T: 10, 20, 40 mg LC: 10 mg/5 mL	20–40	10–60	
Escitalopram (Lexapro)	T: 5, 10, 20 mg	10–20	10–30	
Serotonin-norepinephrine reuptake Inhibitors (SNRIs)				
Venlafaxine (Effexor and generics)	T: 25. 37.5, 50, 75, 100 mg XR: 37.5, 75, 150 mg	75–300	75–450	
Duloxetine (Cymbalta)	C: 20, 30, 60 mg	30–90	30–120	
Desvenlafaxine (Pristiq)	T: 50, 100 mg	50–100	50–400	
Milnacipram (Savella; approved for fibromyalgia in US) (not indicated for depression in the United States)	T: 12.5, 25, 50, 100 mg	100–200	50–300	
Norepinephrine reuptake inhibitors (NRIs)				
Reboxetine (not available in the United States)		4–10	4–12	
Atomoxetine (Strattera) (not indicated for depression)	T: 10, 18, 25, 40, 60 mg	40–80	40–120	
Serotonin receptor antagonists and agonists				
Trazodone (Desyrel and generics)	T: 50, 100, 150, 300 mg	200–500	100–600	
Nefazodone (Serzone and generics)	T: 50, 100, 150, 200, 250 mg	200–450	100–600	
Norepinephrine-dopamine reuptake inhibitors (NDRIs)				
Bupropion (Wellbutrin and generics)	T: 75, 100 mg XR: 100, 150, 200 mg XL: 150, 300 mg	200–300	150–450	

(continued)

TABLE 3.3	Available Preparations of Antidepressants *(continued)*				

Drug	Dose Forms	Usual Daily Dose (mg)	Extreme Daily Dosage (mg)	Therapeutic Plasma Levels (ng/mL)
α_2-Adrenergic receptor antagonists				
Mirtazapine (Remeron and generics)	T: 15, 30, 45 mg T(Soltab): 15, 30, 45 mg	15–45	15–60	
Mianserin (not available in the United States)		30–60	30–90	
Tricyclic antidepressants (TCAs) and other cyclic compounds				
Imipramine (Tofranil and generics)	T: 10, 25, 50 mg C: 75, 100, 125, 150 mg INJ: 25 mg/2 mL	150–200	50–300	>225[a]
Desipramine (Norpramin and generics)	T: 10, 25, 50, 75, 100, 150 mg C: 25, 50 mg	150–200	50–300	>125
Amitriptyline (Elavil and generics)	T: 10, 25, 50, 75, 100, 150 mg INJ: 10 mg/mL	150–200	50–300	>120 (?)[b]
Nortriptyline (Pamelor and generics)	C: 10, 25, 50, 75 mg LC: 10 mg/5 mL	75–100	25–150	50–150
Doxepin (Adapin, Sinequan, and generics)	C: 10, 25, 50, 75, 100, 150 mg LC: 10 mg/mL	150–200	25–300	100–250 (?)
Trimipramine (Surmontil and generics)	C: 25, 50, 100 mg	150–200	50–300	
Protriptyline (Vivactil and generics)	T: 5, 10 mg	20–40	10–60	
Maprotiline (Ludiomil and generics)	T: 25, 50, 75 mg	100–150	50–200	
Amoxapine (Asendin and generics)	T: 25, 50, 100, 150 mg	150–200	50–300	
Clomipramine (Anafranil and generics)	C: 25, 50, 75 mg	150–200	50–250	
Monoamine oxidase inhibitors (MAOIs)				
Phenelzine (Nardil and generics)	T: 15 mg	45–60	15–90	
Tranylcypromine (Parnate and generics)	T: 10 mg	30–50	10–90	
Isocarboxazid (Marplan)	T: 10 mg	30–50	30–90	
Selegiline (EmSam)	Patch: 6, 9, and 12 mg/24 hours	6–9	6–12	

C, capsules; LC, liquid concentrate or solution; T, tablets; CR, controlled release; XR, extended release; XL, ; INJ, injectable form.
[a]Sum of imipramine plus desipramine.
[b]Sum of amitriptyline plus nortriptyline.

TABLE 3.4	Tricyclic Antidepressants and Monoamine Oxidase Inhibitors Side Effect Profile		
Category and Drug	Sedative Potency	Anticholinergic Potency	Orthostatic Hypotensive Potency
Tricyclic and related cyclic compounds[a]			
Amitriptyline	High	High	High
Amoxapine	Low	Moderate	Moderate
Clomipramine	High	High	High
Desipramine	Low	Moderate	Low
Doxepin	High	High	Moderate
Imipramine	Moderate	High	High
Maprotiline	Moderate	Low	Moderate
Nortriptyline	Moderate	Moderate	Low
Protriptyline	Low	High	Low
Trimipramine	High	Moderate	Moderate
Monoamine oxidase inhibitors			
Isocarboxazid	—	Very low	High
Phenelzine	Low	Very low	High
Tranylcypromine	—	Very low	High

[a]All of the tricyclic and related cyclic compounds have well-established cardiac arrhythmogenic potential.

efficacy of the available antidepressants for MDD, including various subtypes, and for other disorders has been described previously. Although there are some differences in efficacy across the class of antidepressants for subtypes of depression, the major clinically significant differences among the antidepressants are in their side effects. All of the TCAs and related compounds (maprotiline and amoxapine) cause some degree of anticholinergic side effects and postural hypotension, and all are potentially cardiotoxic in susceptible individuals or in overdose (Table 3.4). The consensus among experts in formulating depression treatment guidelines is that the first line of treatment should be a newer antidepressant in light of safety and tolerability concerns over the long term. Although most of the newer antidepressants may initially cause agitation, insomnia, nausea, and headache, and, over time, sexual dysfunction, among other side effects, they are generally more tolerable to patients than are the older cyclic compounds. The MAOIs may cause significant side effects, including postural hypotension, and require dietary and drug interaction precautions, thereby raising issues of treatment adherence.

At a minimum, general physicians should be comfortable prescribing at least two of the SSRIs and the SNRIs, and at least one compound of every other class of new antidepressants (NRIs, NDRIs, serotonin receptor antagonists and agonists, and α_2-adrenergic receptor antagonists). Because psychiatrists will often be called on to treat patients who have failed initial treatments, they should have broader experience, including experience with tricyclics and MAOIs. The following are general guidelines for choosing an antidepressant:

1. It is reasonable to prescribe a drug that was clearly effective in the past if it was well tolerated by the patient. It is also reasonable to prescribe an antidepressant that was clearly effective in the past in a first-degree relative of the patient.

2. Avoid drugs (e.g., amitriptyline, protriptyline) with the highest levels of anticholinergic activity to maximize patient comfort and compliance. In addition to bothersome side effects such as dry mouth, dry throat, urinary retention, blurred vision, and constipation, diminished working memory and dental cavities are also considered to be possible side effects secondary to anticholinergic effects. (Despite its relatively high anticholinergic potency, clomipramine is considered useful because of its efficacy in OCD and its superior efficacy for severe and melancholic depression.)

3. For patients with initial insomnia, many clinicians may opt for the temporary use of a short-acting benzodiazepine or other hypnotic combined with SSRIs, SNRIs, or other nonsedating newer antidepressants, with the expectation of tapering and discontinuing the hypnotic when the depression has improved. Both benzodiazepines and nonbenzodiazepine hypnotics such as zolpidem and eszopiclone have been shown to be more effective than placebo in treating insomnia during antidepressant treatment. Benzodiazepines with relatively long half-lives increase the risk of unwanted somnolence and sleepiness during the day. Other clinicians may select a sedating secondary-amine tricyclic compound (e.g., nortriptyline) given at bedtime. To avoid anticholinergic and cardiovascular side effects, however, the sleep-enhancing, α_2-adrenergic receptor antagonist mirtazapine would be preferred, with the expectation that daytime sedation will abate over time with these medications. The sedating tricyclic drug amitriptyline used to be popular with general physicians, but because it is among the most anticholinergic of the tricyclics, it should not be a first-choice agent. The serotonin receptor antagonist trazodone, which lacks anticholinergic side effects, is very sedating, but its overall efficacy as monotherapy for depression is often questioned by clinicians. Trazodone at lower doses (50 to 300 mg at bedtime) has been used in place of benzodiazepines or other hypnotics to treat insomnia, particularly middle to late insomnia, in patients treated for depression with an SSRI or an SNRI. Although benzodiazepines and hypnotics such as zolpidem are often started either simultaneously with the antidepressant or added later to the treatment, trazodone is typically not started at the same time as the antidepressant but is instead added later on for the management of the insomnia. For most depressed patients, if insomnia is related to depression, the sleep difficulties will improve with any effective antidepressant over time, even those without sedation as a side effect. With more sedating drugs, on the other hand, the side effect may persist after it is helpful and may interfere with daytime function and compliance.

4. All of the tricyclics and most of the SSRIs (e.g., fluoxetine, fluvoxamine, paroxetine, citalopram, and sertraline) are available generically and have the advantage of being the least costly treatments in terms of formulary cost. On the other hand, when one considers the other direct and indirect costs of treatment, however, the financial savings of the generic TCAs diminish.

5. For patients who want to avoid sedation, it is reasonable to prescribe SSRIs, SNRIs, NRIs, and NDRIs, which are usually nonsedating. Among the tricyclics, desipramine and protriptyline are probably the least sedating.

6. In elderly patients, especially those with constipation or glaucoma, and in men with prostate hypertrophy, the least anticholinergic drugs should be used, such as SSRIs or other newer agents.

7. SSRIs, SNRIs, NRIs, NDRIs, and the α_2-adrenergic receptor antagonist mirtazapine generally do not cause postural hypotension, whereas TCAs, MAOIs, and the serotonin receptor antagonists nefazodone and trazodone

have this risk. In the case of TCAs and both nefazodone and trazodone, the blockade of α_1-receptors is thought to be related to the risk of postural hypotension. Nortriptyline, desipramine, and protriptyline may have an advantage among the tricyclics in causing relatively less postural hypotension than the others. The tricyclics have on rare occasion been associated with hypertension, and at higher doses, a small percentage of patients may have blood pressure elevation with venlafaxine.

8. In patients with cardiac disease or significant delay in intracardiac conduction, the tricyclics with their quinidine-like properties should be avoided.

9. Epileptic patients may develop a primary depressive disorder or secondary depression. Because all of the tricyclic and related cyclic antidepressants and the NDRI bupropion may decrease the seizure threshold, these agents should be avoided in these populations. When combining any antidepressant with an anticonvulsant, the clinician must be alert for possible pharmacokinetic interactions, because many of the anticonvulsants may be inducers or inhibitors of cytochrome P450 (CYP) systems.

10. Most antidepressants may cause or worsen sexual dysfunction. In particular, decreased libido, delayed orgasm or anorgasmia, arousal difficulties, and erectile dysfunction have been reported with almost all the classes of antidepressants. Trazodone and nefazodone have been associated with the uncommon occurrence of priapism in both men and women. Two recent studies by Clayton et al. suggest that the NDRI bupropion and the NRI reboxetine may be the least likely antidepressants to cause sexual dysfunction.

11. Two cyclic compounds that we do not recommend are, in fact, rarely used. Maprotiline has produced a high incidence of seizures at dosages above 200 mg per day (and occasionally at lower dosages), possibly limiting the prescription of adequate therapeutic doses. A study reported that almost one third of the cases of seizures in the Swedish national database for spontaneous reporting of adverse drug reactions were related to the use of maprotiline. Because 47% of such patients had been concomitantly treated with drugs with potential inhibitory effects on the CYP2D6 system, whenever maprotiline or other TCAs are used, it is important to watch for possible drug–drug interactions because TCAs and maprotiline are substrates of the same system. Amoxapine has antipsychotic drug–like effects in both animal models and humans, making it analogous to a combination drug containing both an antipsychotic and an antidepressant, but one in which the physician has no control over the ratio. In fact, positron emission tomography data show that amoxapine's profile is very similar to that of the established second-generation antipsychotics. In addition, amoxapine has been associated with the emergence of antipsychotic drug–like side effects, such as akathisia and tardive dyskinesia and dystonia. An increased risk for seizures has also been associated with amoxapine.

12. In general, although promising ease of use, fixed combination drugs, such as those older compounds that contained a tricyclic and an antipsychotic drug or a tricyclic and a benzodiazepine, are not recommended because they do not allow optimal titration of the component drugs for any given patient. The exception to our skepticism about fixed combinations may be the olanzapine and fluoxetine combination, which has shown efficacy in psychotic depression.

13. Most patients seeking treatment for depression will have one or more comorbid conditions; the comorbid disorder should influence initial

treatment selection in choosing an agent thought to be efficacious for the comorbid condition as well as the depression, as with SSRIs and OCD or the NDRI bupropion and attention deficit disorder.

SELECTIVE SEROTONIN REUPTAKE INHIBITORS

The recognition that a specific neuronal uptake mechanism for serotonin was found in the brain suggested, as early as the late 1960s, a potential target for new antidepressants. By the early 1970s, the technology existed for the screening of molecules that could selectively inhibit serotonin uptake. In 1972, fluoxetine was shown to produce selective inhibition of serotonin uptake in rat synaptosomes. This drug, the first of a class that includes sertraline, paroxetine, citalopram, escitalopram, and fluvoxamine, was approved for release in the United States in December 1987. The impact of this class of drugs on the treatment of depression has been extraordinary (e.g., it has been estimated that SSRIs have been prescribed to more than 100 million people worldwide). The success of these drugs appeared to derive mainly from side-effect advantages over older agents such as the TCAs and the MAOIs. The absence of anticholinergic, antihistaminergic, anti–α_1-adrenergic, and cardiotoxic effects and their relative safety in overdose compared to the TCAs and the MAOIs generated wide patient and prescriber acceptance. This milder side-effect profile made the delivery of adequate antidepressant doses available to patients for both acute and long-term treatment without the need for dose titration and the endurance of persisting unpleasant or dangerous side effects. **The SSRIs are by no means free of side effects,** but they appear to be more tolerable than the older drugs, and some patients are virtually free of any daily medication-related discomfort. During the acute phase of treatment, the side effects of SSRIs include nausea (which tends to be worst during early treatment) and other gastrointestinal symptoms, reduced appetite, weight loss, excessive sweating, tremor, flushing, headaches, insomnia, anxiety, agitation, jitteriness, sedation, dizziness, and sexual dysfunction. Other, less common, adverse events associated with SSRI treatment include diarrhea, rash, syndrome of inappropriate antidiuretic hormone (SIADH) and hyponatremia, galactorrhea and hyperprolactinemia, dry mouth, prolonged bleeding time and abnormal bleeding, bruxism, and hair loss. There have also been reports of postoperative bleeding among SSRI-treated patients and, in some cases, of upper gastrointestinal bleeding, particularly when the SSRIs were combined with nonsteroidal antiinflammatory drugs (NSAIDs). There have also been reports linking the chronic use of SSRIs with bone fractures in the elderly, but further studies are needed. During long-term treatment with SSRIs, weight gain, sleep disturbances, sleepiness, apathy, fatigue, cognitive and memory symptoms, and sexual dysfunction are possible side effects Although these are class-related side effects, some patients will tolerate one agent better than another or not suffer a particular adverse effect with a different SSRI. Most patients who report a history of treatment nonresponse due to intolerance of one SSRI may actually respond to treatment with a second SSRI. Despite this, most head-to-head comparisons of the SSRIs have failed to show significant differences among them in rates of treatment-emergent adverse events, with the exception perhaps of a greater risk for weight gain during long-term treatment with paroxetine (see later). Most of the SSRI-related adverse events are transient and short-lived or, if they persist, are usually tolerated well and do not require pharmacologic management. However, there are some side effects that may require pharmacologic interventions.

SSRI-Related Agitation and Anxiety

As mentioned earlier, anxiety, agitation, jitteriness, and nervousness are common side effects during treatment with SSRIs (occurring typically in more than 10% of the patients) and tend to arise primarily during acute treatment. Dividing the dose of the antidepressant could be a helpful option in the event that these side effects are related to peak plasma concentrations. More commonly, however, adjunctive drug treatments are used for the pharmacologic management of these side effects: benzodiazepines [e.g., lorazepam 0.5 to 1 mg twice a day (b.i.d.) to three times a day (t.i.d.) as needed (p.r.n.), alprazolam 0.25 to 1 mg b.i.d. to four times a day (q.i.d.) p.r.n., or clonazepam 0.25 to 0.5 mg b.i.d. p.r.n.], β-blockers (e.g., propranolol 10 to 30 mg b.i.d. to t.i.d. p.r.n.) anticonvulsants (e.g., gabapentin 100 to 300 mg b.i.d.,), second-generation antipsychotics (e.g., quetiapine 25 to 300 mg per day), mirtazapine [15 to 60 mg at bedtime (q.h.s.)], and TCAs (e.g., clomipramine 25 to 50 mg q.h.s.).

SSRI-Related Sexual Dysfunction

Up to 30% to 40% of the patients on SSRIs may experience changes in libido or delayed ejaculation or anorgasmia. Although these side effects occasionally remit spontaneously, they frequently persist over time. As an alternative to switching drugs, placebo-controlled trials have suggested the efficacy of phosphodiesterase-5 inhibitors such as sildenafil (50 to 100 mg p.r.n.) and of NDRIs such as bupropion [100 to 150 mg sustained release (SR) b.i.d.], with the benefit of the latter being primarily evident in improving libido. Among patients nonresponding to SSRIs, augmentation with the dopamine-D_2 partial agonist aripiprazole has led to a greater improvement in libido than do placebo augmentation. Anecdotal or uncontrolled reports have also touted an array of other sexual dysfunction antidotes, including yohimbine (ranging from 2.7 mg p.r.n. to 5.4 mg t.i.d.), amantadine (100 to 200 mg per day), cyproheptadine (4 to 8 mg per day, although this risks transient loss of antidepressant effect), mirtazapine (15 to 30 mg q.h.s.), buspirone (10 to 30 mg b.i.d.), psychostimulants (e.g., methylphenidate 10 to 20 mg p.r.n. or b.i.d.), dopamine D_2 and D_3 receptor agonists (e.g., pramipexole 0.125 to 0.5 mg b.i.d. to t.i.d.), gingko biloba, and even cholinergic drugs (e.g., bethanechol 10 to 50 mg p.r.n.).

SSRI-Related Weight Gain

Although the SSRIs as a class tend to be weight neutral, especially over the short term, some weight gain may occur over the long term in 5% to 20% of the patients. The likelihood of significant weight gain ($\geq$7% increase in body weight over baseline) appears significantly higher with paroxetine than with sertraline, citalopram, or fluoxetine. Although there have been no placebo-controlled studies, anecdotal reports and open trials suggest the usefulness of adding phentermine (15 to 30 mg b.i.d.), bupropion [150 mg b.i.d. or 300 mg extended release (XL) every day (q.d.)], sibutramine (5 to 15 mg per day), modafinil (200 to 400 mg per day), histamine-2 (H_2) receptor antagonists (e.g., nizatidine 15 to 300 mg per day, famotidine 20 to 40 mg q.d.), dopaminergic agents (e.g., amantadine 100 to 300 mg per day, pramipexole 0.125 to 0.25 mg t.i.d.), and the anticonvulsant drugs zonisamide (100 to 300 mg per day) or topiramate (100 to 300 mg per day) to SSRIs to manage weight gain.

SSRI-Related Sleep Disturbances

Sleep disturbances are rather common side effects during treatment with SSRIs and may arise during both acute and long-term treatment. Changes in daytime dosing schedule of the antidepressant are tried to manage both insomnia (by shifting the timing of antidepressant administration to early in the morning) and hypersomnia (by shifting to bedtime dosing) due to antidepressants. Many adjunctive drug treatments have been used for the pharmacologic management of insomnia: benzodiazepines (e.g., temazepam 15 to 30 mg q.h.s.), zolpidem (5 to 20 mg q.h.s. or 12.5 mg of the SR formulation), zaleplon (10 to 20 mg q.h.s.), eszopiclone (1 to 3 mg q.h.s.), mirtazapine (15 to 60 mg q.h.s.), trazodone (50 to 200 mg q.h.s.), quetiapine (25 to 100 mg q.h.s.), antihistaminic drugs (e.g., diphenhydramine 25 to 100 mg q.h.s.), and

TCAs (e.g., trimipramine 25 to 50 mg q.h.s.). In some cases, the patient may report daytime tiredness and oversleeping in the morning, which may be due to poor night sleeping; in that case, sedative drugs (like the ones used for the management of insomnia) prescribed at bedtime may help with the problem. In the case of hypersomnia or daytime sedation, augmentation with psychostimulants (e.g., methylphenidate 10 to 40 mg b.i.d.), modafinil (100 to 400 mg q.d.), activating antidepressants [e.g., bupropion (100 to 150 mg q.d. or b.i.d.), atomoxetine (25 to 40 mg b.i.d.) indicated for attention deficit/hyperactivity disorder, reboxetine (2 to 4 mg b.i.d.), or protriptyline (10 to 30 mg q.d.)], and dopaminergic agents (e.g., pramipexole 0.125 to 0.25 mg t.i.d.) may be helpful.

SSRI-Related Fatigue
Fatigue occurs during long-term treatment with SSRIs in 10% to 30% of the patients. As noted, fatigue could be improved with bedtime dosing of the antidepressant. Particular attention should be paid to assessing whether this side effect is the result of a poor or bad sleep quality; in this case, augmentation with sedating antidepressants (e.g., mirtazapine or trazodone) at bedtime could offer benefit. Daytime pharmacologic management of fatigue, supported by anecdotal reports, can be accomplished by augmentation with psychostimulants (e.g., methylphenidate 10 to 40 mg b.i.d.), modafinil (100 to 400 mg q.d.), dopaminergic agents (e.g., pramipexole 0.125 to 0.25 mg t.i.d.), thyroid hormone [e.g., triiodothyronine (T_3) 25 to 50 μg per day], bupropion (100 to 150 mg q.d. or b.i.d.), atomoxetine (25 to 40 mg b.i.d.), reboxetine (2 to 4 mg b.i.d.), or protriptyline (10 to 30 mg q.d.). However, a recent pooled analysis of two placebo-controlled studies has provided support for the use of modafinil (200 mg per day) in the management of fatigue in SSRI-treated patients with incomplete response.

SSRI-Related Cognitive and Memory Symptoms
Cognitive and memory symptoms (such as difficulties with focusing and recall, and trouble finding words) are reported in 10% to 30% of the patients on SSRIs despite the overall improvement in depressive symptoms. Caffeine, donepezil (5 to 10 mg per day), dopaminergic agents (e.g., pramipexole 0.125 to 0.25 mg t.i.d.), modafinil (100 to 400 mg q.d.), and psychostimulants (e.g., methylphenidate 10 to 40 mg b.i.d.) are the suggested augmenting treatments for this side effect, based only on anecdotal or uncontrolled reports.

Before Beginning SSRIs
A comprehensive medical and psychiatric history and, only if deemed appropriate, laboratory work including liver function tests and thyroid function tests should be performed for any patient newly diagnosed with depression. However, there are no medical tests specifically required before administering SSRIs. It is important to discuss fully with patients the common side effects that might occur; informing and reassuring the patient in this manner will help the individual understand the physical symptoms that may be experienced and will enhance compliance. As with all antidepressants, it is important to stress to patients that onset of therapeutic benefit is most often delayed by several weeks and that the drugs are not effective if taken on an as-needed basis.

After Starting SSRIs
Close monitoring of side effects and therapeutic response is useful, because the emergence of poorly tolerated side effects may require the use of concomitant medications. Plasma levels of SSRIs have not been shown to correlate with efficacy and thus are not useful for therapeutic monitoring other than for compliance or to rule out the presence of fast or ultrarapid metabolism in patients without reported

benefit and side effects. Plasma levels can also be used to establish the safety of beginning an MAOI trial following treatment discontinuation of an SSRI.

Drug Interactions with SSRIs

SSRIs should **never be used concomitantly with MAOIs,** because there have been a number of reports of fatal cases of serotonin syndrome due to the simultaneous use of these classes of drugs or to the inadequate period of wash-out between the two.

Patients should be cautioned about the risk of bleeding associated with the concomitant use of SSRIs and NSAIDs, aspirin, or other drugs that affect coagulation. Given the similarities in efficacy across the SSRIs, the drug interaction profile has been marketed by some companies as a basis for determining the agent of first choice within the class. Concern about drug interactions, however, is pertinent to patients taking medications of narrow therapeutic margins that are metabolized by isoenzymes inhibited by the SSRI and if the prescriber is unfamiliar with or unable to determine the appropriate dose adjustment. Reports of clinically significant interactions with the SSRIs are remarkably rare, given their vast availability. Among the SSRIs, citalopram, escitalopram, and sertraline have the most favorable profile with respect to inhibition *in vitro* of CYP isoenzyme systems. Of the isoenzymes of most interest in predicting psychiatric drug–drug interactions (e.g., with tricyclics, antipsychotics, β-blockers) the CYP2D6 isoenzyme is moderately inhibited by paroxetine and by fluoxetine and its metabolites. However, for all of the SSRIs, some vigilance is reasonable concerning the possibility of increased therapeutic or toxic effects of other coprescribed drugs metabolized by P450 2D6. In particular, if combining a tricyclic with an SSRI, the tricyclic should be initiated with low doses, and plasma levels should be monitored. Given the high capacity of the CYP3A3/3A4 system, inhibition of this isoenzyme is not a major concern for the SSRIs, although fluvoxamine and less so fluoxetine can inhibit it to some extent. Of little importance to drug interactions is the high rate of protein binding of the SSRIs because, if other drugs are displaced from carrier proteins, the result is simply an increase in the rate and amount of free drug being metabolized.

Use in Elderly Patients

Elderly patients generally tolerate the side effects of the SSRIs (and other newer agents) better than they tolerate the anticholinergic and cardiovascular side effects of the tricyclic and related cyclic antidepressants. However, elderly patients may have alterations in hepatic metabolic pathways, especially the so-called phase I reactions including demethylation and hydroxylation, which are involved in the metabolism of both SSRIs and cyclic antidepressants. In addition, renal function may be decreased, and there may be increased end-organ sensitivity to the effects of antidepressant compounds. Because the elimination half-life of the SSRIs can be expected to be significantly greater than what it is in younger patients, accumulation of active drug will be greater and occur more slowly. Clinically, this means that elderly patients should be started on lower doses, that dosage increases should be slower, and that the ultimate therapeutic dose may be lower than in younger patients. However, given the wide margin of safety of the SSRIs, full-dose treatment in older patients, if tolerated, is required before considering treatment to have failed. As mentioned earlier, there have also been reports linking the chronic use of SSRIs with bone fractures in elderly populations, but further studies are needed.

Use in Pregnancy

Whenever possible, unnecessary exposure to any drug during pregnancy should be minimized, and thoughtful prepregnancy treatment planning and consideration of alternative interventions such as psychotherapies (e.g., CBT) are to be recommended.

However, there is accumulating information about the use of all the SSRIs in pregnancy, although the bulk of available data is on fluoxetine. One prospective study of 128 pregnant women who took fluoxetine, 10 to 80 mg per day (mean 25.8 mg), during their first trimester did not find elevated rates of major malformations compared with matched groups of women taking tricyclics or drugs thought not to be teratogenic. There was a higher, albeit not statistically significant, rate of miscarriages in the fluoxetine (13.5%) and tricyclic (12.2%) groups compared with the women exposed to known nonteratogenic drugs (6.8%). Whether this increased rate of miscarriages is biologically significant and, if so, whether it relates to the drugs or to the depressive disorder could not be determined from this study. Decisions on continuing antidepressant drugs during pregnancy must be individualized, but it must be recalled that the effects of severe untreated depression on maternal and fetal health may be far worse than the unknown risks of SSRIs or tricyclic drugs. A large registry of fluoxetine exposure during pregnancy is consistent with generally reassuring data from the tricyclic era that antidepressant agents are not evidently teratogens.

Infants exposed to SSRIs during late pregnancy may be at increased risk for serotonergic CNS adverse effects, although the incidence of these events has not been well established. Recently, the FDA has issued a warning for all SSRIs, reporting an increased risk for neonatal toxicity and recommending cessation of treatment prior to delivery. However, in clinical practice, the risk of postpartum depression often warrants continued treatment and close monitoring of the newborn.

An alternative for severe depression that also appears to be safe is ECT.

SSRIs are secreted in breast milk. Because their effects on normal growth and development are unknown, breast-feeding should be discouraged for mothers who are on SSRIs.

Specific Drugs

Overall, the SSRIs have similar side-effect profiles and spectrum of efficacy. However, there are some slight differences meriting individual discussion.

Fluoxetine

Fluoxetine is usually begun at a dosage of 20 mg per day given in a single daily dose. It is generally given in the morning because for some patients it may have an activating profile, although initial sedation is actually as likely as activation. Doses greater than 20 mg may be given in a single dose. Although an initial antidepressant effect usually emerges within 2 to 4 weeks, remission will often require 6 to 12 weeks. **Fluoxetine has a long half-life** (2 to 4 days on average for fluoxetine and 7 to 9 days for its active metabolite norfluoxetine).

Some patients may respond to dosages as low as 5 mg per day. Therefore, patients with poorly tolerated side effects on 20 mg may use 10-mg capsules or use the liquid formulation for even lower dosages. Dosages of 20 or 40 mg per day are considered adequate, although some patients may require 60 to 80 mg per day. Use of the lowest effective dose will minimize side effects and therefore increase patient compliance. There is evidence that maintenance treatment for some patients can be accomplished with a single weekly dose of 90 mg (weekly formulation). Fluoxetine was the first antidepressant to demonstrate efficacy in the treatment of depression in children and adolescents. It is now available in generic formulations.

The potential for drug–drug interactions should be recalled because it may remain a consideration for several weeks after treatment discontinuation given the drug's long half-life. Fluoxetine should be discontinued 5 weeks before starting an MAOI because of its long half-life. Its long half-life minimizes the risk of the emergence of symptoms induced by abrupt discontinuation, which have been reported with shorter acting SSRIs.

Sertraline

Sertraline's efficacy and side effects in general clinical practice suggest a similar profile to other SSRIs. The half-life of sertraline is shorter than that of fluoxetine, approximately 25 hours; it has a less potently active metabolite with a half-life of approximately 56 hours.

Sertraline is typically begun at 50 mg per day with a target dosage of at least 100 mg per day in healthy adults. The dosage range is 50 to 200 mg in single or divided daily doses. The recommended washout period before starting an MAOI is 14 days. For some prescribers, sertraline offers a reasonable choice because of its intermediate half-life and relatively favorable drug interaction profile.

Paroxetine

Paroxetine was the third SSRI approved in the United States for MDD, but the first to obtain approval by the FDA for use in the treatment of panic disorder. Although some clinicians perceive paroxetine to have greater anxiolytic effects than some of the other SSRIs, double-blind studies in anxious depression have not shown significant differences in efficacy across SSRIs. As with other SSRIs, its relative efficacy, compared with the dual-action tricyclics, for the most serious cases of MDD with melancholia has been called into question (e.g., when clomipramine proved superior in one study of severely depressed inpatients). Paroxetine is typically begun at 20 mg in a single morning dose; elderly patients or those with serious hepatic or renal dysfunction should start at 10 mg daily. For patients who do not respond after 4 weeks, the dosage can be increased to up to 50 mg per day and for elderly patients to up to 40 mg per day. A controlled-release formulation has been introduced especially to reduce the risk of gastrointestinal side effects. Paroxetine has a side-effect profile similar to that of other SSRIs in clinical trials, but many clinicians report the anecdotal impression that this agent may be somewhat **more sedating** than the other SSRIs. As mentioned earlier, the potential for weight gain appears to be slightly greater with paroxetine than with other drugs of the class. As an SSRI with a relatively shorter half-life and perhaps because it has nonlinear kinetics (it is a substrate and **inhibitor of CYP2D6,** thereby inhibiting its own metabolism at higher doses), paroxetine is the SSRI most associated with difficulties due to abrupt discontinuation; therefore, slow taper (over 3 to 4 weeks) on termination after chronic treatment is essential to prevent patient distress when patients have been exposed to it for more than 2 months. Paroxetine may enhance the effects of anticoagulants such as warfarin, suggesting the need for close monitoring of such patients. The washout period before starting an MAOI is 14 days.

Citalopram

Citalopram was introduced to the U.S. market in late 1998, although it had been widely available for several years in the rest of the world. It is a racemic mixture of two enantiomers: R-citalopram and S-citalopram. Preclinical studies suggest that the therapeutic activity of citalopram primarily resides in the S-isomer and that the S-citalopram binds with high affinity to the human serotonin transporter. Conversely, R-citalopram is approximately 30-fold less potent than the S-isomer (escitalopram) at this transporter. As the most selective of the SSRIs (lacking meaningful other pharmacodynamic effects besides uptake inhibition of the serotonin transporter), it is considered by many to have a favorable SSRI side-effect profile, even though double-blind comparisons with other SSRIs have not provided consistent support for this view. Its interaction with the CYP systems suggests that, together with sertraline and escitalopram, it is the least likely of the SSRIs to be associated with pharmacokinetic drug–drug interactions; its intermediate half-life of more than 30 hours and linear kinetics predict that discontinuation syndromes will be somewhat less than those with shorter half-lives. The washout period before starting an MAOI is 14 days.

The dose range for citalopram is 20 to 60 mg. Dosing of citalopram usually begins with a single daily dose of 20 mg, but this can be reduced to 10 mg in the event of significant side effects. An adequate antidepressant daily dose for some will be 20 mg, but others may do better on or require 40 mg. The daily dosing range in the elderly population is typically 20 to 40 mg.

Acceptance of citalopram was initially influenced by concerns about cardiac and overdose toxicity. The cardiac concern was based on observations of chronic high-dose toxicity studies in beagles that on investigation turned out to be a breed-specific issue of no relevance to humans, as evidenced by citalopram's FDA approval. The rare overdose deaths reported on very high dose ingestion, on review of all SSRIs, also did not implicate a citalopram-specific concern.

Fluvoxamine

Although fluvoxamine has been introduced into the United States with the labeled indication for OCD only and for social anxiety disorder in its extended-release formulation, this SSRI is marketed for depression in other countries and clinical trial data and clinical experience would predict a spectrum of efficacy similar to that of other SSRIs, including efficacy for MDD. It is usually initiated in a single dose beginning with 50 mg, building up to a usual therapeutic range of 150 to 250 mg. In its XL formulation, it is usually initiated with a dosage of 100 mg per day. It has a half-life of 15 hours. Like all SSRIs, it is likely to cause sexual dysfunction but possibly to a lesser degree. Fluvoxamine may offer some drug–drug interaction challenges because it **inhibits CYP1A2, CYP2C9, and CYP3A4.** As with all the other SSRIs (except fluoxetine), the washout period before starting an MAOI is 14 days.

Escitalopram

Escitalopram is the S-enantiomer of the racemic compound citalopram; it was introduced to the U.S. market in 2002. Because of its high selectivity, as with citalopram, it is considered by many to have a favorable SSRI side-effect profile. Its interaction with the CYP systems suggests that, together with sertraline and citalopram, it is the least likely of the SSRIs to be associated with pharmacokinetic drug–drug interactions. Escitalopram has linear pharmacokinetics, so that plasma levels increase proportionately and predictably with increased doses, and its half-life of 27 to 32 hours predicts that discontinuation syndromes will be somewhat less than with the SSRIs with shorter half-lives.

Clinical trials of escitalopram in depressed patients indicate that escitalopram, 10 mg per day, is as effective as 20 or 40 mg per day of its parent compound citalopram. The typical dose range for escitalopram is therefore 10 to 20 mg. Dosing of escitalopram usually begins with a single daily dose of 10 mg. An adequate antidepressant daily dose for most will be 10 mg. The washout period before starting an MAOI is 14 days.

Augmentation and Combination Strategies with SSRIs

When one takes into consideration the number of patients who fail to achieve full remission with an initial adequate antidepressant trial, added to those who do not improve at all plus those who lose benefit in the continuation or maintenance phase of treatment, it is evident that most depressed patients will require a next step in their treatment. Whereas for some patients higher doses or medication switches will be effective, many clinicians will use instead an augmentation or combination strategy. Although the usual goal of augmentation or combination treatment is to convert partial responders or nonresponders to full response or remission, some strategies have also been used to enhance therapeutic efficacy or accelerate response, that is, to diminish the latency to response, or to manage side effects. Many of the strategies favored by clinicians are not supported by published clinical trials. Some commonly used strategies are briefly reviewed here.

G. V. GRAVES

Second-Generation Antipsychotics

SSRI augmentation with second-generation antipsychotic agents is, by far, the best studied strategy in resistant depression. Risperidone, olanzapine, quetiapine, ziprasidone, and aripiprazole have all shown good responses both in some small trials in SSRI nonresponders and in large, adequately powered, placebo-controlled studies. The typical dosages in augmentation of antidepressants are 0.5 to 2 mg per day for risperidone, 5 to 20 mg per day for olanzapine, 25 to 300 mg per day for quetiapine, 40 to 160 mg per day for ziprasidone, and 5 to 20 mg per day for aripiprazole. The rapid onset of the effect of this strategy has made it relatively popular among clinicians in the treatment of SSRI-resistant depressed patients. Ariprazole was the first drug to receive from the FDA an indication as augmenting agent for SSRI nonresponders.

Lithium

Lithium augmentation is not as popular currently as it was in the 1980s, although there are a few studies that have clearly shown that the addition of a dose of 600 mg or more of lithium a day, typically in divided doses and with reasonably good blood levels, leads to a robust increase in the chances of response in patients who have not responded to SSRIs. While most of the positive double-blind controlled trials of lithium augmentation concerned TCA-treated patients, in several studies lithium did not do particularly well when added to SSRIs, including the Sequenced Treatment Alternatives to Relieve Depression (STAR*D) study. Therefore, despite the relative robust findings concerning lithium augmentation of TCAs in the literature, the role of lithium in managing nonresponse among MDD patients treated with the SSRIs remains to be established.

Thyroid Hormone

In treatment-resistant depression studies, T_3, typically in dosages of 25 to 50 μg per day, has been used in preference and has been shown to be superior to thyroxine (T_4). Among four randomized double-blind studies of T_3 augmentation of antidepressants, pooled effects were not significant, but one study with negative results accounted for most of the intertrial heterogeneity in results. Because all the published, placebo-controlled studies of T_3 augmentation involved the use of TCAs, the efficacy of this strategy in SSRI-resistant patients is primarily supported by the open, randomized STAR*D study, where T_3 was nonsignificantly more efficacious than lithium.

Buspirone Augmentation

Buspirone is typically a well-tolerated antianxiety drug with serotonin (5-HT_{1A}) partial agonist properties. Open-label studies using 5 to 15 mg b.i.d. of buspirone have shown significant improvement in SSRI-resistant patients. Although the first placebo-controlled study in refractory depression comparing buspirone against placebo augmentation did not find any statistically significant difference in response rates between these two treatments (51% vs 47%, respectively), another double-blind study showed that among the SSRI-resistant patients with severe depression, buspirone was more effective than placebo augmentation. In the STAR*D study, buspirone augmentation of citalopram was slightly (significantly only on secondary outcome measures) less efficacious than the combination of bupropion and citalopram.

Pindolol

Pindolol augmentation is rarely used in clinical practice in the United States, but it is relatively more popular in Europe and Canada in the management of resistant depression. Pindolol is a β-blocker and a serotonin 5-HT_{1A} antagonist. A dosage of

2.5 mg t.i.d. has been used in most depression studies. This agent has generated a lot of interest because it has been shown to accelerate antidepressant response when combined with SSRIs in some but not all the studies. An earlier study found no response among 10 refractory depressed patients, and two studies showed no difference from placebo in clinical trials of augmentation in refractory depressed populations.

Dopaminergic Drugs
Augmentation of SSRIs with dopaminergic drugs is an interesting strategy. In an open trial, Bouckoms and Mangini used with some success the antiparkinsonian drug pergolide, 0.25 to 2 mg per day, in resistant depression. Similarly, there are reports of the usefulness of antidepressant augmentation with the dopaminergic drugs amantadine (100 to 200 mg b.i.d.), pramipexole (0.125 to 0.50 mg t.i.d.), and ropinirole (0.5 to 1.5 mg t.i.d.). Unfortunately, these studies concerning the augmentation of antidepressants with dopaminergic agents are uncontrolled and have relatively small sample sizes.

Psychostimulants
In line with the potential role of dopaminergic agents as augmentors of antidepressants, psychostimulants, which have significant effects on dopamine neurotransmission, have been used to augment SSRIs. Clinicians typically use methylphenidate, 20 to 80 mg per day, or dextroamphetamine, 10 to 40 mg per day, in divided doses. Two recent placebo-controlled studies of methylphenidate augmentation were negative. In addition to the lack of positive controlled studies, the main issues concerning the use of psychostimulant augmentation are the potential for abuse in some patients with history of substance abuse, the possible emergence of anxiety and irritability, and their relatively short half-life.

Modafinil
Modafinil is a wakefulness-promoting agent with pharmacologic actions somewhat different from those of the amphetamines. A recent pooled analysis of two multicenter, placebo-controlled studies has shown the efficacy of modafinil (200 mg q.d.) augmentation of SSRIs among depressed patients with incomplete response and fatigue and sleepiness. In addition, the somewhat greater ease of use of this agent, compared with the psychostimulants, has made it a relatively popular augmentor of antidepressants for the management of these residual symptoms among SSRI-treated depressed patients.

Folate and S-Adenosyl-Methionine
Folate, in particular its active form methyltetrahydrofolate, and SAMe are compounds closely involved in the one carbon cycle and in methylation processes of the brain. These compounds have been studied extensively in depression, and the literature suggests that they may have antidepressant properties. An open trial of methylfolate (up to 30 mg per day) in SSRI-refractory patients suggested its usefulness as an adjunct, and an open study with SAMe (800 mg b.i.d.) has also shown the usefulness of this augmenting agent in SSRI nonresponders. The availability of SAMe over the counter has made this agent a relatively popular augmentation agent among MDD patients not responding to SSRIs. Similarly, the relative lack of adverse events with methyltetrahydrofolate has also made this compound a popular adjunct with clinicians.

Riluzole and Other Glutamergic Agents
There is some evidence, mostly based on open-label studies, for augmentation of SSRIs with the glutamergic drugs riluzole (150 to 200 mg per day) and amantadine

(100 to 200 mg b.i.d.). Given the dramatic effects of the ketamine intravenous administration in resistant depression, there is increasing interest among clinicians in the use of orally available glutamergic agents.

Inositol

Despite initial anecdotal positive reports of the usefulness of augmentation of antidepressants with dosages of inositol up to 12 g per day, a controlled, double-blind augmentation trial did not support its use in SSRI treatment nonresponders, and a study showed no difference in outcome between patients treated with SSRIs and placebo versus those treated with SSRIs and inositol.

Opiates

There is very modest evidence, mostly based on case reports and case series, for augmentation of antidepressants with opiates in severe refractory patients, using oxycodone, oxymorphone, tramadol, and buprenorphine. The lack of adequate studies on the usefulness in depression of these highly controlled agents with significant potential for abuse markedly limits their use.

Estrogen

There is mostly anecdotal evidence for the efficacy of estrogen augmentation of SSRIs in resistant depression among postmenopausal women. In addition, there are no guidelines on how to optimize antidepressant administration with estrogen, especially in women insufficiently responsive to antidepressants.

Dehydroepiandrosterone and Testosterone

Dehydroepiandrosterone, a major circulating corticosteroid in humans, has an unclear physiologic role. In addition to serving as a precursor to testosterone and estrogen, dehydroepiandrosterone and its sulfated metabolite, dehydroepiandrosterone-S, most likely have important biological roles and have been hypothesized to be involved in regulating mood and sense of well-being. A very small, preliminary, double-blind study suggests its usefulness (up to 90 mg per day) as an adjunct to antidepressants in refractory depression. Further studies are necessary, given the small number of patients studied. Similarly, in an 8-week randomized, placebo-controlled trial of testosterone transdermal gel among 23 men aged 30 to 65 years who had resistant depression and low or borderline testosterone levels, testosterone was significantly better than placebo in treating depressive symptoms.

Adding a Second Antidepressant to the SSRI (Combination Therapies)

Although there are numerous double-blind studies of augmentation strategies, there are fewer than five double-blind studies of combination strategies, reflecting the need for further studies in this area. It appears that the improvement following the combination of antidepressants tends to occur within 4 to 6 weeks, so it may be premature to decide after a few days or weeks whether or not a combination strategy is working. Almost all the studies on the efficacy of these strategies have focused on the short-term outcome, and very little is known about the minimum duration of the combination trial in responders to such strategy. In the event of therapeutic response, it is typically difficult to determine what is due to the combination (the synergy between the two antidepressants) and what is due to the second antidepressant itself. In fact, most combination strategies use full doses of both antidepressant agents.

Bupropion Plus SSRIs

Bupropion SR (100 to 150 mg q.d. or b.i.d.) or its XL formulation (150 or 300 mg q.d.) combined with SSRIs is a very popular strategy among clinicians. On the other hand, the evidence for this combination is primarily based on the STAR*D study findings, which showed that bupropion added to citalopram was slightly (significantly only on secondary outcome measures) more efficacious than buspirone added to citalopram.

Mirtazapine Plus SSRIs
Mirtazapine is a dual-action antidepressant that (a) increases both serotonergic and noradrenergic activity by blocking the α_2-adrenergic auto- and heteroreceptors and (b) blocks the serotonergic 5-HT$_2$ and 5-HT$_3$ receptors (see later). Mirtazapine (15 to 30 mg q.h.s.) combined with SSRIs has been reported to be helpful in an open study of nonresponders to SSRIs and to be more effective than placebo plus SSRIs in a subsequent double-blind study among 20 SSRI-resistant depressed patients. A recent study by Debonnel et al. showed a significantly higher response rate to the combination of paroxetine and mirtazapine than to monotherapy with either drug and a 64% response rate to the switch to combination therapy for patients not responding to monotherapy. All these studies suggest the potential usefulness of combining mirtazapine with SSRIs in patients with MDD with partial or nonresponse.

Desipramine or Other TCAs Plus SSRIs
An early study by Nelson et al. showed that the TCA plus SSRI combination may produce a more rapid onset of action. A more recent study by the same author has shown that remission rates are significantly higher on desipramine plus fluoxetine than on either drug alone in severe depression. This is consistent with the reports that desipramine and other TCAs were effective in combination with SSRIs in small cohorts of patients. The main issue related to combining TCAs with SSRIs is that TCAs are substrates of the CYP2D6, so there may be TCA level increases when coadministered with SSRIs inhibiting this pathway, raising the risk of toxicity. Low dosages of TCAs (25 to 75 mg per day) are therefore typically used, and monitoring of the TCA blood levels is necessary. The efficacy of the combination of low-dose TCAs with SSRIs has been put in question by two studies that showed that adding low-dose desipramine to fluoxetine was less effective than raising the dose of fluoxetine in patients who had not responded to 8 weeks of treatment with fluoxetine 20 mg per day.

Reboxetine/Atomoxetine Plus SSRIs
Three open trials, using dosages up to 8 mg per day, have suggested the usefulness of adding reboxetine to SSRIs in resistant depression. Because reboxetine is not available in the United States, a number of clinicians have been using atomoxetine in combination with SSRIs. Atomoxetine is a relatively selective NRI approved in the United States for the treatment of attention deficit disorder with hyperactivity (see later). A placebo-controlled study of atomoxetine augmentation of SSRIs was negative, although a post-hoc analysis using pharmacogenetic data showed a positive signal in a subgroup with a specific polymorphism of the serotonin transporter.

Venlafaxine Plus SSRIs
There have been only anecdotal reports suggesting the efficacy of combining SSRIs with venlafaxine. Venlafaxine is a substrate of the CYP2D6, and there have been reports of accumulation of venlafaxine when coadministered with some SSRIs, which inhibits the 2D6 pathway and leads to marked blood pressure elevation and severe anticholinergic side effects. Rare anecdotes of serotonin syndrome–like symptoms when combining venlafaxine with SSRIs (or the overlap of use of two SSRIs together) are difficult to understand in terms of mechanism because the effect should be similar to raising the dose of a single SSRI.

OTHER NEWER ANTIDEPRESSANTS

Serotonin-Norepinephrine Reuptake Inhibitors

Venlafaxine
Introduced in the United States in 1994, venlafaxine at higher doses inhibits the uptake of both norepinephrine and serotonin. **At lower doses (≤150 mg), the drug acts essentially like an SSRI** with a very short half-life. At higher doses, venlafaxine appears to recruit its noradrenergic mechanism and is therefore considered an SNRI. Venlafaxine lacks significant cholinergic, antihistaminergic, and α_1-adrenergic blocking effects. Venlafaxine is metabolized by CYP2D6, of which it is also a very weak inhibitor. Drugs that inhibit this enzyme may increase venlafaxine concentrations. Venlafaxine has a most favorable profile with respect to the CYP system in that it is not a meaningful inhibitor of the isoenzymes pertinent to drug metabolism. The half-lives of venlafaxine and its active metabolite O-desmethylvenlafaxine are about 5 and 11 hours, respectively. The drug and its metabolite reach steady state in plasma within 3 days in healthy adults, and discontinuation among those exposed to this drug for more than 2 months must be accompanied by a very gradual taper (over at least 4 weeks) to reduce the risk of intense **discontinuation symptoms.** Although many patients find that the recently introduced extended-release preparation reduced initial treatment-emergent adverse effects (e.g., nausea), the newer formulation would not be expected to extend the half-life or reduce the need for vigilance when discontinuing treatment.

The usual dosage range is 75 to 225 mg given in divided doses on a b.i.d. schedule [for the IR formulation] or once per day with the extended-release formulation. Dosages as high as 450 mg per day have been used in seriously ill depressed inpatients. Although the extended-release form has only been labeled for use of up to 225 mg per day, there is no pharmacologic reason to limit treatment below the range of the IR preparation (e.g., up to 375 to 450 mg per day if necessary).

The safety and side-effect profile of venlafaxine is generally similar to that of the SSRIs. Anxiety or nervousness may emerge or worsen on initiation of treatment. Other side effects include nausea, insomnia, sedation, sexual dysfunction, headache, tremor, dizziness, and constipation. Unlike the SSRIs, but more like the tricyclics, venlafaxine may cause **excessive sweating, tachycardia,** and palpitations. At the higher doses, 5% to 7% of the patients may develop a modest but persisting increase in blood pressure. Thus, baseline blood pressure screening and periodic rechecks after upward titration of the dose should be performed. Like other newer agents, venlafaxine is safer in overdose than older agents such as the TCAs. Patients should be cautioned about the risk of bleeding associated with the concomitant use of venlafaxine and NSAIDs, aspirin, or other drugs that affect coagulation. Hyponatremia may occur as a result of treatment with SNRIs, including venlafaxine. In many cases, this hyponatremia appears to be the result of the SIADH secretion.

Some treatment-resistant depressed patients with well-documented treatment failures on prior antidepressant therapies have done well in open and double-blind studies with venlafaxine treatment. Venlafaxine represents an alternative to tricyclics and is considered to have a similar efficacy profile but a more favorable acute and long-term side-effect burden. Some clinical trial data suggest that the rate of remission with venlafaxine can be higher than that for some of the SSRIs for populations with relatively more severe and melancholic depression. Its effects on blood pressure have not proven to be an obstacle to its use in clinical practice. There is some evidence in support of the use of this drug in pain–depression syndromes as an alternative to tricyclics. For partial and nonresponders to venlafaxine, for those who lose benefit on it, or for those who have significant difficulties tolerating it, the same augmentation strategies as described for SSRIs can be considered (e.g., addition of benzodiazepines for agitation and of mirtazapine for resistance to respond). Venlafaxine should be stopped 14 days prior to initiating therapy with an MAOI, and, again, stopping should always be done with a gradual taper.

Duloxetine

Introduced in the United States in the second half of 2004, duloxetine binds selectively with high affinity to both norepinephrine and serotonin (5-HT) transporters and lacks affinity for monoamine receptors within the CNS. It appears that the dual effect on both serotonin and norepinephrine systems is present at the lower dosages as well (40 to 60 mg per day). Duloxetine is therefore considered an SNRI. Duloxetine lacks significant cholinergic, antihistaminergic, and α_1-adrenergic blocking effects. Duloxetine is extensively metabolized to numerous metabolites primarily excreted into the urine in the conjugated form. The major metabolites in plasma are glucuronide conjugates of 4-hydroxy duloxetine (M6), 6-hydroxy-5-methoxy duloxetine (M10), 4,6-dihydroxy duloxetine (M9), and a sulfate conjugate of 5-hydroxy-6-methoxy duloxetine (M7). Duloxetine is metabolized by CYP1A2 and by CYP2D6, of which it is also a moderate inhibitor, intermediate between paroxetine and sertraline. Drugs that inhibit this enzyme may increase duloxetine concentrations. The half-life of duloxetine is about 12.5 hours. In a pooled analysis of six short-term treatment trials, in which treatment was stopped abruptly, discontinuation-emergent adverse events were reported by 44.3% and 22.9% of duloxetine- and placebo-treated patients, respectively ($p < 0.05$), in a fashion that is consistent with the discontinuation reactions observed by SSRIs and other SNRIs such as venlafaxine and desvenlafaxine. We suggest that discontinuation among those exposed to this drug for more than 2 months should be accompanied by a **gradual taper** (over at least 2 to 4 weeks) to reduce the risk of discontinuation-emergent adverse events.

The usual daily dosage range is 60 to 120 mg given in single or divided doses. The starting dosage is 60 mg per day, although some patients may require a lower starting dosage (20 or 30 mg per day). The safety and side-effect profile of duloxetine is generally similar to that of the SSRIs. Side effects include nausea, anxiety, dry mouth, insomnia, sedation, sexual dysfunction, urinary hesitancy, headache, excessive sweating, and dizziness. Unlike venlafaxine, it does not appear to be associated with a significant risk of sustained elevated blood pressure at higher doses, although in clinical trials across indications, relative to placebo, duloxetine treatment was associated with mean increases of up to 2.1 mm Hg in systolic blood pressure and up to 2.3 mm Hg in diastolic blood pressure. Because it is possible that duloxetine and alcohol may interact to cause liver injury or that duloxetine may aggravate preexisting liver disease, duloxetine should ordinarily not be prescribed to patients with substantial alcohol use or evidence of chronic liver disease. Like other newer agents, duloxetine is safer in overdose than older agents such as the TCAs. Patients should be cautioned about the risk of bleeding associated with the concomitant use of duloxetine and NSAIDs, aspirin, or other drugs that affect coagulation. Hyponatremia may occur as a result of treatment with SNRIs, including duloxetine. In many cases, this hyponatremia appears to be the result of the SIADH secretion.

Some SSRI-resistant depressed patients have done well in a large open trial with duloxetine treatment. Similar to venlafaxine, some clinical trial data suggest that the rate of remission with duloxetine may be higher than for some of the SSRIs, particularly in more severe and anxious depression, but further studies are needed to confirm these preliminary observations. As with the other SNRI venlafaxine, there is some evidence in support of the use of this drug in pain–depression syndromes as an alternative to tricyclics, and duloxetine is FDA-approved for diabetic peripheral neuropathic pain and generalized anxiety disorder. For partial responders to duloxetine, for those who lose benefit on it, or for very resistant cases, the same augmentation strategies as described for SSRIs can be considered. Duloxetine should be stopped 14 days prior to initiating therapy with an MAOI.

Desvenlafaxine

Introduced in the United States in May 2008, desvenlafaxine at higher doses inhibits the uptake of both norepinephrine and serotonin. Desvenlafaxine (O-desmethylvenlafaxine) is the major active metabolite of the antidepressant venlafaxine. Desvenlafaxine lacks significant cholinergic, antihistaminergic, and α_1-adrenergic blocking effects. Desvenlafaxine is metabolized by CYP3A4 and has minimal inhibitory effects on CYP2D6. Desvenlafaxine has a most favorable profile with respect to the CYP system in that it is not a meaningful inhibitor of other isoenzymes pertinent to drug metabolism. The mean terminal half-life, $t_{1/2}$, is approximately 11 hours. With once-daily dosing, steady-state plasma concentrations are achieved within approximately 4 to 5 days. At steady state, multiple-dose accumulation of desvenlafaxine is linear and predictable from the single-dose pharmacokinetic profile. Discontinuation among those exposed to this drug for more than 2 months must be accompanied by a **very gradual taper** (over at least 2 to 4 weeks) to reduce the risk of intense discontinuation symptoms.

The usual dosage range is 50 to 100 mg given once per day, and desvenlafaxine is available as 50 and 100 mg tablets. Dosages as high as 400 mg per day have been used in clinical studies and were shown to be effective, although no additional benefit was demonstrated at doses greater than 50 mg per day and adverse events and discontinuations were more frequent at higher doses.

The safety and side-effect profile of desvenlafaxine is generally similar to that of the SSRIs. Anxiety or nervousness may emerge or worsen on initiation of treatment. Other side effects include nausea, insomnia, sedation, sexual dysfunction, headache, tremor, dizziness, and constipation. Desvenlafaxine may cause excessive sweating, tachycardia, and palpitations. Between 0.7% and 1.3% of patients may develop a modest but persisting increase in blood pressure. Thus, baseline blood pressure screening and periodic rechecks should be performed. Like other newer agents, desvenlafaxine is safer in overdose than older agents such as the TCAs. Patients should be cautioned about the risk of bleeding associated with the concomitant use of desvenlafaxine and NSAIDs, aspirin, or other drugs that affect coagulation. Hyponatremia may occur as a result of treatment with SNRIs, including desvenlafaxine. In many cases, this hyponatremia appears to be the result of the SIADH secretion. Dose-related elevations in fasting serum total cholesterol, low-density lipoprotein cholesterol, and triglycerides were observed in the controlled studies of desvenlafaxine.

Anecdotal reports suggest that some treatment-resistant depressed patients with well-documented treatment failures on prior antidepressant therapies may do well with desvenlafaxine treatment, but systematic studies in this population are needed. For partial and nonresponders to desvenlafaxine, for those who lose benefit on it, or for those who have significant difficulties tolerating it, one would expect that the same augmentation strategies as described for SSRIs can be considered (e.g., addition of benzodiazepines for agitation and of mirtazapine for resistance to respond). Desvenlafaxine should be stopped 14 days prior to initiating therapy with an MAOI, and, again, stopping should always be done with a gradual taper.

Milnacipran

Milnacipran is an SNRI approved in early 2009 by the FDA (under the brand name "Savella") for the treatment of fibromyalgia and available in Europe for the treatment of depression. Milnacipran inhibits the noradrenaline and serotonin neuronal reuptake. Milnacipran has virtually no relevant affinity for any neurotransmitter receptor studied, in particular postsynaptic α_1-adrenergic, muscarinic, and histamine receptors. Milnacipran is metabolized only to a limited extent, and therefore circulates in the body principally as the unchanged parent drug, which is the only pharmacologically active compound at clinical doses. The pharmacokinetic profile of milnacipran is characterized by rapid absorption, high bioavailability, low protein binding, and rapid elimination, both by hepatic glucuronidation and renal excretion. Its elimination half-life is 6.1 or 8.1 hours. The drug does not appear to be metabolized by the hepatic CYP system. Daily doses range from 50 to 200 mg, often in divided doses. A rapid dose titration from 12.5 mg b.i.d. to 50 mg b.i.d. is recommended in practice. Common side effects reported during treatment with milnacipran include headaches, excessive sweating, hot flushes, dry mouth, dysuria, tremor, tachycardia, sedation, and weight gain. Since milnacipram treatment has been associated with elevations of both heart rate and blood pressure, blood pressure should be measured prior to initiating treatment and periodically measured throughout treatment. There have been cases of increased liver enzymes and reports of severe liver injury with milnacipram, which should therefore be discontinued in patients who develop jaundice or other evidence of liver dysfunction and should ordinarily not be prescribed to patients with substantial alcohol use or evidence of chronic liver disease.

Norepinephrine Reuptake Inhibitors

Reboxetine

Reboxetine is an NRI available in Europe for the treatment of depression. Reboxetine is a highly selective antagonist of the presynaptic norepinephrine transporter, with little or no affinity for other noradrenergic receptors or other neurotransmitter transporters or receptors. Early clinical studies comparing reboxetine to fluoxetine suggested that the noradrenergic agent might offer certain advantages in improving motivation, energy, and social interaction, despite comparable antidepressant effect. This observation requires further study. Reboxetine, a morpholine compound, is chemically unrelated to the other antidepressants. It is highly protein bound and has a plasma half-life of about 13 hours. The drug does not appear to be a meaningful inhibitor of the CYP system and is metabolized itself by CYP3A4 isozyme with two inactive metabolites. Clinical data indicate that reboxetine has comparable efficacy to the TCAs and SSRIs but has some different side effects, particularly increased heart rate, urinary hesitancy, constipation, headache, dry mouth, excessive sweating, and some insomnia. The incidence of nausea, fatigue, headache, and sexual dysfunction appears to be lower with reboxetine than with the SSRIs. Increased blood pressure has been reported to be a problem for some patients, particularly those with a genetic variant of the norepinephrine transporter (SCL6A2). The urinary hesitancy and constipation do not reflect anticholinergic but rather are noradrenergic effects. The usual dosage range for reboxetine is 4 mg q.d. to 5 mg b.i.d. Lower dosages (2 mg b.i.d.) are recommended in those with hepatic or renal insufficiency and in elderly patients. There is some preliminary evidence in favor of combining this selective noradrenergic agent with selective serotonergic agents for treatment-resistant depression.

Atomoxetine

Atomoxetine is an NRI available in the United States with an FDA-approved indication of attention deficit disorder with hyperactivity and is occasionally used off-label for the treatment of depression. *In vitro, ex vivo,* and *in vivo* studies have shown that atomoxetine is a highly selective antagonist of the presynaptic norepinephrine transporter, with little or no affinity for other noradrenergic receptors or other neurotransmitter transporters or receptors (with the exception of a weak affinity for the serotonin transporter). Atomoxetine is rapidly absorbed, with peak plasma concentrations occurring 1 to 2 hours after dosing, and its half-life hovers around 3 to 4 hours. The most common drug-related events reported in trials have been decreased appetite, insomnia, and an initial period of weight loss followed by an apparently normal rate of weight gain. Atomoxetine has also been associated with mild increases in blood pressure and pulse that plateau during treatment and resolve on discontinuation. There have been no effects seen on the Q-T interval. It is a substrate of CYP2D6 and its biotransformation involves aromatic ring hydroxylation, benzylic oxidation, and *N*-demethylation. At high therapeutic doses, atomoxetine inhibits CYP2D6 and CYP3A activity, although *in vivo* studies clearly indicate that atomoxetine administration with substrates of CYP2D6 and CYP3A does not result in clinically significant drug interactions. Severe liver injury has been reported with atomoxetine in a small percentage of patients; therefore, the medication should be **discontinued immediately in patients who develop jaundice or laboratory evidence of liver injury.** No controlled trials of atomoxetine in MDD have been published, although an open trial from the early 1980s had suggested its efficacy in this population. Therefore, the efficacy and dosing of atomoxetine in depression have not been determined, but clinicians may use dosages ranging from 40 to 120 mg per day alone or in combination with SSRIs. A placebo-controlled study of atomoxetine augmentation of SSRIs was negative, although a post-hoc analysis using pharmacogenetic data showed a positive signal in a subgroup with a specific polymorphism of the serotonin transporter.

Norepinephrine-Dopamine Reuptake Inhibitors

Bupropion

As mentioned earlier, there is no consensus on whether bupropion is a true NDRI, although there is evidence for this compound's effects on norepinephrine and dopamine neurotransmission. Bupropion in its immediate-release (IR) formulation was marketed in the United States in the late 1980s for the treatment of depression, but its use in clinical practice was fairly limited until bupropion SR formulation was developed and marketed in 1996 on the basis of demonstration of bioequivalence to the IR formulation. The SR formulation allowed for twice daily dosing up to 400 mg per day versus the t.i.d. dosing required by the IR formulation. An XL formulation of bupropion was developed to provide for once daily dosing and was marketed in September 2003. Similar to the SR formulation, bupropion XL was approved on the basis of bioequivalence to the IR formulation and also was demonstrated to be bioequivalent to the SR formulation. Bupropion is a phenethylamine compound that is effective for the treatment of MDD. Bupropion is structurally related to amphetamine and the sympathomimetic diethylpropion and primarily blocks the reuptake of dopamine and norepinephrine and has minimal or no affinity for postsynaptic receptors. Although some researchers have argued that the NDRI bupropion's effect on norepinephrine is primarily through an increase in presynaptic release, there is still convincing evidence for the binding of both norepinephrine and dopamine transporters. Bupropion is rapidly absorbed after oral administration and demonstrates biphasic elimination, with an elimination half-life of 11 to 14 hours. It is converted to two active metabolites, hydroxybupropion, threohydrobupropion, and erythrohydrobupropion, all of which have been demonstrated to have antidepressant activity in animal models.

Patients are generally begun on 100 mg b.i.d. of the IR or 150 mg q.d. of its two extended-release formulations (SR and XL). A significant proportion of patients may respond to the initial dosage, although the dosage is typically increased to 300 mg per day (once daily in the XL formulation or in divided doses) and in some cases up to 450 mg per day in divided doses. Although the agent is usually well tolerated, patients may develop agitation, dry mouth, restlessness, diminished appetite, weight loss, headache, constipation, insomnia, anxiety, or gastrointestinal distress during the acute phase of the treatment. For those who have significant difficulties tolerating it, the same augmentation strategies as described for SSRIs can be considered (e.g., addition of benzodiazepines for agitation). In addition, a recent report from the Massachusetts General Hospital suggests that low doses of bupropion may act synergistically with low doses of buspirone in the treatment of depression. **Rates of sedation appear to be lower on bupropion than on SSRIs, and bupropion appears to be relatively weight neutral even after long-term treatment.** Rare adverse events reported with bupropion are blood pressure elevations, cognitive side effects, and dystonias. The major medically important adverse event associated with bupropion is seizure. With the IR formulation, the rate is 0.4% (4/1,000) at dosages up to 450 mg per day, whereas with bupropion SR, the rate is 0.1% (1/1,000) at dosages up to the target antidepressant dosage of 300 mg per day, a rate comparable to those of other antidepressants. Patients who do not improve may have their bupropion dosage increased to as high as 450 mg per day. Because of the risk of seizures, it is recommended that the total daily dose of bupropion not be higher than 450 mg (in any formulation) and that no individual dose of the original bupropion formulation be higher than 150 mg in the IR formulation or 200 mg in the SR formulation, whereas single doses of 300 mg can be administered in the XL formulation.

Bupropion lacks anticholinergic properties and does not cause postural hypotension or alter cardiac conduction in a clinically significant manner. It is a substrate of CYP2B6 and **appears to have CYP2D6 inhibition potential**, which suggests that when it is combined with fluoxetine or paroxetine (both 2D6 substrates), levels of the SSRI may increase. Compared with SSRIs, bupropion has the advantage of being significantly less likely to be associated with sexual dysfunction and weight gain. Bupropion is contraindicated for use in patients with anorexia or bulimia because these patients were reported to have a very high incidence of seizures in prerelease studies. Its stimulant-like appetite-suppressing properties, however, may make it particularly useful for depressed patients who have hyperphagia or who have atypical depression features. Under a different brand name (Zyban), bupropion is marketed as a treatment to enhance smoking cessation, and it appears to be more efficacious for this indication than the nicotine patch. The recent STAR*D trial has demonstrated that bupropion combined with SSRIs is an effective treatment for SSRI nonresponders.

Serotonin Receptor Antagonists and Agonists

Nefazodone

Nefazodone is a phenylpiperazine compound chemically similar to trazodone but with less α_1-adrenergic blocking properties and also less sedation. Nefazodone weakly inhibits serotonin (and somewhat norepinephrine) uptake but is principally a blocker of postsynaptic 5-HT$_2$ serotonin receptors. The half-life of nefazodone is approximately 5 hours. It also may have additional psychoactive properties through one of its major metabolites, m-CPP, a postsynaptic serotonin agonist of the 5-HT$_{2C}$ receptors that may be able to release serotonin presynaptically. Nefazodone has been found to **inhibit CYP3A4 and to result in serotonin syndrome when combined with SSRIs**. Its most common side effects are headache, somnolence, dizziness, dry mouth, asthenia, constipation, headache, and nausea. Amblyopia, blurred vision, and visual disturbances (e.g., palinopsia) are uncommon adverse events reported with nefazodone. Rare but serious adverse events related to nefazodone are priapism of both penis and clitoris and, in a single case report, one incident of torsades de pointes. In addition, an increasing number of reports suggest that treatment with nefazodone may be associated with hepatotoxicity, often severe and typically appearing during the first 6 months of treatment. Because of these cases (according to one estimate, 29 cases per 100,000 patient-years), nefazodone was removed from the market in 2003 in both Europe and Canada. Although still available in the United States, its use is minimal, given the concerns about this potentially serious adverse event.

The usual starting dosage is 50 mg per day q.h.s. or b.i.d., titrated up in the absence of daytime sedation as rapidly as tolerated to achieve a usually effective antidepressant dosage in the 450 to 600 mg per day range in divided doses. Slower dose titration is recommended in elderly patients. Anxiety symptoms and insomnia often improve before the onset of an antidepressant effect. Sedation interferes most with rapid attainment of an effective antidepressant dose. Unusual but occasional adverse effect is irritability (possibly related to its m-CPP metabolite, which may occur in higher levels in the presence of a CYP2D6 inhibitor). The drug is helpful for depression-associated insomnia and is significantly less likely than SSRIs to cause sexual dysfunction or weight gain.

Trazodone

Trazodone, a triazolopyridine derivative, very weakly inhibits serotonin reuptake and appears to act mainly postsynaptically as a 5-HT$_2$ antagonist. It also may have additional psychoactive properties through its major metabolite, m-CPP, a postsynaptic serotonin agonist of the 5-HT$_{2C}$ receptors. Trazodone is also an α_1-adrenoceptor blocker, which likely contributes to such side effects as sedation and postural hypotension.

Trazodone is rapidly absorbed following oral administration, achieving peak levels in 1 to 2 hours. It has a relatively short elimination half-life of 3 to 9 hours and is excreted mainly in urine (75%); m-CPP has a similar pharmacokinetic profile. Despite the short half-life, once-daily dosing at bedtime is the usual route of administration because of its sedating properties.

The therapeutic range for trazodone is 200 to 600 mg per day, although this has not been clearly delineated. Therapeutic blood levels have not been established. Generally, a patient can be started on 100 to 150 mg daily either in divided doses or in a single bedtime dose and gradually the dosage can be increased to 200 to 300 mg per day. For optimal benefit, doses in the range of 400 to 600 mg may be needed. Most clinicians question whether trazodone is as effective as other antidepressants and see it **mainly as an adjunctive agent for sleep.** Trazodone does appear to be useful in the treatment of SSRI-, bupropion-, and MAOI-induced insomnia in a dose range from 50 to 200 mg. Patients combining SSRIs or MAOIs with trazodone occasionally complain of mental clouding. Common side effects of trazodone include sedation, orthostatic hypotension, headaches, and less commonly nausea. Side effects may be lessened if the drug is taken in divided doses and with meals.

Trazodone lacks the quinidine-like properties of the cyclic antidepressants but has been associated in rare cases with cardiac arrhythmias, which may be related to trazodone's ability to inhibit potassium channels. Thus, **trazodone should be used with caution in patients with known cardiac disease.** The most common cardiovascular toxicity of trazodone is postural hypotension. Rare cases of hepatotoxicity have been associated with the use of trazodone and fatal cases of trazodone overdose have been reported.

Priapism may rarely occur with trazodone, most commonly early in therapy. Men given trazodone should be instructed to report abnormally prolonged erections to their physician or go to an emergency room. Should priapism occur, the drug should be permanently discontinued.

Gepirone

Gepirone is a full agonist of the serotonin 5-HT$_{1A}$ autoreceptors and a partial agonist of postsynaptic serotonin 5-HT$_{1A}$ receptors. It also has weak affinity for α_1-adrenergic receptors. Gepirone is currently under development for the treatment of depression, and double-blind, placebo-controlled studies have supported its efficacy in this condition.

Tandospirone

Tandospirone is another partial agonist of the serotonin 5-HT$_{1A}$ receptors. It is available in Japan for the treatment of anxiety and depression.

α₂-Adrenergic Receptor Antagonists

Mirtazapine

Mirtazapine, a piperazino-azepine compound, is a tetracyclic agent with a unique pharmacologic mechanism of action profile. As an antagonist at 5-HT$_{2A}$ and 5-HT$_{2C}$ receptors and at α₂-adrenergic auto- and heteroreceptors, the molecule increases both serotonergic and noradrenergic neurotransmission. It also blocks 5-HT$_3$ and histamine receptors but does not inhibit serotonin or norepinephrine reuptake, muscarinic cholinergic receptors, or α₁-adrenergic receptors. Mirtazapine shows linear pharmacokinetics over a dose range of 15 to 80 mg and its elimination half-life ranges from 20 to 40 hours, consistent with its time to reach steady state (4 to 6 days). Biotransformation is mainly mediated by the CYP2D6 and CYP3A4 isoenzymes. Inhibitors of these isoenzymes, such as paroxetine and fluoxetine, cause modestly increased mirtazapine plasma concentrations, whereas **mirtazapine has little inhibitory effects on CYP isoenzymes** and, therefore, the pharmacokinetics of coadministered drugs are hardly affected by mirtazapine.

It is an efficacious antidepressant with some data to assert a somewhat faster onset of action than SSRIs based on comparison trials. It is not associated with adverse cardiac effects and has been safe in overdose. It is quite sedating and thus generally administered at bedtime, but residual sedation is for some a limiting side effect, although typically diminishing with patient accommodation over days. Presumably because of its histamine-blocking effects, it is associated with increased appetite and **weight gain**. If weight gain is not observed in the first few months of therapy, it is unlikely to emerge later as a problem. Other side effects reported with mirtazapine are dizziness, dry mouth, and constipation. Perhaps because of its antagonist properties at the level of 5-HT$_2$ and 5-HT$_3$ receptors, there is evidence that sexual dysfunction, headaches, and nausea may be less common with mirtazapine than with the SSRIs. Severe neutropenia has been rarely reported (1 in 1,000) with uncertain relationship to the drug, but as with other psychotropics, the onset of infection and fever should prompt the patients to contact their physician. The drug is most efficacious at doses of 30 to 45 mg (although 60 mg per day has been used in refractory cases) usually given in a single bedtime dose. Available in 15-, 30-, and 45-mg scored tablets and in an orally soluble tablet formulation (Soltab) at 15, 30, and 45 mg, the lower dose may be suboptimal, and compared with the 15-mg dose, the 30-mg dose also may be less or at least not more sedating, possibly as a consequence of the noradrenergic effects being recruited at that dose. Mirtazapine has been successfully combined with SSRIs and venlafaxine for partial responders or nonresponders to the other drugs. In addition to enhanced efficacy with the combination, some SSRI side effects (e.g., sexual dysfunction, nausea) have been observed to improve as a likely consequence of the 5-HT$_2$– and 5-HT$_3$–blocking properties of mirtazapine. As with the SNRIs, there is interest in the use of this drug in pain–depression syndromes as an alternative to tricyclics.

Mianserin

Mianserin is another antagonist of α₂-adrenergic auto- and heteroreceptors and of serotonin 5-HT$_2$ receptors. It is available in Europe for the treatment of depression. Its most common side effects include somnolence, weight gain, dry mouth, sleep difficulties, tremor, and headaches. Effective daily doses of mianserin range from 30 mg to 60 mg, usually given at bedtime.

TRICYCLIC AND RELATED CYCLIC ANTIDEPRESSANTS

Chemistry

The tricyclic compounds were first developed in the 1950s. The antidepressant properties of imipramine, a structural analog of chlorpromazine, were discovered fortuitously when it was being tested as a potential antipsychotic compound.

A number of tricyclic and closely related tetracyclic compounds have been developed since.

Pharmacology

Most of the antidepressants are available only as oral preparations, although amitriptyline, imipramine, and clomipramine are also available for parenteral use. The parenteral forms are not clearly established as more rapidly acting or more effective than oral preparations; their advantage lies in the possibility of administering them to patients who cannot or will not take oral medication. For such patients, they may provide an alternative to ECT.

Oral preparations of tricyclics and related drugs are rapidly and completely absorbed from the gastrointestinal tract; a high percentage of an oral dose is metabolized by the liver as it passes through the portal circulation (first-pass effect). The tricyclics are metabolized by the microsomal enzymes of the liver; the tertiary amines are first monodemethylated to yield compounds that are still active. Indeed, the desmethyl metabolites of amitriptyline and imipramine are nortriptyline and desipramine, respectively, and are marketed as antidepressants. Other major metabolic pathways include hydroxylation (which may yield partially active compounds) and conjugation with glucuronic acid to produce inactive compounds.

Tricyclic drugs are highly lipophilic, meaning the free fraction passes easily into the brain and other tissues. They are also largely bound to plasma proteins. Given their lipophilicity and protein binding, they are not removed effectively by hemodialysis in cases of overdose. The time course of metabolism and elimination is biphasic, with approximately half of a dose removed over 48 to 72 hours and the remainder, strongly bound to tissues and plasma proteins, slowly excreted over several weeks. There is considerable variation among individuals in their metabolic rate for cyclic antidepressants based on genetic factors, age, and concomitantly taken drugs. In fact, when metabolic differences are combined with variation in the degree of protein binding, as much as a 300-fold difference in effective drug levels may be found among individuals.

Method of Use

Before Beginning Cyclic Antidepressants

A medical history and examination are indicated before beginning cyclic antidepressants, particularly to determine whether the patient has cardiac conduction system disease, which is the major medical contraindication to tricyclic use. An electrocardiogram (ECG) should be obtained for any patient with a history of cardiac symptoms or known cardiac disease; it is also reasonable as a screening test for patients older than 40 years. Although it appears that minor conduction system disease, such as first-degree heart block, does not increase the risk of serious sequelae from cyclic antidepressants, the **presence of conduction system abnormalities relatively contraindicates the use of TCAs.** Aside from the ECG, no other tests are generally indicated in healthy adults before starting a tricyclic.

Prescribing Cyclic Antidepressants

Tricyclics are started at a low dose with gradual increase until the therapeutic range is achieved. Finding the right tricyclic dose for a patient often involves a process of trial and error. The most common error leading to treatment failure is inadequate dosage. In healthy adults, the typical daily starting dose is 25 to 50 mg of imipramine or the equivalent. Nortriptyline and protriptyline are relatively more potent; thus, their daily starting dose is 10 to 25 mg. In some clinical situations, especially in elderly patients and patients with panic disorder, it may be necessary to start with lower doses (as low as 10 mg of imipramine or the equivalent) because of intolerance to side effects.

Generally, tricyclics are administered **once a day at bedtime** to help with compliance and, when the sedating compounds are used, to help with sleep. Divided doses are used if patients have side effects due to high peak levels. The dosage can be increased by 50 mg every 3 to 4 days, as side effects allow, up to a dose of 150 to 200 mg of imipramine or its equivalent at bedtime, with the exception of nortriptyline and protriptyline, which require lower doses (Table 3.3).

If there is no therapeutic response in 3 to 4 weeks, the dosage should be slowly increased, again as side effects allow. The maximum dosage of most tricyclics is the equivalent of 300 mg per day of imipramine, although rare patients who metabolize the drug rapidly may do well on higher dosages. The final dosage chosen is that at which the patient has a therapeutic response without severe side effects. If the patient has been on a maximal dose for 6 to 12 weeks without response, the drug trial should be considered a failure. Discontinuation of treatment should be done with a taper to minimize the risk of discontinuation symptoms, including gastrointestinal distress and dizziness.

Blood Levels

There has been considerable interest in antidepressant blood levels because of the marked interindividual differences in steady-state blood levels produced by any given oral dose. The literature on the relationship between antidepressant blood levels and therapeutic response often has been inconclusive or conflicting.

Of the currently available cyclic antidepressants, only four drugs have been studied well enough to make generalizations about the value of their blood levels in treatment of depression: imipramine, desipramine, amitriptyline, and nortriptyline. Serum levels of the other cyclic antidepressants have not been well enough investigated to be clinically meaningful at present except generally to confirm presence of the drug or to document extremely high serum levels.

Most studies of imipramine suggest a linear relationship between therapeutic response and blood levels of the parent compound and its desmethyl metabolite, desipramine; patients with a combined level of imipramine and desipramine greater than 225 ng/mL are believed to improve more than patients below that level. Desipramine given as a parent compound also appears to have a linear relationship to clinical improvement with a level greater than 125 ng/mL, producing a better response than lower levels.

Nortriptyline levels have been the best studied of the antidepressants. Some researchers believe that such studies reveal a more complex pattern than do imipramine or desipramine studies—an inverted U-shape correlation with clinical improvement, which is sometimes referred to as a therapeutic window. Clinical improvement correlates with levels of 50 to 150 ng/mL. The reason for poorer response above 150 ng/mL is not known, but it does not appear to relate to any measurable toxicity. On the other hand, the number of subjects in well-designed studies that indicate a therapeutic window is small, so not all researchers believe there is adequate evidence in favor of a therapeutic window. Studies of amitriptyline levels have resulted in disagreement about the utility of levels, with linear, curvilinear, and lack of relationship reported by different investigators.

Although clinical observation and judgment are still the best method to achieve maximal therapeutic benefit without producing intolerable side effects, blood levels for imipramine, desipramine, and nortriptyline might be useful in the following limited situations:

1. To assess compliance
2. To confirm rapid metabolism, resulting in lack of both therapeutic efficacy and side effects, often due to genetic differences or to induction of hepatic enzymes by anticonvulsants, cigarette smoking, or other agents

3. To discover slow metabolizers (i.e., patients with severe side effects at low oral doses as a result of high blood levels rather than somatization)
4. To document that a substantial level was obtained before terminating a drug trial

When used, blood levels should be drawn when the drug has achieved steady-state levels (at least 5 days after a dosage change in healthy adults; longer in elderly patients) and 10 to 14 hours after the last oral dose. One final caveat regarding tricyclic blood levels is the variability that is evident among laboratories. It is worth establishing the reliability of local laboratories if tricyclic blood levels are to be used.

Discontinuation
As with all psychotropic drugs, it is good practice to taper cyclic antidepressants gradually rather than to discontinue them abruptly. The reasons for tapering are to prevent withdrawal symptoms and to catch reemergence of depressive symptoms so that effective doses for treatment can be rapidly restored if necessary. Withdrawal symptoms may in part represent cholinergic rebound and include gastrointestinal distress, malaise, chills, coryza, and muscle aches.

Use During Pregnancy
There are limited data on the use of cyclic antidepressants during pregnancy. There have been reports of congenital malformations in association with tricyclic use, but no convincing causal association. Overall, the tricyclics may be safe, but given the lack of proven safety, the drugs should be avoided during pregnancy unless the indications are clearly compelling. Pregnant women who are at risk for serious depression might be maintained on tricyclic therapy. This decision should always be made very carefully and with extensive discussion of the risk–benefit factors. Because of greater clinical experience, older agents, such as imipramine, may be preferred to newer TCAs during pregnancy.

Tricyclics appear to be secreted in breast milk. Because their effects on normal growth and development are unknown, breast-feeding should be discouraged for mothers who are on tricyclics.

Augmentation of Tricyclics
As with the SSRIs, clinicians have used a number of augmentation or combination strategies for poor responders to a tricyclic.

Lithium
As with the SSRIs, lithium is combined with tricyclics in treatment nonresponders. For augmentation, lithium is generally added to an established tricyclic regimen at a daily dosage of 600 mg or more. Although initial reports found a high percentage of responders within 24 to 48 hours regardless of lithium level, later reports suggest a more variable response, with a delay of up to 2 weeks before improvement was evident. A small percentage of patients relapse despite initial improvement. A study from the Massachusetts General Hospital has put into question the efficacy of lithium augmentation of TCAs.

T_3
The strategy in using T_3 with tricyclics is similar to that described for its use with SSRIs. When patients have failed adequate trials of a cyclic antidepressant, 25 to 50 µg per day of T_3 may be added to their regimen. The mechanism of action does not appear to be an increase in tricyclic blood levels. Most responders are said to have had normal thyroid function at baseline. When this treatment is successful, some improvement is usually seen within 2 weeks and maximal improvement within 4 weeks.

Methylphenidate or Dextroamphetamine
The psychostimulants methylphenidate and dextroamphetamine have occasionally been used to augment a tricyclic regimen. For example, dosages of methylphenidate, 10 mg b.i.d. to 20 mg t.i.d., have been used; although these dosages produce a small increase in tricyclic levels, this does not seem to be the mechanism by which patients improve. This augmentation is successful in a small number of patients and is usually well tolerated. Patients should be monitored for onset of insomnia or agitation. This strategy is not recommended for patients with a history of psychostimulant abuse.

Side Effects and Toxicity of Cyclic Antidepressants
In general, the side effects of the tricyclics and related cyclic antidepressants are more difficult for patients to tolerate than the side effects of the newer drugs (see Table 3.4.). It should be recognized, however, that many patients tolerate tricyclic drugs well, especially the less anticholinergic and less sedating compounds such as desipramine and nortriptyline. In addition to side effects occurring with therapeutic use, another difficulty with the cyclic antidepressants (as well as the MAOIs) lies in their potential for lethality in overdose.

At therapeutic levels, tricyclics may produce **sedation, postural hypotension, anticholinergic (antimuscarinic) effects** (e.g., dry mouth, dry throat, urinary retention, blurred vision, constipation, diminished working memory, and dental cavities), and **quinidine-like effects** on cardiac conduction and may decrease the seizure threshold. In addition, cyclic antidepressants cause weight gain that may be significant. Cyclic antidepressants may cause sexual dysfunction, most frequently erectile dysfunction in men. Also, patients may experience excessive sweating. Most side effects of cyclic antidepressants worsen with increased doses, although some may manifest even at lower doses (e.g., dry mouth, constipation, postural hypotension). Elderly patients are generally more susceptible to these side effects. The major medical contraindication to the use of cyclic antidepressants is serious cardiac conduction disturbances.

Complaints of side effects should be taken seriously; often, however, reassurance and symptomatic treatment (e.g., stool softeners for constipation, mouthwashes or sugar-free hard candies for dry mouth) are the best course. It is certainly better to help the patient tolerate side effects or to change to a different drug than to administer subtherapeutic doses.

Orthostatic Hypotension
Orthostatic hypotension is the **most serious common side effect** of the TCAs. In elderly patients, there is an increased risk of falls, with subsequent increased risks of fractures and head injuries. Severe postural hypotension may limit therapy.

Postural hypotension is largely due to the α_1-adrenergic receptor antagonist properties of these drugs, although the exact mechanism is unclear. This side effect is not always dose related, as one would expect; it often occurs at low doses and may not always worsen with higher doses. In addition, patient factors are very important—depressed patients have a higher incidence of orthostatic symptoms than do normal controls on an equivalent dose of drug.

None of the cyclic antidepressants is free of this hypotensive side effect. As mentioned earlier, there are conflicting reports as to whether nortriptyline is less likely to cause hypotension. All patients beginning tricyclics should be warned to arise slowly from recumbency or sitting positions, especially on arising in the morning. Postural blood pressures should be obtained when a patient complains of dizziness, blackouts, or falling.

| | Symptoms and Signs of Anticholinergic Toxicity |
Systemic	Neuropsychiatric
Tachycardia	Agitation
Dilated, sluggishly reactive pupils	Motor restlessness
Blurred vision	Confusion
Warm dry skin	Disturbance of recent memory
Dry mucous membranes	Dysarthria
Fever	Myoclonus
Reduced or absent bowel sounds	Hallucinations (including visual)
Urinary retention	Delirium
	Seizures

Anticholinergic Effects

Mild anticholinergic effects are common with therapeutic doses of cyclic antidepressants. These effects include symptoms such as dry mouth, blurred near vision, constipation, and urinary hesitancy. More severe anticholinergic effects may occur in older patients even at therapeutic dosages. These include agitation, delirium, tachycardia, urinary retention, and ileus. A common reason for the appearance of a severe anticholinergic syndrome (Table 3.5) is the concomitant use of more than one anticholinergic drug. This often is seen in clinical situations when cyclic antidepressants are used in combination with low-potency typical antipsychotics (especially thioridazine), antiparkinsonian drugs, antihistamines, and over-the-counter sleep medications. It is important to be aware of the possibility of precipitating an attack of narrow-angle glaucoma. Patients with open-angle glaucoma can be treated with cyclic antidepressants so long as their intraocular pressures are checked by their ophthalmologist and their glaucoma medications are adjusted as needed.

If mild to moderate anticholinergic symptoms interfere with treatment, bethanechol chloride, a cholinergic agent that does not cross the blood–brain barrier, may be prescribed. Effective dosages range from 10 to 25 mg orally t.i.d. For acute urinary retention, bethanechol chloride, 2.5 to 5.0 mg, may be given subcutaneously; rarely, a urinary catheter may be temporarily required. If an anticholinergic delirium or severe anticholinergic syndrome is suspected, the medication should be stopped. Although the use of physostigmine can be diagnostically useful in these situations, its short half-life and toxicity limit its therapeutic use. An alternative remedy to the anticholinergic side effects of TCAs is the use of cholinesterase inhibitors such as donepezil (5 to 10 mg q.d.).

Cardiac Toxicity

The cardiac toxicity of tricyclic and related cyclic antidepressants may limit their clinical use (Table 3.6). The toxicity is due to the quinidine-like effects of these drugs and slowing intracardiac conduction and to a lesser extent to their anticholinergic effects. Patients at risk of serious cardiac toxicity are those with significant underlying conduction system disease. Except in overdose, major cardiac complications are extremely rare in patients with normal hearts (although benign ECG changes may occur).

In general, use of tricyclic and related cyclic antidepressants should be avoided in patients with bifascicular block, left bundle branch block, or a prolonged Q-T interval. Because the cyclic antidepressants slow intracardiac

TABLE 3.6	Cardiac Toxicity of Cyclic Antidepressants

Sinus tachycardia
Supraventricular tachyarrhythmias
Ventricular tachycardia and fibrillation
Prolongation of P-R, QRS, and Q-T intervals
Bundle branch block
First-, second-, and third-degree heart block
ST- and T-wave changes

conduction, they are actually mildly antiarrhythmic, tending to decrease ventricular premature beats. Despite early reports to the contrary, cyclic antidepressants appear to have little, if any, clinically significant effects on cardiac contractility.

Overdoses with TCAs

Acute doses of **more than 1 g of TCAs are often toxic and may be fatal.** Death may result from cardiac arrhythmias, hypotension, or uncontrollable seizures. Serum levels should be obtained when overdose is suspected both because of distorted information that may be given by patients or families and because oral bioavailability with very large doses of these compounds is poorly understood. Nonetheless, serum levels of the parent compound and its active metabolites provide less specific information about the severity of the overdose than one might hope. Serum levels of greater than 1,000 ng/mL are associated with serious overdose, as are increases in the QRS duration of the ECG to 0.10 seconds or greater. However, serious consequences of a TCA overdose may occur with serum levels under 1,000 ng/mL and with a QRS duration of less than 0.10 seconds.

In acute overdose, **almost all symptoms develop within 12 hours.** Antimuscarinic effects are prominent, including dry mucous membranes, warm dry skin, mydriasis, blurred vision, decreased bowel motility, and often urinary retention. Either CNS depression (ranging from drowsiness to coma) or an agitated delirium may occur. The CNS depressant effects of cyclic antidepressants are potentiated by concomitantly ingested alcohol, benzodiazepines, and other sedative-hypnotics. Seizures may occur, and in severe overdoses, respiratory arrest may occur. Cardiovascular toxicity presents a particular danger (Table 3.6). Hypotension often occurs, even with the patient supine. A variety of arrhythmias may develop, including supraventricular tachycardia, ventricular tachycardia or fibrillation, and varying degrees of heart block including complete heart block.

Treatment of Overdose

Basic management of overdose includes induction of emesis if the patient is alert and intubation and gastric lavage if the patient is not. Because bowel motility may have been slowed, it is worth giving 30 g of activated charcoal with a cathartic, such as 120 mL of magnesium citrate, to decrease the absorption of residual drug.

Basic cardiorespiratory supportive care should be administered if needed. Patients with depressed respiration will require ventilatory assistance. Hypotension will require the administration of fluid (however, this must be done cautiously if heart failure is present). In refractory hypotension, or if heart failure is present, pressors such as epinephrine or phenylephrine would be the agents of choice because they counteract the anti–α_1-adrenergic effects of the antidepressant.

Any patient with arrhythmias, a QRS duration of more than 0.10 seconds, or a serum tricyclic level greater than 1,000 ng/mL requires continuous cardiac monitoring, preferably in an intensive care unit setting. It is sound practice to monitor levels serially and to continue cardiac monitoring until the QRS interval has normalized.

Sinus tachycardia usually requires no treatment. Supraventricular tachycardia contributing to myocardial ischemia or hypotension may be treated with direct current cardioversion. Digoxin should be avoided because it might precipitate heart block, but propranolol appears to be safe in treating recurrent supraventricular tachycardia. Cardioversion is the treatment of choice for ventricular tachycardia or fibrillation. Administration of phenytoin may curtail ventricular arrhythmias. If lidocaine is administered, the likelihood of seizures may increase. If lidocaine fails to prevent further arrhythmias, propranolol and bretylium are the next agents of choice. Because quinidine, procainamide, and disopyramide may prolong the QRS interval and may precipitate heart block in tricyclic-overdosed patients, these agents should be avoided. Second- and third-degree heart blocks can be managed by insertion of a temporary pacemaker. Physostigmine is not generally effective in the treatment of most tricyclic-induced cardiac arrhythmias.

CNS toxicity also can produce significant morbidity or **death in tricyclic overdose.** Generally, delirium is managed with a quiet environment and reassurance; severely agitated patients may need restraints. For patients with uncontrollable delirium that is threatening their medical condition, low doses of benzodiazepines may be effective. Because of its toxicity and short duration of action, physostigmine is not generally recommended as a therapeutic agent.

One of the most troublesome medical complications following overdose with cyclic antidepressants is seizures. First-line pharmacologic treatment for seizures induced by cyclic antidepressants is one of the benzodiazepines, diazepam or lorazepam. Diazepam is given intravenously in a dose of 5 to 10 mg at a rate of 2 mg per minute. The dose may be repeated every 5 to 10 minutes until seizures are controlled. The risk of respiratory arrest can be minimized if intravenous benzodiazepines are given slowly, but resuscitation equipment should be available. Lorazepam is given intravenously in a dose of 1 to 2 mg over several minutes. The advantage of lorazepam is a longer biologic effect than do diazepam in acute usage (hours as opposed to minutes) due to a smaller volume of distribution and perhaps a lesser tendency to respiratory depression. If a benzodiazepine fails, phenytoin should be given in a full loading dose of 15 mg/kg no more rapidly than 50 mg per minute. Overrapid administration of phenytoin causes severe hypotension.

Forced diuresis and dialysis are of no value because of protein and tissue binding of cyclic antidepressants and may exacerbate hemodynamic instability. Hemoperfusion may have a limited role in extremely severe cases, but its use must be considered experimental.

Drug Interactions
The cyclic antidepressants have a variety of important pharmacodynamic and pharmacokinetic drug–drug interactions that may worsen toxicity (Tables 3.7 and 3.8).

MONOAMINE OXIDASE INHIBITORS
Iproniazid, the first of the MAOIs, was synthesized as an antituberculous drug in the 1950s. It was noted clinically to have striking stimulant and antidepressant properties and was subsequently shown to be an inhibitor of the enzyme MAO. Although its hepatotoxicity precluded its continued clinical use, other MAOIs were developed. The four MAOIs currently available in the United States for the treatment of depression are phenelzine, isocarboxazid, tranylcypromine, and selegiline.

MAO is found primarily on the outer membrane of mitochondria and is the enzyme primarily responsible for the intracellular catabolism of biogenic amines. In presynaptic nerve terminals, MAO metabolizes catecholamines that are found outside their storage vesicles. In the liver and gut, MAO metabolizes bioactive amines that are ingested in foods, thus serving an important protective function.

TABLE 3.7   Drug Interactions with Cyclic Antidepressants

Worsen sedation	Alcohol Antihistamines Antipsychotics Barbiturates, chloral hydrate, and other sedatives
Worsen hypotension	α-Methyldopa (Aldomet) β-Adrenergic blockers (e.g., propranolol) Clonidine Diuretics Low-potency antipsychotics
Additive cardiotoxicity	Quinidine and other type 1 antiarrhythmics Thioridazine, mesoridazine, pimozide, ziprasidone

Additive anticholinergic toxicity	Antihistamines (diphenhydramine and others)
	Antiparkinsonians (benztropine and others)
	Low-potency antipsychotics, especially
	  thioridazine
	Over-the-counter sleeping medications
	Gastrointestinal antispasmodics and
	  antidiarrheals (Lomotil and others)

Other	Tricyclics may increase the effects of warfarin Tricyclics may block the effects of guanethidine

It is known that MAO enzyme activity may vary markedly among individuals and appears to increase with age.

Two subtypes of MAO have been described. As mentioned earlier, MAOA preferentially oxidizes norepinephrine and serotonin and is irreversibly inactivated by low concentrations of the acetylenic inhibitor clorgyline. MAOB preferentially oxidizes phenylethylamine and benzylamine and is irreversibly inactivated by low concentrations of pargyline and deprenyl. Dopamine, tyramine, and tryptamine are

TABLE 3.8   Drugs that may Affect Levels of Cyclic Antidepressants

Increase Levels	Decrease Levels
Acetazolamide	Alcohol (chronic use)
Antipsychotics	Barbiturates and similarly acting sedative/
Disulfiram	hypnotics
Paroxetine, fluoxetine,[a] and other SSRIs	Carbamazepine[a]
Duloxetine	Heavy cigarette smoking
Glucocorticoids	Rifampin[a]
Methylphenidate and amphetamines	Phenobarbital[a]
Oral contraceptives	Phenytoin[a]
Salicylates	Primidone[a]
Thiazides	
Thyroid hormone	
Buproprion	

SSRIs, selective serotonin reuptake inhibitors.
[a]Major effect.

substrates for both forms of MAO. Although selective MAOIs have been developed, the four approved for use in depression in the United States affect both the A and B types of the enzyme.

Chemistry

Phenelzine, tranylcypromine, and isocarboxazid are all irreversible blockers of MAOA and MAOB activity. Tranylcypromine is the only available nonhydrazine MAOI antidepressant. It has structural characteristics similar to those of amphetamine and has some stimulant properties (Fig. 3.1). An additional MAOB inhibitor, selegiline, has been approved in its oral form for the treatment of Parkinson's disease. In low dosages ($\leq$10 mg per day), as used in Parkinson's disease, it is a selective inhibitor of MAO type B and therefore does not require a tyramine-free diet. At higher dosages (e.g., 30 mg orally per day), it may have antidepressant effects but becomes a nonselective MAOI; therefore, dietary precautions must be observed. The efficacy of a selegiline transdermal patch in depression has been approved by the FDA in the first half of 2006; because a patch can deliver drug to the bloodstream and thence to the brain while avoiding the gut wall for absorption, there is a potential for a significantly decreased risk of the selegiline patch causing hypertensive crisis by interaction with tyramine-containing foods.

Pharmacology

The MAOIs are well absorbed after oral administration. Parenteral forms are not available. As described, these compounds inhibit MAO in the CNS, peripheral sympathetic nervous system, and nonnervous tissues, such as liver and gut. They also partially inhibit other enzymes, but this effect probably is of little clinical consequence. With repeated dosing, maximal inhibition of MAO occurs in several days. Onset of action for antidepressant effect with MAOIs is 2 to 4 weeks, approximately equivalent to the latency of onset of other antidepressants. Because MAOIs irreversibly inhibit the enzyme, return of enzyme function after discontinuation may require 2 weeks (the time it takes for *de novo* synthesis of the enzyme).

Metabolism

The metabolism of MAOIs is not well understood. Selegiline and tranylcypromine have methamphetamine and amphetamine as metabolites. There is controversy as to whether phenelzine is cleaved and acetylated in the liver. It is known that a sizable number of people are slow acetylators (a high percentage of Asians and about 50% of whites and blacks), but there is little evidence that the rate of acetylation is clinically significant for this class of drugs. Of clinical importance is the observation that metabolism of MAOIs does not seem to be affected by anticonvulsants.

MAO Levels

Although plasma levels of MAOIs are not well studied, the degree of enzyme inhibition produced by these drugs has been investigated. For phenelzine, inhibition of greater than 85% of baseline platelet MAOB activity appears to correlate with therapeutic efficacy. Dosages of phenelzine greater than 45 mg per day are usually necessary to achieve this level of inhibition. This test is not useful for tranylcypromine because it maximally inhibits platelet MAO at subtherapeutic doses.

Interaction with Tyramine and Other Amines

MAOIs inactivate intestinal and hepatic MAO. Thus, when patients taking MAOIs ingest vasoactive amines in foods, they are not catabolized but instead enter the bloodstream and are taken up by sympathetic nerve terminals. **These exogenous amines may cause severe hypertension, hyperpyrexia, and other symptoms** of sympathetic hyperactivity including tachycardia, diaphoresis, tremulousness, and cardiac arrhythmias (the clinical syndrome is described later). A number of amines (especially tyramine, but also phenylethylamine, dopamine, and others) in foods may induce these sympathomimetic crises in MAOI-treated patients. For this reason, foods containing tyramine and other vasoactive amines and sympathomimetic drugs should not be ingested by patients on irreversible MAOIs.

Another potentially life-threatening drug interaction involves MAOIs and agents that are serotonergic, including certain tricyclics (e.g., clomipramine) and SSRIs. The latter agents in combination with MAOIs may result in a serotonin syndrome, which if mild may feature tachycardia, hypertension, fever, ocular oscillations, and myoclonic jerks, but in its severe form may include severe hyperthermia, coma, convulsions, and death. There are similar life-threatening interactions with certain opioid derivatives, including meperidine and dextromethorphan.

Method of Use

Generally speaking, MAOIs are effective treatments for major depressive illness. Older trials in which MAOIs appeared to be less effective than tricyclics suffered from poor patient selection and, more importantly, doses of MAOIs that would now be considered subtherapeutic. More recent controlled studies (e.g., using 45 mg per day of phenelzine) have shown equivalent efficacy of MAOIs compared with tricyclics. In clinical practice, MAOIs are frequently effective when all other agents have failed, and they are particularly robust therapeutic options for atypical depressives.

Nonetheless, given the complexity of their use, including dietary restrictions, MAOIs are usually reserved for patients in whom non-MAOIs have failed or have not been tolerated.

Preparing Patients for Use of MAOIs

Before beginning therapy with MAOIs, it is important to educate the patient about the risks of interactions with amine-containing foods, beverages, and medications. Patients should clearly understand the need for dietary restrictions, and it is recommended that the physician fully describe these issues before medication is prescribed. It is most useful to **have a prepared list of restrictions** (Table 3.9) that can be given to the patient. It may be useful to enlist family support in planning meals that avoid proscribed foods. Symptoms of a hypertensive crisis should be discussed with the patient, with clear instructions to contact the treating physician immediately or proceed to an emergency room if symptoms occur. Patients should be questioned about compliance both with medication dosage and with dietary restrictions at follow-up visits. Any signs of noncompliance should be taken seriously and corrected. If patients report "safe" transgression of dietary rules, clarification should be given that certain foods may vary in tyramine content from portion to portion; thus, successful cheating on one occasion does not rule out the possibility of a hypertensive crisis on another occasion. Given the life-threatening nature of hypertensive crises, repeated or flagrant noncompliance with the prescribed dietary regimen should prompt the physician to consider discontinuation of the MAOI. Patients also should be made aware of prescribed medications and should be reminded to tell their other physicians and dentists that they are taking an MAOI.

In addition to dietary restriction, it is important to educate patients regarding common side effects, especially postural hypotension, insomnia, and possible sexual dysfunction. Informing patients about the latency of onset of therapeutic effects will minimize discouragement and noncompliance.

Choice of Drug

Although phenelzine has been better studied clinically, it has a greater incidence of side effects than do tranylcypromine (most notably weight gain, drowsiness, anticholinergic-like effects such as dry mouth, and a greater incidence of **impotence**

TABLE 3.9 Sample Instructions for Patients Taking Monoamine Oxidase Inhibitors (MAOIs)

1. Certain foods and beverages must be avoided:
   All cheese except for fresh cottage cheese or cream cheese
   Meat
   　Beef liver
   　Chicken liver
   　Fermented sausages
   　Pepperoni
   　Salami
   　Bologna
   　Other fermented sausages
   　Other cured, unrefrigerated meats
   Fish
   　Caviar
   　Cured, unrefrigerated fish
   　Herring (dried or pickled)
   　Dried fish, shrimp paste
   Vegetables
   　Overripe avocados
   　Fava beans
   　Sauerkraut
   Fruits
   　Overripe fruits, canned figs
   Other foods
   　Yeast extracts (e.g., Marmite, Bovril)
   Beverages
   　Chianti wine
   　Beers containing yeast (unfiltered)
   Some foods and beverages should be used only in moderation:
   　Chocolate
   　Coffee
   　Beer
   　Wine
2. If you visit other physicians or dentists, inform them that you are taking an MAOI. This precaution is especially important if other medications are to be prescribed or if you are to have dental work or surgery.
3. Take no medication without a doctor's approval.
   　Avoid all over-the-counter pain medications except plain aspirin, acetaminophen (Tylenol), and ibuprofen.
   　Avoid all cold or allergy medications except plain chlorpheniramine (Chlor-Trimeton) or brompheniramine (Dimetane).
   　Avoid all nasal decongestants and inhalers.
   　Avoid all cough medications except plain guaifenesin elixir (plain Robitussin).
   　Avoid all stimulants and diet pills.
4. Report promptly any severe headache, nausea, vomiting, chest pain, or other unusual symptoms. If your doctor is not available, go directly to an emergency room.

and anorgasmia). In addition, although hepatotoxicity is rare, phenelzine has a greater risk of causing serious or fatal hepatotoxicity than do tranylcypromine. (It is believed that the hydrazine moiety is responsible for hepatotoxicity.)

Although tranylcypromine has a lower incidence of bothersome side effects, it does cause insomnia, which may be severe. Clonazepam 0.5 mg or trazodone 50 mg at bedtime may safely and effectively treat insomnia. Tranylcypromine might be the first-choice MAOI in patients who are intolerant of sedation.

The selegiline patch at the lowest dose (6 mg per day) does not require dietary restrictions and is therefore preferred by patients who are concerned about such restrictions.

Using MAOIs

Initially, oral MAOIs are administered at low doses, with gradual increases as side effects allow. Some tolerance may develop to side effects, including **postural hypotension**. Phenelzine is usually started at 15 mg b.i.d. (7.5 to 15.0 mg per day in elderly patients), isocarboxazid at 10 mg b.i.d., and tranylcypromine at 10 mg b.i.d. (5 to 10 mg per day in elderly patients). Dosages can be increased by 15 mg weekly for phenelzine and 10 mg weekly for isocarboxazid and tranylcypromine (as side effects allow) to 45 to 60 mg per day for phenelzine (30 to 60 mg per day in elderly patients) and 30 to 50 mg per day for the others. Dosages as high as 90 mg per day of these drugs may be required, although these exceed the manufacturer's recommendations. Once depressive symptoms remit, full therapeutic doses are protective against relapse, although in managing patients on MAOIs, dose adjustments over time to manage side effects or clinical response are common. The selegiline patch is typically started at the lowest dose (6 mg per day) and its dose may be titrated up to 9 or 12 mg per day, depending on the response.

Therapeutic effects often are not evident for 4 to 6 weeks. It is prudent to taper MAOIs over 2 to 4 weeks when discontinuing them; rarely, delirium and other discontinuation symptoms have been reported with abrupt discontinuation. When MAOIs are stopped, MAO levels do not immediately return to normal. Thus, it is prudent to wait 2 or more weeks before discontinuing MAOI dietary and drug restrictions after discontinuing MAOIs. During changes from an MAOI to a cyclic antidepressant or an SSRI, similar waiting periods should be observed. Severe and even fatal interactions have been reported when tricyclics or SSRIs have been added to MAOIs. It is generally recommended that tricyclics be stopped for 2 weeks, fluoxetine for 5 weeks, and other agents for 2 weeks before starting an MAOI.

Use in Pregnancy

There is little experience with the use of MAOIs in pregnancy. For this reason, their use should be avoided. If severe depression occurs, alternatives include SSRIs, tricyclics, and ECT.

Side Effects and Toxicity

Fear of MAOI toxicity has severely limited their use. Nonetheless, in compliant patients these drugs can be used safely and effectively.

Postural Hypotension

Postural hypotension is **dose related and may limit therapy.** This side effect may be worsened markedly if patients are also receiving diuretics or antihypertensives. Patients should be advised to arise slowly from sitting positions or recumbency, especially on awakening in the morning, and to lie down if they become dizzy. Except in overdose or combined treatment with antihypertensives, episodes of hypotension almost always respond to a supine position. In the rare event of severe and unremitting hypotension, intravenous fluids are required; pressor amines should be avoided if at all possible.

CNS Side Effects

Intractable insomnia and agitation can be troublesome with MAOIs. When this occurs, a trial on lower dosages should be considered, or a benzodiazepine or trazodone may be prescribed. Daytime somnolence may occur with MAOIs, especially phenelzine, and there are anecdotal reports of "sleep attacks" or "MAOI nods." Patients may develop tolerance to this side effect.

Hyperadrenergic Crises

Hyperadrenergic crises are caused by ingestion of sympathomimetic drugs or pressor amines, such as tyramine, which are found in some foods and beverages. These reactions are serious and may cause stroke or myocardial infarction. All sympathomimetic drugs can lead to crises, as can L-Dopa and TCAs (Table 3.10). Symptoms include severe headache, diaphoresis, mydriasis, neuromuscular irritability, hypertension (which may be extreme), and cardiac arrhythmias.

Patients should be advised to contact their physician and to proceed to an emergency room if any such symptoms occur. For severe reactions, treatment consists of blockade of α_1-adrenergic receptors with phentolamine, 5 mg intravenously, repeated as necessary. Phentolamine can be administered over the next 12 to 36 hours (0.25 to 0.50 mg intramuscularly every 4 to 6 hours) as needed to control blood pressure. Sodium nitroprusside is extremely effective but requires

TABLE 3.10 Interactions of Monoamine Oxidase Inhibitors (MAOIs) with Other Drugs[a]

Drug	Effect
Sympathomimetics [e.g., amphetamines, dopamine, ephedrine, epinephrine (Adrenalin), isoproterenol (Isuprel), metaraminol, methylphenidate, oxymetazoline (Afrin), norepinephrine, phenylephrine (Neo-Synephrine), phenylpropanolamine, pseudoephedrine (Sudafed)]	Hypertensive crisis
Meperidine (Demerol and others)	Fever, delirium, hypertension, hypotension, neuromuscular excitability, death
Oral hypoglycemics	Further lowering of serum glucose
L-Dopa	Hypertensive crisis
Tricyclic antidepressants (e.g., imipramine, desipramine, nortriptyline)	Fever, seizures, delirium, hypertensive crisis
SSRIs	Serotonin syndrome
SNRIs	Serotonin syndrome
Tryptophan	Nausea, confusion, anxiety, shivering, hyperthermia, rigidity, diaphoresis, hyperreflexia, tachycardia, hypotension, coma, death
Bupropion	Hypertensive crisis

SSRIs, selective serotonin reuptake inhibitors; SNRIs, serotonin-norepinephrine reuptake inhibitors.
[a]This may include selegiline even at low doses.

continuous blood pressure monitoring for safe use. The most common strategy for mild to moderate reactions has been the use of the calcium channel blocker nifedipine, which in recent years has been considered controversial because of concerns over extreme decreases in pressure when used emergently for malignant hypertensive events. β-Blockers should not be used because, as in the treatment of pheochromocytoma, a potential clinical effect would be to intensify vasoconstriction and thus worsen hypertension by leaving α-adrenergic effects unopposed. After acute treatment, it is important to identify the cause of the crisis; if the cause is deliberate dietary indiscretion, continuing therapy with MAOIs should be reconsidered. When a serotonergic agent is combined with an MAOI, a serotonin syndrome may occur (see later section on overdose).

Other Side Effects
Patients have reported weight gain on all MAOIs and occasionally weight loss more commonly on tranylcypromine. Anticholinergic-like side effects occur, although they are not due to muscarinic antagonism. These side effects are less severe than those seen with tricyclics, although patients on phenelzine may experience dry mouth. Elderly patients may develop constipation or urinary retention. Alternatively, nausea and diarrhea have been reported by some patients. Sweating, flushing, or chills also may occur. Rarely, hepatotoxicity may occur with phenelzine, which may be serious. Peripheral edema likely reflecting effects of the drug on small vessels may prove difficult to manage. Finally, some patients complain of muscle twitching or electric shock–like sensations. The latter may respond to clonazepam, although the emergence of neurologic or neuropathic symptoms may reflect interference with absorption of vitamin B_6, which should improve with dietary supplementation of pyridoxine (vitamin B_6) 50 to 100 mg per day.

Overdose

MAOIs are extremely dangerous in overdose. Because they circulate at very low concentrations in serum and are difficult to assay, there are no good data on therapeutic or toxic serum levels. Manifestations of toxicity may appear slowly, often taking up to 12 hours to appear and 24 hours to reach their peak; thus, even if patients appear clinically well in the emergency room, they should be admitted for observation after any significant overdose. After an asymptomatic period, a serotonin syndrome may occur, including hyperpyrexia and autonomic excitation. Neuromuscular excitability may be severe enough to produce rhabdomyolysis, which may cause renal failure. This phase of excitation may be followed by CNS depression and cardiovascular collapse. Death may occur early because of seizures or arrhythmias or later because of asystole, arrhythmias, hypotension, or renal failure. Hemolysis and a coagulopathy also may occur and contribute to morbidity and mortality.

Treatment should include gastric emptying followed by oral administration of a charcoal slurry. With the emergence of symptoms such as delirium, hyperpyrexia, and hypertension or hypotension, meticulous supportive care is required. CNS excitation can be treated with lorazepam or diazepam intravenously. These agents should not be used excessively, however, because they may potentiate CNS depression later. If multiple doses are to be used, lorazepam is preferred because of its shorter elimination half-life. Neuroleptics, especially low-potency agents such as chlorpromazine, should be avoided because they can produce or worsen hypotension. Seizures may be treated with lorazepam 1 to 2 mg or diazepam 5 to 10 mg given slowly intravenously and repeated every 10 to 15 minutes as needed. Severe neuromuscular irritability or rigidity may occur and may be so severe as to impair respiration because of decreased chest wall compliance. Muscular irritability and rigidity may contribute to fever, a hypermetabolic state, and rhabdomyolysis. There are several case reports of successful use of dantrolene sodium, a directly acting muscle relaxant, to treat these problems. A dosage of 2.5 mg/kg intravenously every 6 hours for 24 hours was used successfully in one patient; it is prudent to continue therapy with lower doses for several days afterward. A severe serotonin syndrome with hyperpyrexia and muscular rigidity may be best treated with anesthesia and muscle paralysis. Severe hypertension may be treated with phentolamine 5 mg intravenously, repeated as necessary, or with sodium nitroprusside (which requires continuous blood pressure monitoring). Ventricular arrhythmias can be safely treated with lidocaine, but bretylium should be avoided because of its adrenergic effects.

The serotonin syndrome produced by the interaction of MAOIs with meperidine, dextromethorphan, clomipramine, and SSRIs, and occasionally with cyclic antidepressants, may be similar clinically to overdose, with similar principles of management applying.

Drug Interactions
Important drug interactions are listed in Table 3.10.

PSYCHOTHERAPY
Cognitive therapy and interpersonal psychotherapy are probably the most efficacious forms of psychotherapy in the treatment of patients with depressive disorders. Both therapies are short-term and focused on the "here and now." Behavioral therapy and short-term dynamic psychotherapy have also been studied in the treatment of major depression, but their efficacy is less well established. Many other forms of therapy are currently used in the treatment of depressed patients, but more studies are needed to establish their usefulness. It is common practice to treat patients with depressive disorders with a combination of psychotherapy and pharmacotherapy with antidepressants. This combination can be prescribed from the beginning when the depressive disorder emerges in the context of severe psychosocial stressors or in the absence of social support. More typically, psychotherapy is added to pharmacotherapy once the patient has reported a significant clinical improvement, to consolidate the progress, address residual symptoms, and prevent relapses. The usefulness of this combination, particularly when antidepressants are combined with cognitive therapy or modified forms of cognitive therapy (e.g., well-being therapy), has been demonstrated in research studies.

Bibliography

Antidepressant Mechanism of Action
Fava M, Kendler KS. Major depressive disorder. *Neuron* 2000;28:335.
Hyman SE, Nestler EJ. Initiation and adaptation: a paradigm for understanding psychotropic drug action. *Am J Psychiatry* 1996;153:15.
Malberg JE. Implications of adult hippocampal neurogenesis in antidepressant action. *J Psychiatry Neurosci* 2004;29:196.
Nestler, EJ, Hyman, SE, Malenka RJ. *Molecular neuropharmacology: foundation for clinical neuroscience.* New York: McGraw-Hill, 2001.
Sanacora G, Saricicek A. GABAergic contributions to the pathophysiology of depression and the mechanism of antidepressant action. *CNS Neurol Disord Drug Targets* 2007;6(2):127–140.

Antidepressants in Depressive Subtypes
Fava M, Rosenbaum JF. Anger attacks in patients with depression. *J Clin Psychiatry* 1999;60(suppl 15):21.
Fava M, Rosenbaum JF, Hoog SL, et al. Fluoxetine versus sertraline and paroxetine in major depression: tolerability and efficacy in anxious depression. *J Affect Disord* 2000;59:119.
Fava M, Rush AJ, Alpert JE, et al. Difference in treatment outcome in outpatients with anxious versus nonanxious depression: a STAR*D report. *Am J Psychiatry* 2008;165(3):342–351.
Fava M, Uebelacker LA, Alpert JE, et al. Major depressive subtypes and treatment response. *Biol Psychiatry* 1997;42:568.

Guelfi JD, Ansseau M, Timmerman L, Korsgaard S; Mirtazapine-Venlafaxine Study Group. Mirtazapine versus venlafaxine in hospitalized severely depressed patients with melancholic features. *J Clin Psychopharmacol* 2001;21:425.

Quitkin FM. Depression with atypical features: diagnostic validity, prevalence, and treatment. *Prim Care Companion J Clin Psychiatry* 2002;4:94.

Sonawalla SB, Fava M. Severe depression: is there a best approach? *CNS Drugs* 2001;15:765.

Stewart JW, McGrath PJ, Quitkin FM. Do age of onset and course of illness predict different treatment outcome among DSM IV depressive disorders with atypical features? *Neuropsychopharmacology* 2002;26:237.

Therapeutic Use of Antidepressants

Barbui C, Hotopj M, Freemantle N, et al. Selective serotonin reuptake inhibitors versus tricyclic and heterocyclic antidepressants: comparison of drug adherence. *Cochrane Database Syst Rev* 2000;4:CD002791.

Bielski RJ, Ventura D, Chang CC. A double-blind comparison of escitalopram and venlafaxine extended release in the treatment of major depressive disorder. *J Clin Psychiatry* 2004;65:1190.

Bouckoms A, Mangini LP. An antidepressant adjuvant for mood disorders? *Psychopharmacol Bull* 1993;29:207.

Clayton AH, Warnock JK, Kornstein SG, et al. A placebo-controlled trial of bupropion SR as an antidote for selective serotonin reuptake inhibitor-induced sexual dysfunction. *J Clin Psychiatry* 2004;65:62.

Clayton AH, Zajecka J, Ferguson JM, et al. Lack of sexual dysfunction with the selective noradrenaline reuptake inhibitor reboxetine during treatment for major depressive disorder. *Int Clin Psychopharmacol* 2003;18:151.

Debonnel G, Gobbi G, Turcotte J, et al. The alpha-2 antagonist mirtazapine combined with the SSRI paroxetine induces a greater antidepressant response: a double-blind controlled study. 39th Annual Meeting of the ACNP, San Juan, Puerto Rico, 2000.

Detke MJ, Wiltse CG, Mallinckrodt CH, et al. Duloxetine in the acute and long-term treatment of major depressive disorder: a placebo- and paroxetine-controlled trial. *Eur Neuropsychopharmacol* 2004;14:457.

Fava GA, Rafanelli C, Cazzaro M, et al. Well-being therapy. A novel psychotherapeutic approach for residual symptoms of affective disorders. *Psychol Med* 1998;28:475.

Fava M, Rush AJ, Wisniewski SR, et al. A comparison of mirtazapine and nortriptyline following two consecutive failed medication treatments for depressed outpatients: a STAR*D report. *Am J Psychiatry* 2006;163(7):1161–1172.

Gaynes BN, Rush AJ, Trivedi MH, et al. The STAR*D study: treating depression in the real world. *Cleve Clin J Med* 2008;75(1):57–66.

Linder MW, Keck PE Jr. Standards of laboratory practice: antidepressant drug monitoring. National Academy of Clinical Biochemistry. *Clin Chem* 1998;44:1073.

Nelson JC, Mazure CM, Bowers MB, et al. A preliminary open study of the combination of fluoxetine and desipramine for rapid treatment of major depression. *Arch Gen Psychiatry* 1991;48:303.

Nelson JC, Mazure CM, Jatlow PI, et al. Combining norepinephrine and serotonin reuptake inhibition mechanisms for treatment of depression: a double-blind, randomized study. *Biol Psychiatry* 2004;55:296.

Nierenberg AA, Farabaugh AH, Alpert JE, et al. Timing of onset of antidepressant response with fluoxetine treatment. *Am J Psychiatry* 2000;157:1423.

Nierenberg AA, Fava M, Trivedi MH, et al. A comparison of lithium and T(3) augmentation following two failed medication treatments for depression: a STAR*D report. *Am J Psychiatry* 2006;163(9):1519–1530.

Nierenberg AA, Petersen TJ, Alpert JE. Prevention of relapse and recurrence in depression: the role of long-term pharmacotherapy and psychotherapy. *J Clin Psychiatry* 2003;64(suppl 15):13.

Renaud J, Axelson D, Birmaher B. A risk-benefit assessment of pharmacotherapies for clinical depression in children and adolescents. *Drug Safety* 1999;20:59.

Rush AJ, Trivedi MH, Wisniewski SR, et al. STAR*D Study Team. Bupropion-SR, sertraline, or venlafaxine-XR after failure of SSRIs for depression. *N Engl J Med* 2006;354(12):1231–1242.

Thase ME, Entsuah AR, Rudolph RL. Remission rates during treatment with venlafaxine or selective serotonin reuptake inhibitors. *Br J Psychiatry* 2001;178:234.

Trivedi MH, Fava M, Wisniewski SR, et al. STAR*D Study Team. Medication augmentation after the failure of SSRIs for depression. *N Engl J Med* 2006;354(12):1243–1252.

Antidepressant Side Effects and Their Management

Cassano P, Fava M. Tolerability issues during long-term treatment with antidepressants. *Ann Clin Psychiatry* 2004;16:15.

Dording CM, Mischoulon D, Petersen TJ, et al. The pharmacologic management of SSRI-induced side effects: a survey of psychiatrists. *Ann Clin Psychiatry* 2002;14:143.

Fava M. Weight gain and antidepressants. *J Clin Psychiatry* 2000;61(suppl 11):37.

Fava M, Nurnberg HG, Seidman SN, et al. Efficacy and safety of sildenafil in men with serotonergic antidepressant-associated erectile dysfunction: results from a randomized, double-blind, placebo-controlled trial. *J Clin Psychiatry* 2006;67(2):240–246.

Fava M, Rankin M. Sexual functioning and SSRIs. *J Clin Psychiatry* 2002;63(suppl 5):13.

Jick H, Kaye JA, Jick SS. Antidepressants and the risk of suicidal behaviors. *JAMA* 2004;292:338.

Lee KC, Finley PR, Alldredge BK. Risk of seizures associated with psychotropic medications: emphasis on new drugs and new findings. *Expert Opin Drug Saf* 2003;2:233.

Lippman SB, Nash K. Monoamine oxidase inhibitor update. Potential adverse food and drug interactions. *Drug Saf* 1990;5:195.

Lucena MI, Carvajal A, Andrade RJ, et al. Antidepressant-induced hepatotoxicity. *Expert Opin Drug Saf* 2003;2:249.

McElroy SL, Keck PE Jr, Friedman LM. Minimizing and managing antidepressant side effects. *J Clin Psychiatry* 1995;56(suppl 2):49.

Nurnberg HG, Hensley PL, Gelenberg AJ, et al. Treatment of antidepressant-associated sexual dysfunction with sildenafil: a randomized controlled trial. *JAMA* 2003;289:56.

Pacher P, Kecskemeti V. Cardiovascular side effects of new antidepressants and antipsychotics: new drugs, old concerns? *Curr Pharm Des* 2004;10:2463.

Rosenstein DL, Nelson C, Jacobs SC. Seizures associated with antidepressants: a review. *J Clin Psychiatry* 1993;54:289.

Shulman KI, Walker SE. Refining the MAOI diet: tyramine content of pizzas and soy products. *J Clin Psychiatry* 1999;60:191.

Sternbach H. The serotonin syndrome. *Am J Psychiatry* 1991;148:705.

Antidepressant Overdose

Backman J, Ekman CJ, Alsen M, et al. Use of antidepressants in deliberate self-poisoning: psychiatric diagnoses and drugs used between 1987 and 1997 in Lund, Sweden. *Soc Psychiatry Psychiatr Epidemiol* 2003;38:684.

Barbey JT, Roose SP. SSRI safety in overdose. *J Clin Psychiatry* 1998;59(suppl 15):45.

Boehnert MT, Lovejoy FH. Value of the QRS duration versus the serum drug level in predicting seizures and ventricular arrhythmias after an acute overdose of tricyclic antidepressants. *N Engl J Med* 1985;313:474.

Buckley NA, Faunce TA. "Atypical" antidepressants in overdose: clinical considerations with respect to safety. *Drug Saf* 2003;26:539.

Cheeta S, Schifano F, Oyefeso A, et al. Antidepressant-related deaths and antidepressant prescriptions in England and Wales, 1998–2000. *Br J Psychiatry* 2004;184:41.

Graudins A, Dowsett RP, Liddle C. The toxicity of antidepressant poisoning: is it changing? A comparative study of cyclic and newer serotonin-specific antidepressants. *Emerg Med (Fremantle)* 2002;14:440.

Grunebaum MF, Ellis SP, Li S, et al. Antidepressants and suicide risk in the United States, 1985–1999. *J Clin Psychiatry* 2004;65:1456.

Linden CH, Rumack BH, Strehlke C. Monoamine oxidase inhibitor overdose. *Ann Emerg Med* 1984;13:1137.

Antidepressants in Pregnancy

Cohen LS, Nonacs RM, Bailey JW, et al. Relapse of depression during pregnancy following antidepressant discontinuation: a preliminary prospective study. *Arch Women Ment Health* 2004;7:217.

Dennis CL, Stewart DE. Treatment of postpartum depression, part 1: a critical review of biological interventions. *J Clin Psychiatry* 2004;65:1242.

Nonacs R, Cohen LS. Assessment and treatment of depression during pregnancy: an update. *Psychiatr Clin North Am* 2003;26:547.

Neonatal complications after intrauterine exposure to SSRI antidepressants. *Prescrire Int* 2004;13:103.

4

Drugs for the Treatment of Bipolar Disorders

Bipolar disorder is a serious mental disorder in which recurrences of mania, hypomania, and depression are the rule, and in perhaps one third of the patients symptoms become chronic. Bipolar disorder's seriousness is marked by high rates of completed suicide, frequent disability, and premature mortality from medical illness. This chapter will review in detail the drugs used for the treatment of bipolar disorder and conclude with recommendations for drug treatments of acute mania, mixed-states, bipolar depression, and rapid-cycling bipolar disorder.

Mania, along with its counterpart melancholia, has been recognized and discussed through the ages. In its purest form, the manic phase of bipolar disorder is one of the most dramatic conditions in all of medicine. Acute mania is easily recognized because it manifests as a **dramatic change from usual personality** with elevated mood or euphoria, usually mixed with increased activity, excessive talking, and decreased need for sleep. Grandiosity, mistrust, and religious obsession are common psychological symptoms. These psychological and behavioral changes impair judgment that often leads to problematic behaviors and decisions, such as foolish money spending or infidelity. It is not unusual for this changed behavior to lead to serious social, marital, financial, or legal problems. The time course for this change of behavior into the manic state may be gradual over several weeks, or it may be abrupt. Untreated, mania may last weeks to many months. The excess activity and elevated mood of mania is often mixed with irritability, hostility, paranoia, or fluctuations from elation to tearful sadness. This manic pole, thus, is often quite unstable. A significant number of patients experience dysphoric mania, or so-called mixed-states, with mania occurring simultaneously with a major depressive episode. In its extreme form, mania may include psychotic symptoms, such as hallucinations or grandiose delusions, thereby blurring the distinction between acute mania with psychotic features and schizophrenia. Because of this, the definitive diagnosis of bipolar disorder often requires a longitudinal perspective.

The depressed phase of the illness may follow the manic phase or periods of euthymia. While it may be marked by low mood and loss of energy, with patients often taking to the bed and sleeping excessively, it may also be accompanied by subsyndromal symptoms of mania such as racing thoughts and psychomotor agitation. Patients lose self-confidence, become pessimistic, and may consider or attempt suicide during this phase of the illness or during mixed states, often during the transition from mania to depression. In the severe form, the depressed phase may include nihilistic delusions or derogatory auditory hallucinations. The depressed phase of bipolar disorder, unfortunately, frequently accounts for the majority of the ill periods of patient's lives, and is notoriously difficult to treat. Many patients also suffer chronic subsyndromal depressive symptoms. Some patients presenting with so-called **atypical depression** may not disclose their periods of hypomania or mania and thus be incorrectly diagnosed with depression rather than bipolar disorder. Interestingly, some patients with early onset and highly recurrent depression may later go on to develop bipolar disorder.

The less severe form of mania, or hypomania, also represents a distinct change in personality with many of the same features as mania, though it does not include psychosis, behavioral changes sufficiently severe to cause hospitalization, or marked impairment in functioning. Patients with hypomania (but never mania) who also suffer depression are characterized as having bipolar II disorder. While not recognized in the *Diagnostic and Statistical Manual of Mental Disorders*, 4th edition (*DSM-IV*), recent evidence suggests that patients with hypomania may also experience concomitant dysphoric symptoms, or so-called hypomanic-mixed states. Although hypomania may be easy to recognize in person, it is often **difficult to diagnose historically,** with some patients overendorsing past behaviors and other patients denying obvious past behavioral changes. For this reason, gathering information from family members or other reliable sources is critical in diagnosing past hypomania. For depressed patients, gathering history to elucidate a brief period of elevated mood may be difficult, particularly when the patient has a history of substance abuse or personality disorder. While underdiagnosis of bipolar II disorder is a significant problem, we commonly see an **overdiagnosis of bipolar II** disorder resulting in long-term medication treatment of a condition that does not exist. Indeed, in many instances, patients are diagnosed with bipolar II disorder when the evidence of past hypomania is scant or better explained by psychosocial factors, impulsive decisions, or substance abuse.

Making the diagnosis of bipolar disorder should not be done lightly because it represents a lifetime condition for which there is only palliative treatment with medications that are often difficult to tolerate. Family and medical history are critical to be sure of the diagnosis. If a person presents with symptoms consistent with mania or hypomania beyond the usual age of onset, in the late teens or early 20s, it is important to look for other causes to explain the change of behavior. Common explanations in younger adults include illicit drugs such as amphetamine or cocaine as well as glucocorticoids or anabolic steroids. HIV infections or syphilis may present with manic symptoms in younger persons as well. In older persons presenting with **new onset mania,** brain infarctions, brain injuries, brain tumors, or autoimmune diseases may lead to manic behaviors. In addition, steroid hormones, antidepressants, or dopamine agonists used to treat Parkinson's disease may also lead to manic behaviors.

Bipolar disorder is **complicated by multiple factors,** all of which conspire against successful treatment. Although the vast majority of patients have recurrence of both forms of the illness, a small minority experience recurrent unipolar mania, especially psychotic mania, as the prominent form of their illness. Other patients experience frequent episodes of illness (four or more times per year), known as rapid cycling, and these patients are frequently treatment resistant. Bipolar disorder is also frequently complicated by co-occurring mental disorders such as anxiety disorders, attention deficit disorder, substance abuse, personality disorders, infectious diseases (e.g., HIV infection), or traumatic brain injuries that result from risky manic behaviors, all of which mitigate against successful treatment. Patients with bipolar disorder also suffer from a number of medical disorders at higher rates than the general population. These disorders complicate treatment and include obesity, diabetes, smoking, chronic obstructive pulmonary disease, HIV infection, hepatitis C, and migraine headaches. Many patients do not adhere to drug treatment because of side effects, denial of illness, or lack of benefit. Finally, the consequences of long-standing bipolar disorder often lead to demoralizing psychosocial problems that make drug treatment alone insufficient for satisfactory outcomes.

Drug treatments must be only part of the treatment of bipolar disorder. A sound therapeutic alliance with the physician and other treatment members is essential for long-term treatment. This alliance will be tested during the times patients experience paranoia and mistrust. Educating the patient and family about the illness and the early manifestations of illness recurrence is critical to prevent full-blown episodes. Most patients can keep mood records and identify stressors as well as subtle behavior changes that suggest other treatments are needed. When possible, family members should be involved to help with early detection of mood changes, medication nonadherence, or substance abuse. Patients also need to learn about the benefits of medication adherence and treatment of medication side effects. Other behavioral strategies, including sleep hygiene, stress reduction techniques, regular exercise, and avoidance of alcohol and illicit drugs should be part of long-term treatment of bipolar disorder. Regular cognitive behavior therapy, social rhythm therapy, or family-focused therapy may prove helpful for patients with bipolar disorder. Some patients may need substance abuse treatment as an ongoing part of their bipolar disorder treatment. Less ill patients may benefit from vocational training.

GENERAL COMMENTS ON THE USE OF MOOD STABILIZERS

The mood stabilizers are a diverse group of drugs used primarily in the treatment of bipolar disorder (manic-depressive illness); as a class, these drugs are effective in acute mania and generally less effective in acute depression, and they act to increase the time to depression or mania recurrence. The longest established mood stabilizers are lithium and the anticonvulsant valproate. Lamotrigine (Lamictal) and all of the second-generation antipsychotic drugs have also shown benefit in different phases of the illness in randomized controlled trials. Clinical trial data are greatest for lithium, divalproex, and the atypical antipsychotics in acute mania. The data are less impressive for bipolar prophylaxis and rather poor for bipolar depression. Unfortunately, no medication is effective in all phases of bipolar disorder. The ideal agent would treat mania and depression in the short term and prevent relapse of either affective phase. This agent, unfortunately, awaits discovery.

A great weight of evidence favors **long-term prophylaxis** against recurrences after effective treatment of acute episodes. The mainstay of treatment of bipolar disorder for nearly four decades has been lithium. Given its long use, lithium's efficacy, limitations, and side effects are extremely well documented. Despite less documentation of the benefits and risks of therapy with divalproex, especially for maintenance treatment, it has become widely used, likely based on the perception that it has fewer side effects and greater ease of use than lithium. Therefore, it has become a first-line treatment, although greater overall benefit may still rest with lithium, particularly for suicide prevention. Carbamazepine, lamotrigine, and the atypical antipsychotics have good evidence for treatment of particular aspects of bipolar disorder, though no existing treatment of bipolar disorder is fully satisfactory.

From the distance of the classroom, we often teach our trainees to avoid polypharmacy because of the risk of cumulative side effects and drug interactions. Although a patient with bipolar disorder may require only one agent such as lithium as the mainstay of treatment, over time, given the complexity of bipolar illness, interventions are likely to include the addition of adjunctive treatments, which may include antidepressants, antipsychotics, benzodiazepines, and other compounds. Approximately two thirds of the patients in contemporary studies fail to achieve complete remission or long-term stability on lithium monotherapy.

If possible, one drug should ideally be used as the anchor medication for the disease; for example, a fully unsatisfactory response to lithium for prophylaxis should lead the clinician to consider the use of divalproex or lamotrigine alone. In practice, however, the clinician does not have the luxury of sequential pure trials of the many drugs available. Therefore, unless the initial treatment has yielded no benefit and/or is poorly tolerated, usual practice is to add a second mood stabilizer or second-generation antipsychotic to the ongoing treatment with the first agent while watching for possible interactions. When the goal is monotherapy, this can be done by crosstapering treatment: tapering the first drug and gradually increasing the second.

Bipolar illness is often a severe and life-altering, if not life-threatening, disease and, as with other serious medical conditions (cancer, hypertension, etc.), the clinician should not shrink from using combination therapies. The combined use of the anchor medication (e.g., lithium divalproex, lamotrigine, or a second-generation antipsychotic) and an additional mood stabilizer is recommended when a partial response is achieved with one mood stabilizer. However, controlled studies of each of these combinatorial possibilities have not yet been accomplished. Combination therapy always must be administered with caution, watching for **combined toxicities.** Some combined regimens are best managed when the clinician monitors blood levels of both compounds.

Over time, the clinician, in partnership with the patient, should be encouraged to reevaluate doses, adverse effects, and regimens, always searching for the optimal combination. Daily mood charting of longitudinal treatment by bipolar patients, with careful documentation of the effect of specific regimens on the various phases of the affective illness, is critical to optimize outcomes.

LITHIUM

Lithium is the lightest solid element in the periodic table; it is active as a psychopharmacologic agent in the form of its singly charged cation. The therapeutic value of lithium was discovered serendipitously by Cade in 1949 when he noted its calming effect on animals. He then tried it on 10 manic patients and found dramatic improvement. The therapeutic usage of lithium was thereafter rapidly explored in Australia and Europe. Its approval for use in the United States, however, was delayed until 1970 because of severe and sometimes fatal cases of lithium poisoning in the 1940s in patients who had unrestricted use of it as a salt substitute. By the time it was approved in the United States, its efficacy as a treatment of mania had been demonstrated beyond question by research in Europe. Its benefit in reducing suicide attempts and completed suicide may be its greatest contribution to the treatment for persons with bipolar disorder.

PHARMACOLOGY

Absorption

Lithium tablets and capsules (Table 4.1) are available as the carbonate salt, which is less irritating to the gastrointestinal tract than the chloride. Each 300-mg tablet contains 8 mmol of lithium. Because lithium is a monovalent ion, **8 mmol is equal to 8 mEq.** Lithium is also available as lithium citrate syrup, containing 8 mmol of lithium per 5 mL. Lithium is well absorbed after oral administration. Standard preparations produce peak serum levels in 1.5 to 2.0 hours; slow-release preparations that achieve peak levels in 4.0 to 4.5 hours also are available. No parenteral forms are available.

TABLE 4.1 Common Causes of Secondary Mania

Drug Causes	Central Nervous System Causes
Amphetamine	Traumatic brain injury
Methamphetamine	Meningioma
Cocaine	Glioma (esp right hemisphere)
Antidepressants	Neurosyphilis
Anticholinergics	HIV infection
Hallucinogens	Posttemporal lobectomy
Phenylcyclidine	Epilepsy
Levodopa	Systemic Lupus
Glucocorticoids	Stroke
Anabolic steroids	Multiple sclerosis exacerbation

Blood Levels

Lithium therapy must be guided by measurement of serum levels. Serum level, not oral dose, is highly correlated with both therapeutic and toxic effects. Levels may be reported as milliequivalents per liter or millimoles per liter, or millimolar, which are equivalent because lithium ion is monovalent. Lithium levels are accurately measured by flame photometry or atomic absorption methods that are identical to those used for sodium and potassium. Standards for interpreting serum lithium levels are based on measurement 12 hours after the last oral dose (generally prior to the first morning dose). Regimens in which the entire dose is given at bedtime will produce morning levels 10% to 20% higher than regimens with divided dosing.

Distribution

Lithium distributes throughout total body water, although neuronal levels may be slightly lower than serum levels. There is some lag in penetration into the cerebrospinal fluid, but equilibration between blood and brain occurs within 24 hours. Like sodium, lithium circulates unbound to plasma proteins. In elderly patients, there is a reduction in lean body mass (and thus total body water) by 10% to 15%; thus, lithium has a smaller volume of distribution in elderly patients than in younger patients. This reduction, along with age-related decreases in glomerular filtration rate (GFR), contributes to the need for lower oral doses in elderly patients.

Excretion

Lithium is excreted almost entirely (95%) by the kidney. It is filtered by the glomerulus and, like sodium, it is 70% to 80% reabsorbed in the proximal renal tubules; lithium is also reabsorbed to a lesser extent in the loop of Henle but, unlike sodium, it is not further reabsorbed in the distal tubules. Thus, its excretion is not facilitated by diuretics (e.g., thiazides), which act at the distal tubules. In fact, because proximal reabsorption of lithium and sodium is competitive, a deficiency of sodium, as may be produced by thiazide diuretics, dehydration, or sodium restriction, increases retention of lithium by the proximal nephron and thus increases serum lithium levels. Typically, thiazides increase lithium levels by about 30% to 50%, thus requiring dose reductions in lithium if they are coadministered. On the other hand, the diuretic furosemide, which acts proximally to thiazides in the nephron (at the loop of Henle), apparently blocks lithium reabsorption to an adequate degree so that it does not generally elevate serum lithium levels. Nonetheless, lithium levels must be monitored closely in any patient initiating diuretic therapy.

The renal excretion of lithium is maximal in the first few hours after peak levels are achieved and then proceeds more slowly over several days. In healthy adults, the elimination half-life of lithium is approximately 24 ± 8 hours. Lithium excretion is directly related to GFR. In elderly patients, who have a diminished GFR, the elimination half-life may be significantly prolonged; it also may be increased with renal dysfunction. Conversely, conditions that increase GFR, such as pregnancy, increase lithium clearance.

MECHANISM OF ACTION

Lithium has many known actions in the nervous system at concentrations that approximate the therapeutic serum concentration of 1 mM. Lithium has acute and chronic effects on the release of serotonin and norepinephrine from nerve terminals; at higher concentrations, it has effects on transmembrane ion pumps. Chronic lithium administration has been shown to alter the coupling of a number of neurotransmitter receptors to their **signal-transducing G proteins**. The two

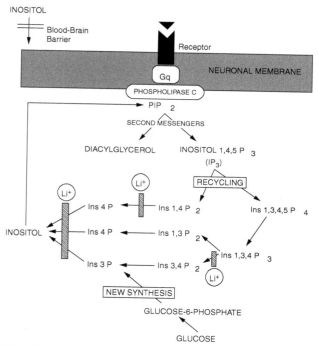

FIGURE 4.1 The effects of lithium (Li$^+$) on the phosphatidylinositol cycle. Lithium blocks the recycling of inositol phosphates and new synthesis of inositol from glucose, thus inhibiting the ability of neurons to generate the second messengers diacylglycerol and inositol 1,4,5-triphosphate (IP$_3$). Gq is the signal-transducing G protein that activates this system. PIP$_2$, phosphatidylinositol 4,5-bisphosphate. (Adapted from Hyman SE, Nestler EJ. *The molecular foundations of psychiatry.* Washington, DC: American Psychiatric Association, 1993:141.)

leading candidate mechanisms of lithium action currently are the inositol depletion hypothesis and the action of lithium on the Wnt signaling pathway. Neither of these hypotheses, however, has a direct link to the therapeutic effect of lithium in bipolar disorder been established.

Inositol Depletion Hypothesis

Many neurotransmitter receptors (e.g., α_1-adrenergic, 5-HT$_2$ serotonin receptors, and muscarinic cholinergic receptors) are linked via the G protein, Gq, to the enzyme phospholipase C, which hydrolyzes the membrane phospholipid phosphatidylinositol 4,5-bisphosphate, to yield two second messengers, diacylglycerol and inositol 1,4,5-triphosphate (Fig. 4.1). Diacylglycerol activates protein kinase C, and inositol 1,4,5-triphosphate binds its receptor on the endoplasmic reticulum to release intracellular Ca^{2+}, itself a critical second messenger. Phosphatidylinositol is synthesized from free inositol and a lipid moiety. Most cells can obtain free inositol directly from the plasma, but neurons cannot, because inositol does not cross the blood–brain barrier. Consequently, neurons must either recycle inositol by dephosphorylating inositol phosphates after they are generated from hydrolysis of phosphatidylinositols or synthesize it *de novo* from glucose-6-phosphate, a product of glycolysis. Lithium, at therapeutically used concentrations, inhibits inositol monophosphatase (IMPase). This blocks the ability of neurons to generate free inositol from recycled inositol phosphates or glucose-6-phosphate. Lithium-exposed neurons, therefore, have a diminished ability to resynthesize phosphatidylinositol 4,5-bisphosphate after it is hydrolyzed in response to neurotransmitter receptor activation. It has been hypothesized that when firing rates of neurons are abnormally high, lithium-treated neurons will become depleted of phosphatidylinositol 4,5-bisphosphate, and neurotransmission dependent on this second messenger system will be dampened.

However, even if this hypothesis is correct, it remains incomplete. The critical cells in the brain that are targets of lithium's therapeutic action remain unknown, and it is unclear which of the many phosphatidylinositol-dependent neurotransmitter systems must be dampened for lithium to have its therapeutic effects.

Regulation of the Wnt Pathway and Glycogen Synthase Kinase 3β
In addition to its antimanic effects, lithium has teratogenic effects on embryos of the African clawed toad, Xenopus laevis. Inhibition of IMPase was thought not only to be a candidate mechanism for mood stabilization (as stated previously) but also to explain the dramatic effects of lithium on early development in some model organisms. The teratogenic effects of lithium have now been found to be due not to inhibition of IMPase but to its ability to inhibit the activity of glycogen synthase kinase 3β (GSK-3β). The GSK-3β pathway is a negative regulator of the cellular signaling pathway in which the key intercellular signaling molecule is a peptide called Wnt. Inhibition of Wnt by molecular means reproduces the teratogenic effects of lithium in several species. The possibility that a pathway involved in brain development might also be involved in brain remodeling in response to pharmacologic agents is an intriguing one. Of note, Wnt signaling also interacts with, and is moderated by, **trophic factors** such as brain-derived neurotrophic factor. Given the continuing difficulty, after more than a decade, of pinpointing a mechanism by which inhibition of IMPase can produce antimanic effects, the implication of GSK-3β has given new impetus to this field.

Lithium Regulation of Adenylyl Cyclase
As mentioned previously, lithium acutely inhibits adenylyl cyclase in most tissues, including those in the brain. Although the concentrations required to exert this effect in the brain appear to be higher than clinically relevant levels, this effect of lithium may account for some of its peripheral side effects. Lithium inhibits the normal activation of adenylyl cyclase by **thyroid-stimulating hormone** (TSH) and **antidiuretic hormone** (vasopressin), which may partly explain its antithyroid effects and its tendency to cause defects in the ability to concentrate urine. These effects on adenylyl cyclase may lead to the clinical conditions of hypothyroidism or nephrogenic diabetes insipidus.

Lithium acts also on a protein involved in circadian rhythms. Because the sleep cycle is frequently disrupted in both the depressive and manic phases of bipolar disorder, this property of lithium has been an appealing area of research. Lithium affects a glycogen synthase known as 3β, and this enzyme is involved in circadian rhythms. Recently it was found *in vitro* that lithium leads to synchronized circadian oscillations by actions on a nuclear receptor known as Rev-erb-α. These studies, though interesting, were performed in cell cultures and further study awaits to determine if this is relevant to unraveling the neurobiologic changes in patients with bipolar disorder.

TABLE 4.2 Available Preparations of Lithium		
Form	**Brand Name**	**How Supplied**
Lithium carbonate	Eskalith	300-mg capsules, tablets
	Lithium carbonate	300-mg capsules, tablets
	Lithonate	300-mg capsules
	Lithotabs	300-mg tablets
Lithium carbonate, slow release	Lithobid	300-mg tablets
	Eskalith CR	450-mg tablets
Lithium citrate syrup	Cibalith-S	8 mEq/5 mL[a]
	Lithium citrate syrup	8 mEq/5 mL[a]

[a]8 mEq of lithium is equivalent to 300 mg of lithium carbonate.

INDICATIONS

Lithium has been shown to be effective in bipolar disorder, both for the treatment of acute mania and for prophylaxis against recurrences. Its usefulness in other psychiatric disorders is less well established (Table 4.2).

Bipolar Disorder

Lithium is one of the best-studied and most broadly effective treatments for bipolar disorder. Approximately 50% to 70% of bipolar patients gain at least moderate benefit from lithium during some stage of their treatment. For most patients, however, lithium is not, by itself, a fully adequate treatment for all phases of their illness. Lithium is most effective in the treatment of acute mania and the prophylaxis of manic recurrences, moderately effective in the prophylaxis of depressive recurrences, and generally inadequate as a sole acute treatment of depressive episodes. In each of these situations, lithium may be supplemented by other drugs. During acute manias, supplementation with antipsychotic drugs or benzodiazepines is often beneficial. During acute depressive episodes, supplemental use of antidepressants has become commonplace, although recent data suggest that there is no benefit to the addition of antidepressants to mood stabilizers in bipolar depression. Bipolar depression is often poorly responsive to all treatments. Because of such complexities, the clinical phases of bipolar disorder are treated separately later.

THERAPEUTIC USE

Before Starting Lithium

Some consensus has developed on the minimum workup of patients prior to starting lithium therapy (Table 4.3). Many clinicians also obtain a pretreatment complete blood count (CBC) because lithium may cause a benign elevation of the white blood cell count. Because lithium may depress sinoatrial node function, patients with sick sinus syndrome probably should be treated only if they have a cardiac pacemaker. There is no need to withhold lithium while waiting for the results of thyroid function tests, because there is no danger to the patient. If the patient proves to have a thyroid abnormality, it can be treated after lithium therapy has commenced. A pretreatment 24-hour creatinine clearance is not needed prior to beginning lithium unless the patient has known renal disease. If a lithium test dose is used for dose prediction and low lithium clearance is discovered or if the patient develops very high lithium levels on low doses when therapy begins, a creatinine clearance should then be performed. Measurement of creatinine clearance is also

TABLE 4.3	Summary: Method of Lithium Use in Acute Mania
Before beginning lithium	Medical history Physical examination Blood urea nitrogen, creatinine T_4, TSH ECG with rhythm strip recommended if patient is older than 40 years or has history of cardiac disease CBC (optional) Human chorionic gonadotropin (pregnancy test), if appropriate
Dosing method	Usually 300 mg two or three times daily. Lower doses in elderly patients or with renal disease (150–300 per day) Increase by 300 mg every 2 d as tolerated to 900 to 1,500 mg in split doses Move dose to bedtime with snack once stable
Blood levels	Draw approximately 12 h after the last oral dose 4 to 5 d after starting. At start of therapy, every 5 d to adjust dose Draw less frequently as levels stabilize For stable long-term patients, draw every 3–6 mo Draw immediately if toxicity suspected
Follow-up monitoring (stable patients)	Creatinine, TSH every 6 mo For patients older than 40 years or with cardiac disease, follow-up ECGs as indicated

CBC, complete blood count; ECG, electrocardiogram; T_4, thyroxine; TSH, thyroid-stimulating hormone.

indicated if during the course of therapy there is a significant increase in the serum creatinine or a significant unexplained increase in lithium levels.

Methods have been developed to predict individual dose requirements using a test dose of lithium. In healthy adults, 600 mg can be given and a blood level is drawn 24 hours later. The expected daily dose requirement can be read from a nomogram.

Lower test doses should be used in elderly patients (Table 4.4). This test can be useful in identifying patients who are at the extremes of the dosage range,

TABLE 4.4	Prediction of Lithium Dose
Level (mEq/L)	**Predicted Total Daily Dose (mg)**
<0.05	3,600
0.05–0.09	2,700
0.10–0.14	1,800
0.15–0.19	1,200
0.20–0.23	900
0.24–0.30	600
>0.30	Use with extreme caution

Dosages required to achieve a serum lithium level of 0.9 ± 0.3 mEq/L predicted from a lithium level drawn 24 hours after a single dose of 600 mg.
Adapted from Cooper TB, Simpson GM. The 24-hour lithium level as a prognosticator of dosage requirements: a two-year follow-up study. *Am J Psychiatry* 1976;133:440.

including some patients with unsuspected renal failure. However, because optimal care requires slow dose increases as side effects allow, dose prediction from a nomogram is no substitute for careful monitoring of side effects and levels.

Prior to starting lithium, patients should be told not to be discouraged if the onset of efficacy is slow and that extra doses are not helpful and may be dangerous. They should also be instructed not to alter their **sodium intake,** embark on a weight reduction diet, or take **diuretics** or **nonsteroidal antiinflammatory agents** (NSAIDs) without medical supervision. This last warning is particularly important now that NSAIDs such as ibuprofen and naproxen are available over the counter.

Blood Levels

Safe and effective lithium therapy is monitored by serum levels; oral dosage is not an adequate guideline. Because lithium levels vary widely from peak to trough with most dosing schedules, it is best to draw blood levels as close to **12 hours after the last oral dose** as possible, usually in the morning prior to the first daily dose. This must be emphasized to patients because a misunderstanding will result in confusing or uninterpretable levels. Regimens in which the entire dose is given at bedtime are being used increasingly. These will produce morning levels 10% to 20% higher than regimens using divided dosing.

Because the half-life of lithium is approximately 24 hours and the time to steady state for any drug is four to five half-lives, levels should be drawn no sooner than 5 days after a change in dosage unless toxicity is suspected. Levels drawn before equilibration is complete can be misleading because they may still be on the rise. In elderly patients and in patients with renal disease, the elimination half-life and hence the time to equilibration is prolonged (often 7 days or more). If toxicity is suspected, lithium should be withheld and a level determined immediately. Interpretation of the level requires that the time since the last dose be taken into account.

Using Lithium

In healthy adults, the usual starting dosage is 300 mg three times daily, but smaller dosages (e.g., 150 mg twice daily) should be used if the patient is elderly or has renal disease, and in less acute circumstances some clinicians will begin at smaller doses in other patients to maximize tolerability initially. At the beginning of therapy, it is useful to draw levels after 5 days and to use results to adjust the dosage upward to the therapeutic range; dosage prediction nomograms, although available, are rarely used. Once the patient is stable, the whole dose can be given at bedtime.

Many side effects that occur early in therapy, such as nausea and tremor, are associated with absolute levels but also may occur at lower levels of lithium if the levels are rising too rapidly. It is best to increase the dosage slowly to avoid such side effects and to maximize patient comfort and eventual compliance. If troublesome side effects emerge at the beginning of therapy, the oral dosage should be temporarily decreased and then slowly increased again after several days as side effects allow. If there is pressure to obtain rapid symptom control, temporary use of antipsychotics or benzodiazepines may be more expedient.

Dosage Forms and Dosing Intervals

One of the major problems with long-term lithium therapy is patient compliance. Compliance is clearly improved when dosing regimens are simplified. Most patients tolerate lithium well on a twice-daily regimen, allowing omission of the often forgotten midday dose. Indeed, there is evidence that lithium may be best tolerated by the kidney in a single nightly dose. Patients taking a single daily dose have less polyuria and fewer renal structural abnormalities than patients taking multiple daily doses (see later section on renal effects). The data suggest that the kidney is able to tolerate higher peak levels reached with single daily dosing but benefits from lower troughs. From the current evidence, it would appear appropriate to treat patients with **single daily doses,** especially if they have compliance problems or severe polyuria. In any case, there appears to be no reason to give lithium more frequently than twice daily unless the patient has serious peak level side effects. Slow-release lithium may help patients who have side effects at peak levels such as severe tremor or nausea, but a minority of patients will only tolerate lithium on a regimen of smaller, more frequent daily doses. The slow-release preparations available in the United States have excellent bioavailability and result in less dose fluctuation during the day than standard lithium. Because their absorption is delayed, however, these preparations have a greater tendency to cause diarrhea than regular lithium preparations.

Target Plasma Levels
As described previously, regimens in which the entire dose is given at bedtime will produce morning levels 10% to 20% higher than regimens with divided dosing. The target levels described in this section are based on divided dosing regimens. For acute mania, a therapeutic response is usually achieved at serum levels of 0.8 to 1.0 mM. There is no convincing justification for levels beyond 1.2 mM; levels greater than 1.5 mM are likely to be toxic. The oral dose that produces therapeutic levels varies with the size of the patient and his or her GFR. In healthy adults, the typical oral dose to produce a level of 1.0 mM is in the range of 1,500 ± 300 mg, but extreme doses range from 300 to 3,000 mg. Some clinicians report that early in the treatment of acute mania the oral doses needed to produce a given level may be higher than later in the treatment. The reasons for this clinical observation are unknown. For prophylaxis, levels of 0.8 to 1.0 mM have been suggested to be more effective than lower blood levels, although they result in more side effects. If side effects are severe and may compromise therapy, the lowest effective serum level for that patient should be determined empirically. If a patient cannot tolerate lithium in the therapeutic range, substitution of another mood stabilizer should be considered.

Monitoring Long-Term Therapy
Following initiation of lithium therapy, patients should have a follow-up serum creatinine drawn after reaching a therapeutic blood level. Follow-up electrocardiograms (ECGs) should be performed as clinically indicated. Lithium can be expected to cause a variety of benign changes in the ECG, including a pattern similar to that of hypokalemia. (It is important to make sure that the patient is not, in fact, hypokalemic.) Therapy should be interrupted only if a potentially dangerous arrhythmia emerges.

During long-term lithium use, serum levels for stable patients can be obtained yearly as indicated (more frequently if toxicity is suspected, if noncompliance is a problem, if medications that affect lithium levels are used, or if mood symptoms emerge). Serum creatinine and TSH should be drawn every 6 to 12 months or if signs of renal or thyroid toxicity emerge. An unexplained increase in serum lithium levels requires an investigation of renal function.

Discontinuation of Lithium Therapy
Both open and controlled trials have documented that there is a substantial risk of new episodes of mania or depression following discontinuation of lithium, or rapid lithium dose change, even after years of stability on lithium. A review of existing studies found a high early risk of recurrent manias in bipolar patients following relatively abrupt lithium discontinuation, with over half of the recurrences occurring within the first 3 months after discontinuation. Depressive recurrences tended to come later. More striking, the survival time for 50% recurrence was 5 months, far shorter than during lithium treatment and even shorter than in

previous untreated cycles (11.6 months) (Suppes et al., 1991). These data suggest a rebound effect with rapid discontinuation. In a prospective study, this group found that gradual (2 to 4 weeks) discontinuation of lithium diminished the risk of early recurrence. Given these data, it would be prudent to taper lithium no more rapidly than 300 mg per month, unless side effects demand a more rapid taper. Concern also has been raised that discontinuation of lithium may cause later unresponsiveness to lithium. However, no evidence of such lithium resistance has emerged in recent follow-up analyses.

USE IN PREGNANCY

Women with bipolar disorder may experience significant affective symptoms during pregnancy and are at elevated risk of developing postpartum manias or depressions. However, use of lithium, divalproex, lamotrigine, or carbamazepine during the first trimester of pregnancy is associated with increased risk of major birth defects. All women with bipolar disorder considering pregnancy or who become pregnant should receive counseling on the relative risks of pharmacologic treatment versus no treatment in their particular case. A contingency plan should be made (and discussed with the family) concerning a course of action, should a severe episode occur, especially during the first trimester of pregnancy.

Use of lithium during the first trimester has been associated with risk of Ebstein's anomaly (right ventricular hypoplasia and tricuspid valve insufficiency). Recent epidemiologic and case-control studies suggest that the rates in the original Lithium Register were likely overestimates due to an overreporting bias. Although there does appear to be an association (with a risk in the general population estimated at 1 in 20,000 births) between first-trimester lithium exposure and risk of Ebstein's anomaly, the revised estimate is about **1 in 2,000 for exposure,** a 10-fold increase over the general population. Thus, the absolute risk is low and certainly does not itself justify a recommendation of termination of pregnancy. Furthermore, modern sensitive fetal ultrasound technology can detect the presence or absence of Ebstein's anomaly by week 16 of gestation. Because of the risks posed by all mood stabilizers, **electroconvulsive therapy** (ECT) is the treatment of choice for severe manic or depressed episodes. Alternatives that appear to be safer than lithium, divalproex, or carbamazepine include high-potency antipsychotic drugs and benzodiazepines.

Lithium use later in pregnancy may pose potential complications for the mother. Regulation of the lithium level may be complicated by changes in maternal blood volume, which increases during pregnancy by 50%, and GFR, which increases by 30% to 50%. At parturition, diuresis may lead to shifts in plasma lithium levels, which must be monitored to avoid lithium toxicity. In addition, therapeutic lithium levels at parturition are associated with significant symptoms in the neonate, but dose reduction of lithium immediately prior to delivery may prevent this.

Lithium is secreted in breast milk at about half the serum levels in the mother. The effects of lithium on growth and development are unknown. Therefore, breast-feeding is typically discouraged among mothers who take lithium to reduce the risk of postpartum illness.

Despite the risks associated with lithium use during pregnancy, they must be balanced against the **risks of untreated or undertreated bipolar disorder** to both mother and fetus. A recent prospective study suggests that the risk of relapse, especially to depression or dysphoric states was double in those who stopped mood stabilizers. In addition, the time to mood recurrence was fourfold shorter, and the time spent ill during pregnancy was five times more in those who stopped mood stabilizers than in those who continued them. Thus, stopping mood stabilizers is risky, and medications such as lithium are reasonably continued during pregnancy after a careful presentation to the patient and family of the risks and benefits.

USE IN ELDERLY PATIENTS
Given the decrease in GFR and the decreased ratio of water to fat that occurs with increasing age, several precautions should be taken when using lithium in elderly patients. Elderly patients should be started at lower dosages (e.g., 150 to 300 mg twice daily) depending on age and presence of renal dysfunction. Level drawing and dose changing should be slower to reflect the increased time to steady state (>7 days). In addition, the physician must be aware of any underlying cardiac disease. Elderly patients are often on drugs, such as diuretics and NSAIDs, that may predispose to lithium toxicity. Finally, elderly patients are more sensitive to the neurologic toxicity of lithium. The physician should carefully document the patient's cognitive function before beginning lithium and then monitor the patient for the emergence of subtle confusional states. Risks of producing confusional states are greater if the patient is on combined therapy with other drugs such as antidepressants, antipsychotics, anticonvulsants, or anticholinergics.

SIDE EFFECTS
Use of lithium is complicated by its low therapeutic index. At serum levels not much higher than therapeutic levels, significant toxicity may occur. Even at therapeutic levels, perhaps 80% of the patients experience some side effects, although only 30% would be characterized as moderate or severe. Mild to moderate side effects can be bothersome enough to patients to limit therapy. The most common side effects include **thirst, increased urination, tremor, and weight gain.** Side effects are often a particular problem at the initiation of therapy when levels are rising or several hours after dosing when peak levels are achieved. Patients who develop bothersome side effects within several hours of a dose may do better on a slow-release preparation; alternatively, the dosage schedule can be altered so that the medication is administered in more frequent smaller doses, but multiple daily dosing makes compliance more difficult.

As serum levels increase, more serious toxic symptoms can be expected, but because patients have varying susceptibility, lithium toxicity is primarily a clinical diagnosis for which serum levels provide confirmation. In general, some toxicity is to be expected at levels above 1.5 mM. Severe toxicity may manifest at levels as low as 2.0 mM and is almost always evident at levels above 3.0 mM. In addition to its dose-related toxicities, lithium may produce several idiosyncratic reactions, such as dermatologic reactions, which may occur at any level.

Gastrointestinal Side Effects
Patients treated with lithium may experience nausea, vomiting, anorexia, diarrhea, or abdominal pain. These symptoms are dose related, emerging at higher serum levels or with rapidly increasing serum levels at the initiation of treatment even if the actual level is not high. Thus, these symptoms are common at the start of treatment and are usually transient. If they occur with rising levels at the start of treatment, the dosage can be temporarily decreased and then increased again more slowly when the symptoms abate. Nausea may be minimized if lithium is given with meals or if slow-release preparations are used. In some cases, cotreatment with a histamine-2 (H_2)-blocker is also helpful in improving tolerability. However, slow-release preparations may result in a higher incidence of diarrhea than regular lithium. Patients who do not tolerate either preparation of the carbonate salt may have less gastrointestinal distress with lithium citrate syrup. Gastrointestinal symptoms that emerge late in treatment suggest the presence of toxic drug levels.

Renal Effects
Although lithium commonly causes defects in urine concentration ability, it rarely causes renal failure in patients whose lithium levels are maintained in the

therapeutic range. An early report of serious abnormalities, including glomeru-losclerosis and interstitial fibrosis on renal biopsies of patients on long-term lithium therapy, however, raised the concern that long-term lithium therapy might lead to renal failure. Longitudinal studies have failed to confirm this fear and have not offered comparable reassurance for patients who have had periods of signifi-cant lithium toxicity. In a naturalistic study, 46 patients who had taken lithium for a mean of 8 years were compared with 16 patients undergoing renal biopsies for other reasons. The number of sclerotic tubules and atrophic glomeruli in the lithium-treated patients were slightly higher than those in controls, but the differences did not achieve statistical significance; changes in glomerular function were not clini-cally significant. However, the proportion of sclerotic glomeruli and atrophic tubules among lithium-treated patients was higher in patients who received lithium in divided daily doses than in those patients taking once-daily dosing.

Polyuria

The most common renal problem due to lithium therapy is polyuria. This may be partly due to the antagonistic effect of lithium on the renal actions of antidiuretic hormone, leading to an inability to produce appropriately concentrated urine; how-ever, other renal processes may contribute. Polyuria may occur in 50% to 70% of the patients receiving long-term therapeutic doses of lithium; about 10% have a urine output greater than 3 L per day, thus qualifying as having nephrogenic diabetes in-sipidus. Currently, lithium therapy is the most common cause of nephrogenic dia-betes insipidus. Whether polyuria progresses with duration of therapy is unclear. One study of 32 patients taking lithium for an average of 10 years found no interval change in polyuria in the final 2-year period of follow-up. Polyuria, nocturia, and thirst can be very troublesome to patients. When severe, these symptoms may in-terfere with normal living habits and sleep. These symptoms may improve with dosage reduction and usually abate entirely when lithium is discontinued. A small number of patients, however, seem to have long-term (many months) or permanent urine-concentrating defects that suggest structural damage to the kidney.

Management of Polyuria. Patients who are symptomatic from polyuria should first be established at the minimum effective lithium levels for them. Second, lithium can be administered as a single bedtime dose. Third, diuretics can be adminis-tered, because diuretics paradoxically decrease urine outputs in lithium-induced polyuria.

The potassium-sparing diuretic amiloride markedly decreases urine volumes without a major effect on lithium or potassium serum levels, so long as the patient has normal renal function. Amiloride is started at 5 mg twice daily and can be in-creased to as much as 10 mg twice daily if the effect is inadequate. Total dosages above 20 mg per day do not have an added benefit. With amiloride, patients can re-main on normal diets with unrestricted sodium. Nonetheless, it is prudent to mon-itor weekly lithium and potassium levels for several weeks after beginning amiloride to be sure that there are no changes.

Should amiloride not be tolerated, hydrochlorothiazide, 50 mg per day, can be substituted; should amiloride be tolerated but prove inadequately effective, hy-drochlorothiazide, 50 mg per day, can be added. However, it must be recalled that thiazides alone or in combination with amiloride may increase lithium levels sub-stantially. Thiazide diuretics reduce extracellular volume, leading to a compensa-tory increase in sodium reabsorption, thereby producing increased lithium reab-sorption and elevation of lithium levels. Typically, thiazides used alone increase lithium levels by 30% to 50%. Thus, if thiazides are used with or without amiloride, the lithium dosage should initially be halved and lithium levels monitored weekly; the needed oral dose to achieve the patient's therapeutic blood level can then be

established. Thiazides have the additional problem of causing potassium depletion; even if the patient is also taking amiloride, potassium levels should be monitored, initially on a weekly basis, until it is determined whether the patient is wasting potassium and needs potassium supplementation. When patients are taking
diuretics, it is prudent to obtain potassium levels when lithium levels are drawn.

Other Renal Problems
Rarely, patients have an acute increase in serum creatinine with the institution of
lithium therapy, usually with a benign urinalysis (i.e., no cells or casts). Such cases
are more common than is reported in the literature. These patients generally do
not require a diagnostic renal biopsy. Most patients have interstitial nephritis
(tubulointerstitial nephropathy). In general, when the creatinine increases significantly in the context of lithium therapy, lithium should be discontinued and a
24-hour creatinine clearance should be performed. Of course, the physician should
be sure that the problem is not due to an episode of lithium toxicity, dehydration,
obstruction, or the addition of another medication. Patients who have acute interstitial nephritis will have markedly decreased creatinine clearance. Fortunately,
when these changes are detected early, they are reversible with permanent discontinuation of lithium.

A small number of patients have been reported to develop nephrotic syndrome in association with lithium therapy. Nephrotic syndrome is usually reversed
by discontinuation of lithium, but occasionally corticosteroids have proved necessary. Renal biopsies have revealed fusion of renal epithelial foot processes (minimal change disease). These patients should not be treated with lithium again.

Edema
A minority of patients develop intermittent edema of the lower extremities or face,
unrelated to any changes in renal function. The edema often resolves spontaneously. If a medical etiology has been ruled out and the edema poses a problem
for the individual, lithium-related edema can be treated with the diuretic spironolactone. If spironolactone is administered, lithium levels and electrolytes should
be monitored (lithium levels may increase with the use of this drug).

Neurologic Side Effects
Mild neurologic side effects may occur with increasing lithium levels at the start of
therapy or with stable therapy, especially at times of peak levels. These complaints
include lethargy, fatigue, weakness, and action tremor. The tremor is a 7- to 16-Hz
action tremor similar to physiologic or essential tremor and unlike the pill-rolling
tremor of parkinsonism. It is aggravated by anxiety and performance of fine motor
movements. It also may be aggravated in some patients by concomitant administration of antidepressants. Tremor may be embarrassing for some patients and
may impair normal daily activities involving delicate motor movements. Tremor
can often be controlled by decreasing the lithium dosage, if possible, and decreasing or stopping caffeine intake and, if these maneuvers fail, by adding a β-adrenergic blocker, such as propranolol. **Propranolol,** 10 to 20 mg, can be taken 30 minutes
prior to an activity in which tremor will be a serious problem. For patients who require suppression of tremor all day, propranolol may be started at 10 to 20 mg
twice daily with the dose titrated upward as needed. Patients who develop central
nervous system side effects from propranolol may do better on the less lipophilic
drug atenolol, 50 mg per day in a single daily dose. Coarsening of the tremor may
be a sign of lithium toxicity.

Lithium may independently cause extrapyramidal symptoms (EPS) in a very
small minority of patients and may worsen neuroleptic-induced EPS in some
patients. The balance of the evidence suggests that lithium neither prevents nor

predisposes to tardive dyskinesia (TD). There have been case reports of lithium causing recurrence of neuroleptic malignant syndrome (NMS) when used in place of antipsychotic drugs in patients recovering from NMS. This may be due to the same mechanisms by which lithium causes EPS. Given the rarity of such reports, lithium may be used safely in patients who have recovered from NMS, but the possibility of recurrence should be kept in mind.

Several cases of benign intracranial hypertension (pseudotumor cerebri) occurring in association with lithium therapy have been reported. Patients presented with headache, blurred vision, and papilledema. If lithium is causally related to pseudotumor at all (perhaps by inhibiting cerebrospinal fluid reabsorption), the problem appears to be extremely rare. Therefore, screening funduscopic examinations appear to be unnecessary. However, it would be prudent to perform a funduscopic examination and to consider this diagnosis in patients who complain of severe headaches or new visual abnormalities while on lithium.

Lithium may produce electroencephalographic changes in a large proportion of patients, but only variable and minor effects on seizure threshold have been reported. Although worsening has been reported in some patients with complex partial (temporolimbic) epilepsy, many other such patients have improved behaviorally without a worsening pattern of seizures. In an open study of bipolar patients with seizure disorders (primary generalized seizures or complex partial seizures), lithium was effective in treating the mood disorder and did not increase the seizure frequency in patients with active seizures or induce seizures in patients whose seizures had remitted (Shukla et al., 1988). Pending new data, lithium should not be withheld from patients who have both mood and seizure disorders, but careful clinical monitoring is needed. Lithium does not affect serum levels of anticonvulsants.

The appearance of new neurologic symptoms during the course of therapy, even if mild, should raise the suspicion of lithium toxicity. A lithium level should be drawn and subsequent doses withheld until the question of toxicity is resolved. Patients may develop moderately severe neurologic symptoms at lithium levels not much higher than therapeutic ones. Some elderly patients or patients with brain lesions or dementia may develop such toxic symptoms even in the conventional therapeutic range. Moderate neurologic toxicity includes neuromuscular irritability, including twitching and fasciculations, EPS, ataxia, coarsening of tremor, dysarthria, incoordination, difficulty in concentrating, confusion, visual disturbance, and altered levels of consciousness. Symptoms of encephalopathy due to lithium, such as confusion or hallucinations, may be difficult to distinguish from the underlying illness, especially in patients who have a concomitant dementia. Lithium combinations with second-generation antipsychotics (commonly used in mania) are more likely to produce EPS and encephalopathy than either drug alone.

Severe neurologic toxicity can cause **ataxia, seizures, hallucinations, delirium, coma, and death.** With lithium poisoning, permanent memory impairment, nystagmus, and cerebellar ataxia may occur.

Cognitive and Psychological Side Effects

Patients taking lithium may complain of dull affect, a sense of depersonalization, a general "graying" of their mental life, or loss of creativity. Patients also may complain of memory disturbance and cognitive slowing. It has been difficult to quantify these complaints, some of which may reflect loss of valued hypomanias or mild depression. Schou (1984) followed artists taking lithium and found that creativity increased, decreased, or was unchanged with lithium treatment, depending on the individual. Several investigators have found that subjective complaints of memory disturbance in their study population were partly explained as effects of aging and depression, although lithium could not be completely exonerated from impairing certain cognitive tasks. Joffe et al. (1988) tested attention, concentration, visuomotor function, and memory in 12 normal controls and 18 patients taking lithium (serum levels 0.7 to 0.9 mM) and on carbamazepine. The lithium and carbamazepine patients did not differ from controls. Further study with larger sample sizes is necessary to decide this issue. Presently, when patients complain of such side effects it makes sense to attempt prophylaxis with the lowest possible lithium level that affords effective treatment. When patients complain of cognitive difficulty, a mental status examination should be performed and symptoms of depression should be elicited to rule out a treatable condition. In some cases, alternative therapies, such as an anticonvulsant, will be necessary.

Thyroid Side Effects

Lithium interferes with the production of thyroid hormones at multiple steps, including iodine uptake, tyrosine iodination, and release of T_3 and T_4. Inhibition of the TSH-responsive adenylyl cyclase in thyroid cells may be responsible. Clinically, patients may develop goiter with or without some degree of hypothyroidism. Overall, approximately 5% of patients receiving long-term lithium therapy develop hypothyroidism (compared with 0.3% to 1.3% in the general population, predominantly women). Perhaps 3% of patients taking lithium will develop goiter. On the other hand, a much larger percentage develops **increased levels of TSH**. The clinical importance of this latter finding is not clear; treatment of TSH abnormalities in the absence of abnormalities in T_3 or T_4 is controversial. Patients with antithyroid antibodies prior to onset of lithium therapy appear to be at higher risk for development of hypothyroidism. The timing of onset of thyroid problems during lithium therapy is extremely variable.

Because of lithium's thyroid toxicities, it is important to perform baseline thyroid studies (TSH, T_4). In follow-up, patients should be observed for development of goiter, and thyroid function tests (at least a TSH, which is the most sensitive for hypothyroidism) should be done every 6 months. Development of thyroid abnormalities does not necessitate a change in lithium therapy but rather treatment of the thyroid problem, usually in consultation with an endocrinologist or general internist. Should hypothyroidism or goiter develop, it can generally be treated by the addition of thyroid hormone (e.g., synthetic T_4). Because hypothyroidism, including lithium-induced hypothyroidism, can present as refractory depression (Yassa et al., 1988), it is important to check thyroid function if the patient's pattern of depressive episodes changes in character or becomes treatment resistant.

Cardiac Toxicity

It is reasonable to question patients about cardiac symptoms or history of cardiac disease before initiating lithium therapy. Patients older than 50 years or those who have a cardiac history should have a baseline ECG with follow-up ECGs as clinically indicated. If there is any question about cardiac disease, a consultation with an internist should be obtained. During follow-up visits, patients should be asked about dizziness, palpitations, or irregular heartbeats when they are asked about other possible side effects of lithium.

Many patients treated with lithium develop ECG changes such as T-wave flattening or inversion. These changes correlate poorly with serum levels, are reversible with discontinuation of lithium, and are almost always benign. It is important, however, that other possible causes of T-wave abnormalities, such as hypokalemia, are not ignored because the patient is taking lithium.

Arrhythmias due to lithium have been described, almost always in patients with preexisting cardiac disease. Sinoatrial node dysfunctions, including sinoatrial block and tachycardia, have been reported. These may present with dizziness, syncope, or palpitations or may be asymptomatic. They are reversible with discontinuation of lithium. Patients with preexisting sinoatrial node dysfunction (sick sinus syndrome) can only be safely treated if they have a cardiac pacemaker. Because the calcium channel blocker verapamil is occasionally used as a treatment of bipolar disorder, there is a possibility that it will be used together with lithium. Cases of serious bradycardia with this combination have been reported.

Ventricular arrhythmias also have been reported, although rarely. In several case reports, patients were also receiving antipsychotic drugs. Now that it is known that some antipsychotics (e.g., thioridazine and trifluoperazine) are calcium antagonists, it is possible that the cause for the arrhythmias should be reassigned to the antipsychotic or to combined toxicity.

Dermatologic Reactions

Dermatologic reactions appear to be idiosyncratic rather than dose related. They include acne and psoriasis (which are the most frequent), maculopapular eruptions, folliculitis, and extremely rare cases of exfoliative dermatitis. This last, a presumed hypersensitivity reaction, may be life threatening; patients who recover should not receive lithium again.

Acne

Acneiform eruptions are probably the most common dermatologic reaction to lithium. They may prove to be a major obstacle to acceptance of lithium by adolescents and young adults unless vigorously treated. The acne usually begins as a monomorphic eruption (all lesions in the same stage) and may occur on the face, neck, shoulders, and back. The eruptions may be new or an exacerbation of preexisting acne. The acne usually responds to vigorous treatment with standard antiacne regimens. If the acne does not respond, a dermatologic consultation might be useful, especially if lithium refusal could result from the patient's cosmetic concerns.

Psoriasis

Lithium may cause exacerbations of preexisting psoriasis or onset of new psoriasis. Psoriasis due to lithium tends to be treatment resistant but usually regresses with discontinuation of the drug. The decision to stop lithium must obviously be balanced with the risks to the patient from affective illness. The anticonvulsants do not appear to have any effects on this skin disorder. The condition of some patients with preexisting psoriasis do not worsen on lithium; thus, a history of psoriasis is not an absolute contraindication to lithium therapy, although patients with severe disease or psoriatic arthritis might be more safely treated with anticonvulsants, including divalproex, carbamazepine, gabapentin, or lamotrigine.

Other Dermatologic Reactions

Maculopapular rashes (usually pruritic) have been reported to occur occasionally early in treatment. These often regress by themselves. Asymptomatic folliculitis, which may occur as hyperkeratotic erythematous follicular papules on extensor surfaces, the abdomen, and the buttocks, has also been reported. It appears to pose little problem for patients and should not require changes in lithium therapy.

Hair loss is a rare side effect of lithium therapy. When hair loss occurs, it is important to check for hypothyroidism and other possible causes of alopecia.

Hematologic Effects

Lithium produces a benign, relative leukocytosis, increasing neutrophil mass without impairing function. There is no known adverse effect; in fact, leukocytosis induced by lithium has been exploited in the treatment of leukopenic patients. It is important to be aware of this effect of lithium to avoid unnecessary medical workups for elevated white blood cell counts. The total white blood cell count rarely exceeds 15,000/μL as a result of lithium therapy alone.

Weight Gain

A side effect that can be extremely troublesome and lead to noncompliance or lithium refusal is weight gain. In some studies, lithium has been associated with weight gain of more than 10 kg in 20% of patients on long-term therapy. Lithium has been reported to have insulin-like effects on carbohydrate metabolism. Antipsychotic drugs and cyclic antidepressants also may cause obesity (a hypothalamic mechanism has been the hypothesized cause for this). Patients who are polyuric should be advised not to replace their fluid losses with high-calorie beverages such as beer or sugary sodas. Some will benefit from dietary consultation. For some patients who have developed severe obesity, substitution of another drug, such as aripiprazole, for lithium might be considered.

Calcium Metabolism

Anecdotal reports and several small studies have associated lithium therapy with mild elevations in calcium and parathyroid hormone. These elevations appear to be rarely, if ever, clinically significant. However, because alterations in calcium level are associated with neuropsychiatric symptoms, serum calcium levels might be obtained if there is a change in a patient's pattern of symptoms, especially depressive symptoms.

EVALUATION AND TREATMENT OF LITHIUM TOXICITY DUE TO ELEVATED LEVELS

For mild toxicity, lithium should be withheld until levels return to the patient's usual therapeutic range. If an obvious cause for the change in level cannot be found, a renal workup should be undertaken, including urinalysis and creatinine clearance.

For moderate to severe lithium toxicity, the patient is best admitted to a hospital. Adequate sodium should be given, and lithium levels should be checked several times a day to make sure that they are decreasing. If the patient does not have congestive heart failure or renal failure, intravenous administration of normal saline at a rate of 150 to 200 mL per hour is often effective in reducing lithium levels rapidly; this is safe as long as urine output is adequate.

Acute Lithium Intoxication

Acute lithium intoxication, manifested by a severe clinical syndrome or levels above 3.0 mEq/L, is a medical emergency. Because the severity and reversibility of toxic symptoms are related both to the serum level and to the duration of high levels, rapid aggressive treatment is necessary even if the patient appears clinically well. Indeed, early in lithium poisoning the patient's symptoms may be relatively mild despite high levels, giving the physician a false sense of security. Symptoms of serious intoxication include both systemic and neurologic symptoms, including nausea, vomiting, diarrhea, renal failure, neuromuscular irritability or flaccidity, ataxia, dysarthria, coarse tremor, confusion, delirium, hallucinations, seizures, and stupor. Protracted coma and glucose intolerance have been reported. Lithium poisoning also may cause death. Survivors of serious toxicity may suffer permanent cerebellar ataxia and severe permanent anterograde amnesia.

In treating acute lithium intoxication, the therapeutic goal is to remove lithium from the body as rapidly as possible. It is important to obtain a toxic screen to know what other agents the patient has ingested, especially if the case appears to be an intentional overdose. If the patient is stuporous or comatose, protection of the airway, with intubation if necessary, and cardiorespiratory support should be the first priority. In overdose cases in which the drug was taken less than 4 hours prior to treatment, induction of vomiting in alert patients or gastric lavage in comatose patients will help diminish the risk of worsening toxicity. Because lithium levels are often high in gastric secretions, continuous gastric aspiration can be helpful.

Despite the fact that most reports of lithium intoxication are either anecdotal or retrospective, there seems to be strong evidence that management should be aggressive. If lithium levels are less than 3 mM and signs of intoxication are mild, fluid and electrolyte abnormalities should be corrected and **normal saline** may be administered at a rate of 150 to 200 mL per hour, as long as urine output is adequate. If the lithium level is greater than 3 mM and signs of toxicity are severe, or if there is poor urine output or renal failure, prompt institution of **dialysis** is indicated. If the lithium level is above 4 mM and does not respond within a few hours to saline diuresis at a rate of 250 mL per hour, dialysis is indicated regardless of the patient's clinical appearance. Hemodialysis is most effective, but where unavailable, peritoneal dialysis may be used. Lithium will reequilibrate from the tissues after a dialysis treatment, so frequent monitoring of the lithium level is important. A reasonable end point is a lithium level of 1.0 mM or less, 6 hours after a dialysis treatment.

Causes of Intoxication

Although overdose is an important cause of toxic serum levels, the most common cause of toxicity among compliant patients is an alteration in sodium balance. Any condition that leads to sodium depletion will elevate lithium levels; thus, dehydration, changes in dietary habits (either with sodium restriction or overall weight reduction diets), or administration of sodium-wasting diuretics will cause elevations in lithium levels. There has been concern that heavy exercise or fever, both of which produce sweating, could result in lithium toxicity. However, it appears that sweat contains enough lithium that heavy perspiration does not elevate lithium levels. Other renal causes of lithium retention include many NSAIDs (not aspirin, however) in susceptible individuals, intrinsic renal disease, and systemic diseases (e.g., congestive heart failure or cirrhosis) that decrease renal blood flow.

DRUG INTERACTIONS

Alcohol and other central nervous system depressants, including prescribed psychotropic drugs and antihypertensive agents, may interact with lithium to produce sedation or confusional states. NSAIDs and thiazide diuretics are probably the most commonly encountered drug interactions that may increase lithium levels with resultant intoxication (Table 4.5). Lithium may be used in combinations with these two drugs, though lower doses are usually needed, and careful attention to toxicity must be taken when using them in combination. Metronidazole has been reported to cause serious renal toxicity when used in combination with lithium. High sodium intake may reduce lithium concentrations and low sodium intake may increase lithium concentrations. Patients in warmer climates should be instructed to take adequate salty foods during warm periods because sweating may cause salt and water loss leading to lithium intoxication.

ANTICONVULSANTS

Three anticonvulsants have proved particularly useful in the treatment of bipolar disorder, whereas others were not superior to placebo in controlled trials. Carbamazepine was the first anticonvulsant used to treat mania, but clinicians have favored valproic acid because it was approved for use many years before carbamazepine, and it is relatively easier to use. Carbamazepine remains a useful, if more complicated, treatment of bipolar disorder. Because of tolerability and drug interaction problems, its use is currently limited. Like lithium, both valproic acid

Pharmacokinetic Interactions with Lithium

Interactions That Increase Lithium Levels	Interactions That Decrease Lithium Levels

Diuretics
  Thiazides
  Ethacrynic acid
  Spironolactone
  Triamterene
	Acetazolamide
	Theophylline, aminophylline
	Caffeine (mild effect)
	Osmotic diuretics

Angiotensin receptor antagonists (e.g., losartan)	
Nonsteroidal antiinflammatory agents (e.g., ibuprofen, indomethacin, naproxen)	
Celecoxib	

Antibiotics
  Metronidazole (Flagyl)
  Tetracyclines	

Angiotensin-converting enzyme inhibitors	
Calcium channel blockers	

and carbamazepine may be more effective in treating and preventing manic episodes than depressive episodes. On the other hand, lamotrigine is better for the prevention of bipolar depression and possibly for the treatment of acute bipolar depression. Topiramate and gabapentin failed to show efficacy in controlled trials in bipolar disorder; other newer anticonvulsants, including oxcarbazepine (Trileptal), tiagabine, levetiracetam, and zonisamide, have not been studied in large trials. These newer anticonvulsants may have adjunctive roles at best. Clonazepam, a benzodiazepine with high enough potency and a long enough half-life to be used as an anticonvulsant, is effective in panic disorder and is a useful adjunct in the treatment of some patients with bipolar disorder or other psychotic conditions who require greater anxiolysis or sedation than is provided by their primary therapeutic agents. Clonazepam is discussed in detail in Chapter 5.

VALPROATE (DIVALPROEX)
Valproic acid was initially approved as an anticonvulsant and is effective in the control of absence (petit mal), myoclonic, and generalized tonic-clonic seizures. It is less effective in partial seizures with or without complex symptomatology. Approved by the Food and Drug Administration (FDA) in 1995 for the treatment of acute mania for up to 3 weeks, divalproex is used widely for the treatment of all phases of bipolar disorder. Although it initially appeared superior to lithium for its efficacy in controlling rapid cycling, a large more recent study suggests otherwise. Maintenance studies have also indirectly suggested efficacy for divalproex, although one large randomized trial failed to show that either lithium or divalproex was superior to placebo for prevention of recurrence.

Pharmacology
Valproic acid is available in several different preparations and dose forms (Table 4.6). Valproic acid is available in capsule or syrup form, including an extended-release form. Divalproex sodium is an enteric-coated form that contains equal parts of valproic acid and sodium. Both valproic acid and divalproex circulate in their

TABLE 4.6	Available Preparations of Valproic Acid and Carbamazepine	
Form	**Brand Name**	**How Supplied**
Valproic acid	Depakene	250-mg capsules
	Depakene	250-mg/5-mL syrup
	Valproic acid	250-mg capsules
Divalproex sodium	Depakote	125-, 250-, 500-mg tablets
	Depakote	125-mg sprinkle capsules
	Depakote ER	250-, 500-mg tablet
Carbamazepine	Atretol	200-mg tablet
	Tegretol	100-, 200-mg tablets
	Tegretol	100-mg/5-mL suspension
	Tegretol XR	100-, 200-, 400-mg tablets
	Carbatrol, Equetro	100-, 200-, 300-mg extended-release capsules
	Carbamazepine	100-, 200-mg tablets
	Carbamazepine	100-mg chewable tablets

ionized form, valproate. Valproic acid is rapidly absorbed after oral administration, achieving peak levels in 1 to 2 hours if taken on an empty stomach and in 4 to 5 hours if taken with food. Divalproex sodium is more slowly absorbed, reaching peak serum concentrations in 3 to 8 hours.

In plasma, valproic acid is **80% to 95% protein bound.** It is rapidly metabolized by the liver; it has no known active metabolites. Interactions with other protein-bound or hepatically metabolized drugs occur. Valproic acid has a short elimination half-life of approximately 8 hours; thus, three times daily dosing is usually recommended for epilepsy. The need for divided dosing in bipolar disorder has not been established.

There is a poor correlation between serum levels and antimanic effects, but levels in the range of 50 to 150 $\mu g/mL$ are generally required. Blood levels are measured by immunoassay or gas chromatography.

The precise mechanism of action in both bipolar disorder and epilepsy is unknown, but valproic acid is known to increase synaptic levels of γ-aminobutyric acid, the principal inhibitory neurotransmitter in the brain. Experimentally, it blocks the convulsive effects of the γ-aminobutyric acid A receptor antagonists picrotoxin and bicuculline. Whether it also shares mechanisms with lithium (e.g., in the GSK-3β/Wnt pathway) is currently a matter of investigation.

Therapeutic Use
There is no standardized workup prior to initiation of valproic acid therapy, but it is optimal to obtain a general medical history and examination, with particular attention to other drugs used by the patient and any history of liver disease or bleeding disorder. Ideally, baseline liver function tests **(LFTs) and a CBC with platelets** should be obtained. Valproic acid should not be administered to patients with known liver disease.

Unlike valproic acid, which had considerable gastrointestinal toxicity, divalproex is generally well tolerated. Divalproex has become the formulation of choice and valproic acid has generally been avoided because of problematic gastrointestinal toxicity, particularly with loading doses. Depending on the severity of symptoms and the age and health of the patient dosing can usually begin at 500 to 1,000 mg per day, in split doses or all at bedtime. The dosage can be increased as tolerated, generally up to 1,500 to 2,000 mg per day. Target levels are generally reached by giving 15 to 20 mg/kg of body weight daily. Some patients may require even higher doses to attain therapeutic concentrations. An alternative approach to initiating valproic acid treatment for inpatients is an oral loading strategy using 20 to 30 mg/kg body weight. The onset of reduction in manic symptoms occurs more quickly, often within a few days of starting treatment, diminishing the need for antipsychotics early in the course of therapy. This more aggressive starting dose should be reserved for younger, generally healthy patients. For some patients, the high initial dose will be intolerable. Neurologic side effects, especially sedation and ataxia, are often rate limiting initial side effects, although weight gain, sometimes to prodigious proportion, is the primary long-term rate-limiting problem. Optimal blood levels for both seizure disorders and mania are debated but appear to be in the range of 50 to 150 µg/mL. Blood levels may be obtained weekly until the patient is stable. Many clinicians also obtain LFTs and a CBC at the same time. Significant antimanic effects are generally seen within 1 to 2 weeks of achieving target levels.

In stable, asymptomatic patients, blood levels, LFTs, and a CBC may be obtained every 6 months. However, the new onset of side effects after stable therapy has been achieved should prompt measurement of drug levels and additional appropriate workup. For example, late onset of nausea, anorexia, or fatigue is an indication for obtaining levels and LFTs, including ammonia levels.

Use in Pregnancy
Although valproic acid has not been well studied in pregnancy, it has been associated with major congenital malformations, including spina bifida. Given reports of neural tube defects as high as 5% in offspring of women treated with divalproex in the first trimester, the drug is not a preferred choice over lithium; although commonly used, supplemental folate does not appear to reduce the risk. Alterations in clotting function may also pose risks to mother and fetus later in pregnancy and at parturition. Alternative treatments for mania that appear to be safer include ECT and high-potency antipsychotic drugs (see earlier section on the use of lithium in pregnancy). Valproic acid that is secreted in breast milk is 1% to 10% of the serum concentration. The effect on the developing child is unknown.

Side Effects and Toxicity
Minor side effects are common at the start of treatment with valproic acid and are often transient. These include gastrointestinal effects (including nausea, vomiting, heartburn, and diarrhea), sedation, tremor, and ataxia (Table 4.7). Administration with food or use of enteric-coated preparations, such as divalproex, usually limits gastrointestinal effects. Histamine H_2 receptor blockers such as ranitidine also may decrease upper gastrointestinal distress but risk possible drug interactions. Approximately half of those treated initially experience some degree of sedation. This tends to diminish with chronic use. Sedation may become a severe problem when valproic acid is coadministered with other anticonvulsants or sedating agents Valproic acid appears to cause mild impairment of cognitive function with chronic use; in this regard, it is slightly inferior to carbamazepine but superior to phenytoin or barbiturates. The other common side effects of valproic acid are alopecia and weight gain. Alopecia is sometimes helped by addition of selenium or zinc, although alopecia may lead to drug discontinuation. Weight gain is almost inevitable. It is not uncommon for patients to gain 20 to 30 pounds if they do not adhere to strict diet control.

TABLE 4.7	Side Effects and Toxicity of Valproic Acid
Common side effects	Gastrointestinal: nausea, vomiting, anorexia, heartburn, diarrhea Hematologic: thrombocytopenia, platelet dysfunction Hepatic: benign elevation of transaminases Neurologic: sedation, tremor, ataxia Other: alopecia, weight gain
Less common side effects	Hematologic: bleeding tendency Metabolic: hyperammonemia Neurologic: incoordination, asterixis, stupor, coma, behavioral automatisms Endocrine: polycystic ovary
Serious idiosyncratic side effects	Hepatitis/hepatic failure Pancreatitis Drug rashes, including erythema multiforme

Hepatotoxicity

Valproic acid may cause transient dose-dependent asymptomatic increases in aspartate and alanine transaminases in 15% to 30% of patients, which are an indication for monitoring but not for stopping treatment. These laboratory abnormalities are generally maximal during the first 3 months of treatment. Some patients may have mildly elevated transaminases for prolonged periods. Isolated hyperammonemia, which may be accompanied by confusion or lethargy, has been reported, generally in older patients. These hepatic effects usually improve with decreased dosage, although sometimes the drug must be stopped. Other patients may have mildly elevated ammonia levels without clinical consequence Rare cases of fatal hepatotoxicity associated with valproic acid have been reported. The rate of fatal hepatotoxicity appears to be very low, the most recent study attributing 29 deaths in 1 million treated patients. Age less than 2 years, multiple anticonvulsant use, and neurological problems are most often associated with death, although rare cases have occurred outside these risk factors. Given the experience with divalproex-lithium combinations in populations with psychiatric rather than seizure disorders, the risk of hepatic toxicity in psychiatric use appears to be very low and certainly far lower than the risk to life from undertreated bipolar disorder. Minor elevations in hepatic transaminases are commonly seen with the use of this medication and should not be viewed as a warning that liver function studies will continue to worsen. Should significant liver function abnormalities or symptoms of hepatitis occur (e.g., malaise, anorexia, jaundice, abdominal pain, or edema), the drug should be immediately discontinued and the patient carefully monitored. Monitoring LFTs at baseline and then every 6 to 12 months is reasonable if there are no other suggestions of liver toxicity.

Neurotoxicity

As noted previously, sedation is the most serious problem, and hand tremor is the most common long-term neurologic side effect. If troublesome, these side effects generally diminish if the dosage is decreased. There are anecdotal reports of tremor responding to β-adrenergic blockers, such as propranolol, but β-blockers have been associated with their own central nervous system side effects, including depression-like symptoms. Ataxia may occur at higher doses of valproic acid. Rarely, asterixis, stupor, coma, and behavioral automatisms have been reported.

Hematologic Toxicity
Valproic acid can cause thrombocytopenia or platelet dysfunction, but only rarely is it associated with bleeding complications. This effect is usually only observed in patients taking high doses. Patients taking divalproex should have their platelet count and bleeding time checked before any surgery. Agranulocytosis is also a rare idiosyncratic side effect.

Other Serious Idiosyncratic Toxicities
Rarely, hemorrhagic pancreatitis may occur, usually in the first 6 months of treatment, and may be fatal. Hepatic failure is another rare complication associated with childhood use. These dangerous toxicities have prompted the FDA to mandate a "black box" warning for divalproex.

Drug rashes, including erythema multiforme, also have been reported. There is concern that the rates of polycystic ovary disease may be increased in women treated with valproic acid, and it is unclear if this is due to drug or weight gain. This association with polycystic ovary disease is strengthened by a recent study, which found that women who stopped valproate experienced reduction in symptoms despite lack of weight change (Joffe et al., 2006). Valproic acid may also cause neural tube defects in the fetus, and the risk of using valproic acid must clearly be weighed against any benefit it may provide for women of childbearing age. Divalproex generally should be avoided in early pregnancy.

Serious Dose-Related Toxicities and Overdoses
Excessive serum levels may occur in the context of drug–drug interactions or intentional overdose. The symptoms of overdose include severe neurologic symptoms. Overdose with valproic acid can be treated with hemodialysis. Only rarely have fatalities been reported, and then in massive doses (e.g., 60 g).

Drug Interactions
Valproic acid may have pharmacodynamic interactions with other psychotropic drugs, including carbamazepine, lithium, and antipsychotic drugs, producing combined central nervous system toxicity. Whenever multiple psychotropic drugs are coadministered, patients must be monitored for deterioration of mental status.

Valproic acid also produces pharmacokinetic interactions with many drugs. It **weakly inhibits several hepatic enzymes** (cytochrome P450 2C9, 2D6, 3A4) and may increase levels of cyclic antidepressants and possibly selective serotonin reuptake inhibitors (SSRIs), phenytoin, phenobarbital, and other drugs. Valproic acid also may increase the effective levels of other protein-bound drugs, or conversely, it may be displaced from protein binding by drugs, such as aspirin, precipitating valproic acid toxicity. Thus, patients who must take other protein-bound drugs, such as warfarin, must be monitored closely at the initiation of combined therapy.

Valproic acid concentrations may be decreased by drugs, such as carbamazepine, that induce hepatic microsomal enzymes. Another important interaction is between valproic acid and lamotrigine. Valproate inhibits the metabolism of lamotrigine. Cotreatment appears to roughly **double levels of lamotrigine** and may increase the risk for serious rash as described later.

It should also be noted that valproic acid is partially eliminated in the urine as a ketometabolite, which may lead to false interpretations of urine ketone tests.

CARBAMAZEPINE

Carbamazepine is an iminostilbene anticonvulsant that is structurally similar to the tricyclic antidepressant (TCA) imipramine. It is generally considered to be the drug of first choice in the treatment of partial epilepsy with or without complex symptomatology; it is also effective for primary generalized seizures. Carbamazepine is also a treatment of choice in trigeminal neuralgia and is used in other neuropathic pain syndromes that have a lancinating component.

Several reports in the neurologic literature suggested that carbamazepine improved mood symptoms in patients treated for epilepsy. It was first reported as a primary treatment of manic-depressive illness in Japan in the early 1970s. Recent studies show extended-release formulations of carbamazepine are more effective than placebo for acute mania. It remains unclear whether it is as effective as lithium. It appears clinically to be useful for some patients in long-term bipolar prophylaxis, but its general utility for this indication has not been established. On the basis of small studies and case reports, some investigators have suggested that carbamazepine may be particularly effective for patients with forms of bipolar disorder that are often relatively refractory to lithium [i.e., patients with mixed bipolar symptoms (both manic and depressed symptoms present), dysphoric mania, and rapid-cycling bipolar disorder]. Carbamazepine may also be helpful for patients with secondary mania related to neurological disorders or impulsivity related to brain injury, or borderline personality disorder. Carbamazepine, however, does not appear to be effective as an antidepressant. Like lithium and divalproex, it may prevent induction of mania in bipolar depressed patients being treated with an antidepressant.

Pharmacology

Carbamazepine is available for oral administration in tablet and suspension form. It is also available in two different extended-release preparations (Table 4.6). No parenteral forms are available. Its absorption is slow and erratic, with peak levels usually achieved in 4 to 8 hours but occasionally later. Slow-release forms appear to produce more stable serum concentrations than regular tablets. Carbamazepine is poorly soluble in gastrointestinal fluids; after oral administration, 15% to 25% is excreted unchanged in the feces. The effect of food on absorption does not appear to be clinically significant. In the blood, it is 65% to 80% protein bound.

Blood levels can be measured by gas-liquid chromatography, high-pressure liquid chromatography, and immunoassays. Therapeutic levels for epilepsy are in the range of 4 to 12 μg/mL (core range 6 to 10 μg/mL), with the lower end of the range typically effective for tonic-clonic seizures and the higher end effective for partial seizures with or without tonic-clonic seizures. For bipolar disorder, initial studies suggested that blood levels in the range of 8 to 12 μg/mL corresponded to therapeutic efficacy. More recently, this correlation has appeared less certain. A therapeutic effect is unlikely with a level of less than 4 μg/mL; however, many clinicians no longer recommend use of blood levels to titrate efficacy in bipolar disorder. Instead, clinical response and toxicity guide dosage.

Carbamazepine is metabolized by the liver. Its 10-, 11-epoxide metabolite (which may reach levels 20% as high as the parent compound) is an effective anticonvulsant; it is unknown whether it is also an active antimanic agent. The elimination half-life of carbamazepine in a single dose in healthy volunteers is 18 to 55 hours; however, with repeated dosing the half-life decreases to 5 to 20 hours (longer in elderly persons). This reduction in half-life with repeated dosing is due to the drug inducing its own metabolism by hepatic P450 enzymes. This induction may be clinically significant. An oral dose, which is effective early in therapy, often becomes ineffective owing to decreasing levels after several weeks. This autoinduction effect generally plateaus within 3 to 5 weeks. Carbamazepine metabolism also can be induced by other drugs, especially the anticonvulsants phenytoin, phenobarbital, and primidone, resulting in lower serum levels.

The 10-keto analog of carbamazepine, oxcarbazepine, does not induce its own metabolism as does carbamazepine and may have less risk of other toxicities. Although at least one contemporary treatment guideline allows the substitution of oxcarbazepine for carbamazepine, the efficacy of oxcarbazepine in bipolar disorder has not been established.

Mechanism of Action

Carbamazepine has two known mechanisms that may be relevant to its antiepileptic effect. Opening of voltage-sensitive sodium channels is central to the mechanism of neuronal action potentials. These channels become temporarily inactive after use. Carbamazepine binds to an inactivated state of sodium channels, resulting in use-dependent and voltage-dependent block. Thus, carbamazepine inhibits repetitive firing of action potentials. This effect of carbamazepine seems particularly to affect sodium channels localized on neuronal cell bodies. Carbamazepine also appears to block presynaptic sodium channels, thus inhibiting depolarization of presynaptic terminals in response to action potentials propagated down the axon. Because the depolarizing effect of the sodium action potential is blocked, voltage-gated calcium channels are secondarily inhibited. The result is decreased calcium entry into the presynaptic terminal and a decrement in neurotransmitter release. Mechanisms of this type could have widespread effects on neural function in addition to treating epilepsy. Their relevance to mood disorder is not known.

There are a variety of animal models in epilepsy. Carbamazepine appears to be the most active anticonvulsant in blocking the development of seizures in the kindling model. Kindling involves the repetitive application of subthreshold electrical or chemical stimuli to produce an autonomous epileptic focus. The effectiveness of carbamazepine in this model has led to a great deal of theorizing that mood disorders and other psychiatric disorders may represent a kindling process. Although no convincing mechanistic models of kindling in mood disorders have emerged to date, speculation about kindling has produced valuable reexaminations concerning the course of psychiatric disorders, focusing attention on the observation that episodes may become more frequent and more autonomous (less related to environmental precipitants) over time in a subset of patients.

Method of Use

At present, the effective oral dose for each patient must be determined empirically by upward dosage titration, using the attainment of therapeutic effects and the emergence of side effects to guide dosing. For acute mania, an average effective dosage is approximately 1,000 mg per day (range 200 to 1,800 mg per day). Carbamazepine must be **started slowly** primarily because of initial neurologic toxicity. For carbamazepine, an initial dose of 100 to 200 mg at bedtime is usually tolerated. Depending on sedation or other neurological side effects, the dose can be increased by 100 to 200 mg per day, as tolerated, in split doses. For the extended-release preparation, higher initial doses (e.g., 400 mg per day, split in two doses) are possible, though the higher starting dose may not be well tolerated. After a therapeutic dosage is established, patients must be carefully observed because after several weeks carbamazepine may induce its own metabolism, requiring a dosage increase. Therapeutic dosage levels for bipolar disorder have not been established; many clinicians use the levels that have been established for epilepsy (e.g., 4 to 12 μg/mL) as a general guide. Although not established by clinical trials, the prophylaxis dose should be the same as the final well-tolerated acute mania dose.

This limited evidence needs further investigation before recommending carbamazepine for rapid cycling considering that evidence exists supporting the use of lithium, valproic acid, and olanzapine.

Therapeutic Use

Preliminary Workup

Patients who are candidates for carbamazepine treatment should have a medical history and physical examination with emphasis on prior history of blood dyscrasias or liver disease. Laboratory tests should include a **CBC with platelets and liver and renal function tests.** Patients with hematologic abnormalities should be considered at high risk for serious blood dyscrasias if treated with carbamazepine; they therefore deserve closer follow-up than usual. Patients with significant hepatic disease should not receive this drug unless there are no better alternatives; they should be started on one third to one half of the normal starting dosage, with longer than usual time (5 to 7 days) between dosage adjustments.

Beginning Carbamazepine

In patients older than 12 years, carbamazepine is begun at 100 to 200 mg once or twice a day. Some patients are exquisitely sensitive to the neurologic adverse effects and require **very slow titration.** The dosage is increased by no more than 200 mg every 2 to 4 days until therapeutic effects or toxicity ensues. The clinical situation determines how aggressively the dosage may be increased. Extended-release preparations generally allow for easier titration. In hospitalized patients with acute mania, the dosage might be increased daily in 200-mg increments up to 800 to 1,400 mg unless side effects develop, with slower increases thereafter as indicated. In less acutely ill outpatients, dosage adjustments should be slower. Rapid dosage increases may cause patients to develop nausea and vomiting or mild neurologic toxicity such as drowsiness, dizziness, ataxia, clumsiness, or diplopia. Should such side effects occur, the dosage can be decreased temporarily and then increased again more slowly once they have passed. As noted previously, therapeutic blood levels for bipolar disorder have not been established.

Some clinicians use the core range for epilepsy, 6 to 10 μg/mL, as a guide. Blood levels are typically observed to decrease after 2 to 4 weeks of treatment, resulting from carbamazepine's autoinduction of cytochrome P450 3A4 isoenzymes; carbamazepine induces its own metabolism and, when this occurs, an upward adjustment of dose is required. Should blood levels be obtained to document a therapeutic trial or to establish an effective level for a given patient, trough levels are most meaningful and are conveniently drawn prior to the first morning dose. Given its elimination half-life, carbamazepine levels should be drawn no more frequently than 5 days after a dosage change. Maintenance dosages for both bipolar and epileptic patients average about 1,000 mg per day, but the dosage range in routine clinical practice is large (400 to 1,800 mg per day). The manufacturer recommends dosages no higher than 1,600 mg per day.

Combinations with Lithium

Carbamazepine is used most often for bipolar patients who prove resistant to treatment with lithium or valproic acid. In many situations, therefore, the patient will already have a pharmacologic treatment of bipolar disorder that has been judged to be inadequate. In acute mania, carbamazepine can be either substituted for lithium or valproic acid or added to the initial drug. The primary danger of adding carbamazepine to lithium or valproic acid (and, in these situations, often a neuroleptic and perhaps an antiparkinsonian or benzodiazepine) is risk of an acute combined central nervous system toxicity, for example, producing a confusional state. However, if the manic symptoms are severe enough to create pressure for rapid treatment, the physician may choose to add carbamazepine to the existing regimen because some patients respond only to combined therapy. If the patient's condition improves, an attempt should be made to taper the lithium (or valproic acid) once the patient's condition has stabilized. Some patients' condition will worsen and require resumption of combined treatment. When such a combined regimen is undertaken, it is also essential to minimize the dose of any antipsychotic drug (e.g., in the range of 8 to 10 mg of haloperidol or the equivalent). Unneeded anticholinergics and sedatives should also be decreased or omitted. In addition, it is important to have a clear idea of the patient's mental status and to consider the possibility of drug toxicity if the mental status worsens.

In elderly patients and in patients whose mania is not so severe, it is preferable to substitute carbamazepine for lithium or valproic acid rather than add it. If the patient remains unresponsive, lithium or valproic acid can be added later. Whether a patient responds to carbamazepine alone or in combination with another mood stabilizer, it is good practice to taper and discontinue antipsychotic drugs once the acute episode has abated to minimize the risk of TD.

Use in Pregnancy
Carbamazepine and other anticonvulsants cross the placenta. Fetal malformations caused by phenytoin (fetal hydantoin syndrome) have been well documented, and carbamazepine had been thought to be safer. However, carbamazepine is also teratogenic. A prospective study of 35 children exposed to carbamazepine alone *in utero* found that 11% had craniofacial defects, 26% had fingernail hypoplasia, and 20% had developmental delay, similar to the abnormalities found with phenytoin. Pending further clarification, carbamazepine should be avoided if possible during pregnancy. Carbamazepine is secreted in breast milk at about 60% of the level found in the mother. Nursing children have been reported to become excessively drowsy. All anticonvulsants, including carbamazepine, are cleared more rapidly in pregnant women, leading to a decrease in serum levels.

Side Effects and Toxicity
Although carbamazepine is associated with several serious toxicities (e.g., hepatitis, severe blood dyscrasias, and exfoliative dermatitis), these are fortunately extremely rare. In general, this drug is well tolerated, with fewer than 5% of patients discontinuing the medication because of side effects. Most of carbamazepine's side effects (Table 4.8) are neurologic or gastrointestinal symptoms due to too rapid a dosage increase or excessively high serum levels. These side effects can usually be avoided by increasing dosages slowly and using the minimum effective dosage. Newer formulations of carbamazepine such as Tegretol XR and Equetro are often better tolerated, especially on initial use.

Neurologic Side Effects
Neurologic side effects are relatively common and may limit the dosage that patients can tolerate. The most common are drowsiness, **vertigo, ataxia, diplopia,** and blurred vision. When such side effects occur, a decrease in dosage is indicated, but these side effects do not represent a reason to stop therapy. When such side effects occur at the initiation of therapy, a temporary dosage decrease with a slower subsequent increase is often successful in permitting achievement of a therapeutic dosage. Carbamazepine can also produce confusion, the risk of which is higher when this drug is combined with antipsychotic drugs or lithium. Risk factors for confusional states include old age or underlying organic brain disease. In the absence of frank confusional states, carbamazepine appears to have little effect on memory or other cognitive functions and is better than phenytoin in this regard.

TABLE 4.8	Side Effects and Toxicity of Carbamazepine
Common dosage-related side effects	Dizziness
	Ataxia
	Clumsiness
	Sedation
	Dysarthria
	Diplopia
	Nausea and gastrointestinal upset
	Reversible mild leukopenia
	Reversible mild increases in liver function tests
Less common dosage-related side effects	Tremor
	Memory disturbance
	Confusional states (more common in elderly patients and in combination treatments with lithium or neuroleptics)
	Cardiac conduction delay
	Syndrome of inappropriate antidiuretic hormone secretion
Idiosyncratic toxicities	Rash (including cases of exfoliation)
	Lenticular opacities
	Hepatitis
	Blood dyscrasias
	Aplastic anemia
	Leukopenia
	Thrombocytopenia

Hematologic Toxicity

Carbamazepine has both benign and severe hematologic toxicities. It is frequently associated with clinically unimportant decreases in white blood cell counts and is rarely associated with serious or irreversible depression of red blood cells, white blood cells, platelets, or a combination of these. Estimates of the rate of severe blood dyscrasias suggest this is a rare event, with an incidence of about 1 in 150,000 patients treated. Because carbamazepine often produces minor hematologic effects, it is important to monitor blood counts, particularly at the beginning of treatment. A CBC should be obtained at the start of treatment and rechecked periodically, particularly if there is any sign of infection or bleeding soon after starting treatment.

Of special importance, however, is the recommendation that patients should be instructed to report fever, sore throat, pallor, unaccustomed weakness, petechiae, easy bruising, or bleeding. Concomitant use of lithium could potentially mask (but not reverse) carbamazepine-induced leukopenia. Thus, lithium should not be added to carbamazepine at times when a potentially serious decrease in the white blood cell count has occurred. Clozapine, because of its propensity to cause agranulocytocis, should not be given to patients taking carbamazepine.

Cardiovascular Effects

Carbamazepine **slows intracardiac conduction** and may worsen preexisting cardiac conduction disease. Both sinus bradycardia and varying degrees of atrioventricular block have been reported. Carbamazepine is less dangerous in this regard than TCAs, but the existence of a high degree of heart block is a relative contraindication to its use. Other cardiovascular side effects listed by the manufacturer (e.g., congestive heart failure) are rare and may not be causally related to the drug.

Gastrointestinal Effects
Nausea and vomiting are relatively common dose-related side effects that do not necessitate termination of therapy. They are common at the start of therapy and, like dose-related neurologic side effects, can be minimized by increasing the dosage slowly or using slow-release preparations. Mild, nonprogressive elevations of LFTs are also relatively common and require follow-up. LFTs should be obtained at the starting of the treatment. The decision to continue the medication in the presence of mild LFT abnormalities must be individualized and should involve consultation with an internist or gastroenterologist.

Rarely, idiosyncratic, non–dose-related hepatitis may occur, usually in the first month of treatment. Patients generally manifest other signs of a hypersensitivity reaction, including fever and rash. Deaths from hepatotoxicity are extremely rare. Young age and multiple anticonvulsants are risk factors for severe toxicity or death. Older patients are more likely to suffer reversible hepatic toxicity. Patients experiencing hepatic toxicity should not be rechallenged with carbamazepine.

Dermatologic Effects
Rashes may develop in up to 3% of patients taking carbamazepine. Patients with urticaria and pruritic erythematous drug rashes should have the medication discontinued. Rarely, patients have developed Stevens-Johnson syndrome, which may be fatal.

Effects on Electrolytes
Carbamazepine has antidiuretic properties that can lead to decreases in serum sodium. These are usually clinically unimportant, but on rare occasions more severe **hyponatremia** may occur. Risk is highest in elderly patients and in patients with a low serum sodium level at baseline. Appearance of new mental symptoms during carbamazepine treatment merits a check of serum electrolytes. Carbamazepine does not appear to be helpful in reversing lithium-induced polyuria. Serum electrolytes should be obtained at the start of treatment.

Effects on Thyroid
Although long-term studies of patients taking carbamazepine show decreases in free T_3 and T_4, reports of clinical hypothyroidism are anecdotal and rare. Carbamazepine is much less likely to produce significant effects on the thyroid than lithium, but hypothyroidism should be considered if a patient develops refractory depression.

Drug Interactions
Carbamazepine, like most anticonvulsants, **induces hepatic microsomal enzymes.** It potently induces P450 3A4, 1A2, 2C9, and 2C19, resulting in increased metabolism and reduced plasma concentrations of many compounds that undergo hydroxylation or demethylation during elimination. Significant drug interactions are listed in Table 4.9.

Overdose
Because of carbamazepine's slow absorption, peak levels in overdose may not be reached until the second or third day after the ingestion. Although it has a tricyclic structure, carbamazepine appears to be less dangerous in overdose than the TCAs. The major concerns in carbamazepine overdose are the development of high

TABLE 4.9	Drug Interactions with Carbamazepine			
Diminishes Effects of	**Unpredictable Effects on**	**May Augment Effects of**	**Carbamazepine Levels Decreased by**	**Carbamazepine Levels Increased by**
Warfarin	Phenytoin	Digitalis (may induce or exacerbate bradycardia)	Phenobarbital	Erythromycin (marked increase)
Ethosuximide			Primidone	Isoniazid (marked increase)
Valproic acid			Phenytoin	Propoxyphene
Tetracycline				Cimetidine
Haloperidol (probably)				SSRIs
Cyclic antidepressants (probably)				
Benzodiazepines, including clonazepam				
Fluoxetine				
Proton pump inhibitors				
mirtazapine				
cyclosporin				

SSRIs, selective serotonin reuptake inhibitors.

degrees of atrioventricular block (meriting cardiac monitoring) and stupor and coma, with risk of aspiration pneumonia. At higher doses, depression of respiration may occur, but it is usually relatively mild. Other symptoms and signs of overdose that have been reported include nystagmus, tremor, ballistic movements, mydriasis, ophthalmoplegia, orofacial dyskinesias, myoclonus, hypo- or hyperreflexia, rigidity, and seizures.

Management of carbamazepine overdoses is supportive. Because the drug is highly protein bound, hemodialysis is of no benefit. Hemoperfusion confers uncertain benefit and does not appear to be indicated.

Oxcarbazepine

Oxcarbazepine (Trileptal) is the 10-keto analog of carbamazepine that has proved efficacy as an add-on treatment in epilepsy. Despite limited clinical study, primarily in the form of small comparison studies with lithium, without a placebo-control group, it has been adopted by some as substitute for carbamazepine. Although it has advantages of being better tolerated that carbamazepine and not causing blood dyscrasias or requiring blood levels, it lacks data clearly suggesting its efficacy. In addition, a recent study in young outpatients (age 7 to 18 years) with bipolar I disorder found that it was no more effective than placebo for controlling manic symptoms. Although oxcarbazepine does not induce as many cytochrome enzymes to the extent that carbamazepine does, it does induce hepatic enzymes, and the clinician who uses it must be aware that drugs metabolized by the 3A4 enzyme may be decreased to clinically significant extent. In particular, oxcarbazepine has been shown to decrease concentrations of hormonal contraceptives by nearly 50%. In addition, usual neurological and gastrointestinal adverse effects associated with anticonvulsants are common with oxcarbazepine. Common adverse effects of oxcarbazepine include dizziness, sedation, ataxia, psychomotor slowing, double vision, nausea, and vomiting. Not uncommonly, patients may develop hyponatremia; monitoring serum sodium is necessary for the first few months of treatment. Rash is also an uncommon side effect and, rarely, patients may develop a toxic epidermal necrolysis. Patients who develop a rash should not be restarted. The dose for oxcarbazepine is not established, though dosing used in epilepsy has sometimes been adopted for use in bipolar patients. Common dosing starts at 300 mg twice daily and is gradually increased to 1,800 to 2,400 mg per day in two doses. In all, although there are some appealing aspects of oxcarbazepine, at this point there is no proven justification for its use in bipolar disorder.

LAMOTRIGINE

Lamotrigine (Lamictal), a phenyltriazine originally approved for adjunctive use in the treatment of partial seizures, has been shown in controlled studies to be effective for the prevention of recurrence in bipolar disorder (Table 4.10). It appears more effective for the treatment or prevention of depression than of mania, though it may be useful for prevention of both manic and depressive episodes. Lamotrigine is the only anticonvulsant approved for the maintenance phase of bipolar disorder. Although acute bipolar depression trials were less strongly positive, lamotrigine provides an important alternative for the treatment of bipolar depression. A trial of lamotrigine in rapid-cycling bipolar disorder also suggested efficacy for lamotrigine, although only in subjects with bipolar II disorder. A randomized, controlled trial in mania, however, found no benefit with lamotrigine.

Pharmacology

The mechanism of action of lamotrigine in bipolar disorder is not known. At the cellular level, lamotrigine inhibits the release of the excitatory amino acid glutamate, thus diminishing central nervous system excitation, and *in vitro* it also inhibits low-voltage sodium channels. Effects on calcium channels are not established. Lamotrigine does not appear to have conduction effects in the human heart, although an N-methyl metabolite causes cardiac conduction delay in dogs.

TABLE 4.10	Available Preparations of Other Anticonvulsants Used in Bipolar Disorders	
Form	Brand Name	How Supplied
Lamotrigine	Lamictal	25-, 100-, 150-, 200-mg tablets 2-, 5-, 25-mg chewable dispersible tablets
Topiramate	Topamax	25-, 100-, 200-mg tablets 15-, 25-mg sprinkle capsules
Oxcarbazepine	Trileptal	150-, 300-, 600-mg tablets 300-mg/5-mL suspension
Gabapentin	Neurontin	100-, 300-, 400-mg capsules 600-, 800-mg tablets 250-mg/5-mL oral solution
Tiagabine	Gabitril	2-, 4-, 12-, 16-, 20-mg tablets

Lamotrigine also appears to modulate the reuptake of serotonin and dopamine, though it is unclear if these properties confer antidepressant benefits.

Lamotrigine is rapidly absorbed by oral administration and reaches peak concentration within 2 to 4 hours. It is only partially bound to plasma proteins, thereby making interaction with drugs that compete tightly for protein binding unlikely to have clinical significance. It is metabolized primarily by glucuronide addition in the liver and excreted through the kidney. Elimination half-life is approximately 24 hours, although this is affected significantly by the presence of hepatic enzyme inducers or inhibitors and is well established with the other commonly used anticonvulsants. For example, with carbamazepine, the elimination half-life of lamotrigine is reduced to approximately 12 hours, although with divalproex, the elimination half-life may rise three- or fourfold and reach 100 hours with some patients. Hence, dosing of lamotrigine must be carefully done in combination with valproic acid, necessitating slow titration and lower than expected final dose. Lamotrigine used in combination with carbamazepine, on the other hand, will require approximately twice the dose to reach the same plasma concentration. Unfortunately, a therapeutic plasma concentration range is not established for epilepsy or bipolar disorder, so a balance must be struck between adverse effects and the desired clinical effect. Doses used in bipolar disorder are generally between 100 and 400 mg per day in a single evening dose.

Although side effects are generally mild, rash may occur in 10% of individuals. Stevens-Johnson syndrome or toxic epidermal necrolysis, which may be fatal, has also been reported (incidence in adult bipolar trials of 0.08%). Rashes appear to depend at least partly on starting dose and rate of increase; therefore, **slow dosage increments are recommended** ("no rush, no rash"), particularly when the drug is used in combination with divalproex, which inhibits the metabolism of lamotrigine. Except in rare cases, when rash occurs, the drug should be stopped and not restarted. The risk of severe or fatal rashes is much higher in the pediatric than in adult age group. Patients who develop rash involving mucous membranes, with or without other systemic signs, should stop the drug immediately and seek emergency evaluation by an internist or dermatologist. Other side effects of lamotrigine include headache, central nervous system symptoms (sedation, diplopia, ataxia, blurred vision,), and nausea and vomiting. The central nervous system adverse effects are generally dose dependent and most patients tolerate lamotrigine quite well. Lamotrigine is generally tolerated better than the other anticonvulsants. Cognitive complaints are lesser for valproate or carbamazepine (Table 4.11). Pregnancy registries

TABLE 4.11	Side Effects and Toxicity of Lamotrigine
Common dosage-related side effects	Dizziness
	Ataxia
	Headache
	Sedation/somnolence
	Diplopia
	Nausea and gastrointestinal upset
	Rash (with or without itching)
Less common dosage-related side effects	Insomnia
	Anxiety
	Memory impairment
	Tremor
	Nystagmus
	Anorexia
	Severe rash (Steven's Johnson syndrome)

suggest that lamotrigine may be somewhat safer than other anticonvulsants, though oral facial cleft has been reported. Teratogenicity, though rare, appears to be dose related. Lamotrigine's therapeutic use in pregnancy is complicated by doubling to tripling in clearance via glucuronidation and renal excretion.

Lamotrigine appears relatively well tolerated in overdose. In cases of single drug overdose, patients suffer gastrointestinal and central nervous system toxicity, though outcomes are generally good and supportive treatment is all that is needed for recovery. Sedation and delirium are the most likely consequences of significant overdose. There have been some reports of prolonged cardiac conduction in lamotrigine overdoses, though none has been of serious cardiac consequence. There have been no confirmed cases of death caused by drug overdose with lamotrigine.

Method of Use
Lamotrigine requires **very slow titration** to minimize rash risk. Lamotrigine is generally begun at 25 to 50 mg per day. The daily dose may be increased by 25 mg every week or two to minimize side effects, especially rash. After reaching 100 mg daily, the dose can generally be increased by 50 mg per week. The typical (studied) maintenance range is 100 to 400 mg per day, although some patients may require greater dosages. The dose of lamotrigine is generally about twofold higher when combined with carbamazepine, because the latter induces enzymes that metabolize lamotrigine; conversely, doses of lamotrigine may need to be halved when combined with divalproex because it inhibits the metabolism of lamotrigine. Dosing must be made in accordance with accompanying anticonvulsant drugs (Table 4.12). Lamotrigine does not affect P450 hepatic enzymes itself, nor does it affect the pharmacokinetics of lithium salts. Lamotrigine is available in starter packs: one for patients taking valproate, another for patients taking enzyme-inducing drugs such as carbamazepine or phenobarbital, and another for patients taking neither enzyme-inducing drugs nor valproate.

OTHER ANTICONVULSANTS
A number of other anticonvulsants have also entered the acute mania fray, though none has proved of benefit in placebo-controlled trials. Most notably, gabapentin

TABLE 4.12   Summary: Method of Lamotrigine Use

Monotherapy lamotrigine	Initial dose 25 mg daily for 1 to 2 weeks Then 50 mg daily for 1 to 2 weeks Then 100 mg daily for 2 weeks Then 150 mg daily for 2 weeks Then 200 mg for 1 week. This is the usual target dose Further increases should be by a maximum of 100 mg/d/week, up to 500 mg
Lamotrigine with valproate	Initial dose 25 mg every other day for 1–2 weeks Then 25 mg daily for 2 weeks Then increase by 25 mg per week until dose of 100–150 mg/d)
Lamotrigine with carbamazepine or other cytochrome P450 inducers	Initial dose of 50 mg/d for 1 to 2 weeks Then 100 mg daily for 2 weeks Then 200 mg daily for 1 week Then 300 mg daily for 1 week Then 400 mg daily for 1 week (If carbamazepine is discontinued, decrease dose by 50%)

was used widely for a period, but benefits were marginal with the exception of treating some anxiety symptoms at high doses, it clearly was not effective for core manic signs and symptoms in placebo-controlled trials. (In fact, placebo was statistically significantly better than adjunctive gabapentin in one trial.) A related drug, pregabalin, which has proved effective for treating anxiety has not been studied in acute mania, though its similarity to gabapentin suggests that it is also ineffective. Similarly, topiramate, leviteracitam, and zonisamide have proven ineffective in acute mania. Topiramate may prove useful as an add-on treatment to reduce appetite often associated with lithium, valproate, or olanzapine, but its significant sedation and cognitive side effects often limit its use. If topiramate is used, it should be started slowly, at 25 mg at bedtime and gradually increased every few days as tolerated to a target dose of 100 to 200 mg at bedtime.

BENZODIAZEPINES

Clonazepam, a potent benzodiazepine FDA approved for the treatment of panic disorder, has been used primarily as an anxiolytic but was originally labeled as an anticonvulsant drug, especially in the treatment of some childhood epilepsies. Clonazepam has gained favor with clinicians as a safe, easily administered, and well-tolerated alternative for antipsychotic drugs, though it is unclear if its benefits are more for sedation than for core manic signs and symptoms. Some patients may become intoxicated, though remain quite manic. One must carefully monitor the manic patient, particularly after the first few doses of clonazepam, to ensure the effect on the patient is not **overly sedating** (drunklike quality), possibly predisposing the patient to falls or other accidents. Some manic patients may become more angry or disinhibited taking clonazepam. Typically, 2 to 5 mg per 24 hours will help with agitation, insomnia, and anxiety. Lorazepam may be just as useful as clonazepam as an adjunctive agent in acute mania, and it has the advantage of being more rapidly absorbed orally and readily available in parenteral form. As with clonazepam, it is best used for anxiety and insomnia rather than for core manic signs and symptoms. Typical lorazepam doses in acute mania are 2 to 6 mg per day. Doses higher than this range generally lead to ataxia, mental clouding, and sedation. The benzodiazepines, though useful in acute mania, do not have a significant role in bipolar prophylaxis or bipolar depression, though some patients with coexisting anxiety disorders (e.g., panic disorder) may benefit from benzodiazepines following acute mania treatment. Clonazepam and lorazepam are discussed in detail in Chapter 5.

OMEGA-3 FATTY ACIDS

Omega-3 fatty acids are hypothesized to dampen signal transduction pathways in a manner similar to the more established mood stabilizers. In a preliminary trial, Stoll et al. (1999) found a combination of the two main omega-3 fatty acids in high doses (9.6 g per day) to be superior to placebo in preventing an acute illness episode and on a variety of symptom-rating scale measures during 4 months of maintenance treatment of 30 patients with mild bipolar disorder. With a range of initial mood states, the continuation of previous medications during the trial in most subjects, and the apparently unsuccessful effort at blinding the fishy aftertaste of the active fatty acid capsules, these findings must be accepted with caution. Moreover, subsequent studies have been negative or only shown modest benefit for bipolar depression, making this option questionable. Given the likely overall health benefits of omega fatty acids, we would not discourage their use, but make it clear that the supplements are not likely to provide a direct benefit in treating the primary symptoms of bipolar disorder.

PRAMIPEXOLE

Pramipexole is a dopamine agonist primarily used in Parkinson's disease. It has been used as adjunctive treatment for patients with treatment resistant depression, and one study found it effective for unipolar depression. There are also two very small placebo-controlled studies, in which it was effective for bipolar depression, one when used in combination with therapeutic concentrations of lithium or divalproex, and one as monotherapy. In these studies approximately 50% of patients responded, whereas only 20% of placebo-treated patients improved. Conclusions must be tentative because both studies had approximately 10 patients per treatment group. Only one patient developed mania or hypomania, though caution must be taken with any dopamine agonist in bipolar disorder because of their potential to induce psychosis or mania. The mean dose in the studies was approximately 1.5 mg daily.

Pharmacology

Pramipexole is an agonist at dopamine-type 2 and 3 receptors. It is readily absorbed in the gastrointestinal system, and like other dopamine agonists may cause nausea at first. It reaches peak concentration within 2 hours and has an elimination half-life of approximately 8 to 10 hours per day. It is excreted unchanged in the urine. Patients with renal compromise will have prolonged effects and dose adjustments should be made accordingly. The most common dose-related side effects are postural hypotension, **somnolence or "sleep attacks,"** nausea and vomiting, and anorexia. Less common side effects include urinary frequency, impotence, disturbed vision, and hallucinations. There are no serious drug–drug interactions, though use of pramipexole could reduce the effects of antipsychotics. Food does not affect maximal concentrations, but may delay peak concentration. It is available in tablet strengths of 0.125, 0.25, 0.5, 1, and 1.5 mg.

Method of Use

Although pramipexole is better tolerated than other dopamine agonists used in Parkinson's disease, titration must be slow to tolerate gastrointestinal toxicity. The initial dose is 0.125 mg two to three times daily. The dose can be increased by 0.125 mg per day every few days as tolerated to a target dose of 1.5 mg per day, generally in two doses. Although some patients can tolerate higher doses, sleep attacks become more problematic at higher doses. Some patients will be intolerant of a 1 mg dose, and a balance must be struck between therapeutic benefit and toxicity. If a patient is on pramipexole for a prolonged period, withdrawing the drug should be done slowly because of the possibility of a condition similar to the NMS that has been reported with abrupt withdrawal or other dopamine agonists used in the treatment of Parkinson's disease.

ANTIPSYCHOTICS

Antipsychotic drugs have long played an important role in the treatment of bipolar disorder. They have been used as either monotherapy or adjunctive treatment in the acute phase of manic episodes and may be required for prevention of recurrences in some cases. Although first-generation drugs, such as haloperidol and fluphenazine, have long been found useful in the treatment of acute mania, the second-generation antipsychotics (aripiprazole, olanzapine, quetiapine, risperidone, and ziprasidone) have been extensively studied as monotherapy in placebo-controlled trials, and all are FDA approved for the treatment of acute mania. Several of the antipsychotics have also been shown to have additional benefit when used for acute mania in combination with therapeutic doses of lithium or valproate. Clozapine has not been studied in acute mania, though it merits consideration for patients with a known history of treatment nonresponse with standard agents. The **dosing** of antipsychotics in **acute mania** is much the same as in schizophrenia, and otherwise healthy patients often tolerate rapid titration and high doses (e.g., 600 mg quetiapine or 30 mg olanzapine within 3 days). Oral dissolvable tablets are available for olanzapine, risperidone, and aripiprazole and these may be useful for paranoid patients or patients without insight. The long acting injectable form of risperidone may be preferable for patients with known noncompliance. The pharmacology of the antipsychotics is covered in Chapter 2.

In addition to acute mania, some of the second-generation antipsychotics have proven efficacy for bipolar prophylaxis and bipolar depression. Two of the drugs, aripiprazole and olanzapine, have shown benefit and are FDA approved for long-term prophylaxis of bipolar disorder. Both aripiprazole and olanzapine, unfortunately, provide efficacy only for manic relapse. Much like valproate, they do not prevent depression relapse. The maintenance dosing for aripiprazole and olanzapine was much the same as for acute mania. Risperidone, quetiapine, and ziprasidone have not been studied for prophylaxis, though it would not be surprising if they also prevented manic relapse.

Two second-generation antipsychotics, olanzapine (in combination with fluoxetine) along with quetiapine, are also effective for treating the depressed phase of bipolar disorder. The effective doses for bipolar depression are olanzapine 6 mg/fluoxetine 25 mg at bedtime or quetiapine 300 to 600 mg at bedtime. The other second-generation antipsychotics have not been well studied for this use, but may well be helpful.

The choice of second-generation antipsychotic must be governed by tolerability factors in both acute and long-term use, as well as by which phase of bipolar disorder is being treated. The choices are unfortunately not simple, and individual factors must be considered. For example, although olanzapine appears a best choice because of its benefits in all phases of the illness, and is particularly well tolerated during acute mania, and may prevent manic relapse it is often problematic in the end for other reasons. Many patients complain of chronic sedation, and weight gain along with elevation of lipids and the propensity to worsen or induce diabetes make it a problematic option for many. The choice of antipsychotic alone or in combination is not simple and is considered in the section below.

TREATMENT OF EACH PHASE OF BIPOLAR DISORDER

Acute Mania

There are many compounds currently available to treat acute mania, and often several in combination are required. Although mild episodes of mania or hypomania can usually be treated in the outpatient setting with lithium, divalproex, or a second-generation antipsychotic drug, if time is more pressing or when mania is accompanied by psychosis or dangerous behavior requiring rapid treatment, second-generation antipsychotic drugs often prove useful, usually in combination with lithium or divalproex. Not only do the antipsychotics improve the rate of response, but they also improve the overall benefit in the short term (Tables 4.13 and 4.14).

At present, there are nine drugs that are FDA approved for acute mania, and likely a number of others that would work as well. Lithium and divalproex as well as the second-generation antipsychotics (risperidone, olanzapine, aripiprazole, ziprasidone, and quetiapine) are generally considered first-line treatments for acute mania. Although extended-release carbamazepine is also FDA approved for acute mania, it is generally considered a second-line treatment because of drug–drug interactions and tolerability problems. In addition, lithium or divalproex combined with quetiapine, risperidone, or olanzapine are also considered first-line options because placebo-controlled studies have shown benefit for these combinations. The same added benefit for acute mania may be true for adding

TABLE 4.13	Drugs Effective for the Treatment of Bipolar Disorder

Acute Mania	Bipolar Prophylaxis	Bipolar Depression
Lithium	Lithium	Olanzapine/fluoxetine combination
Divalproex	Lamotrigine	Quetiapine
Carbamazepine ER	Olanzapine	Lamotrigine
Chlorpromazine	Aripiprazole	Lithium
Haloperidol		
Olanzapine		
Quetiapine		
Risperidone		
Aripiprazole		
Ziprasidone		
Asenapine		

aripiprazole or ziprasidone to lithium or divalproex, though aripiprazole has not been studied as an add-on treatment, and ziprasidone failed to add additional benefit when added to lithium.

In clinical practice, it is common for any of these antipsychotics to be added to lithium or divalproex. Unfortunately, it is also somewhat common for multiple different antipsychotics to be combined when patients do not rapidly respond. This "piling-on" technique is not only unstudied and unsound from a pharmacodynamic perspective but also fraught with the problems of accumulated toxicity. By rushing to add drugs or rapidly escalating the dose, the clinician obscures the benefit that could be obtained from a simpler regimen by being more patient. As in the treatment of psychosis, the benefits of drug treatment of mania take time, often weeks for full effects. In fact, patients are often discharged from the hospital on high doses that are intolerably sedating, and doses need to be lowered following hospitalization.

The choice of antipsychotic or other mood stabilizer is not readily obvious, and there have been no comparison trials to help clarify the issue. When possible, it is best to use medications that have proved useful in the past, for while studies find little differences among agents, individuals are often responsive variably to

TABLE 4.14	Drug Doses Used in Acute Mania

Drug	Starting Dose (mg)	Usual Target Range (mg)
Lithium	600–900 mg split dose	900–1,800 mg/h
Divalproex	15–20 mg/kg split dose	750–2,500 mg/h
Carbamazepine ER	400 mg split dose	1,000–1,600 mg/d
Risperidone	2–3 mg/h	4–8 mg/h
Aripiprazole	15 mg/h	15–45 mg/h
Olanzapine	15 mg/h	15–30 mg/h
Quetiapine	200 mg/h	500–1,000 mg/h
Ziprasidone	40–60 mg b.i.d.	160–200 mg/h
Chlorpromazine	100–200 mg/h	600–1,000 mg/h
Haloperidol	5 mg/h	5–10 mg/h
Loxapine	25 mg/h	25–100 mg/h

drugs. Some patients are historically known to respond only to lithium. Because the second-generation antipsychotic drugs appear generally of equal efficacy in acute mania, long-term tolerability appears to be a reasonable criterion for selecting acute treatment. Although olanzapine and quetiapine may be more desirable for their sedating properties at first, this could be problematic later, even though some patients accommodate to initial sedative effects. Severe manic presentations with marked agitation and florid psychotic symptoms are optimally treated as an acute psychosis with second-generation antipsychotic drugs and often the concomitant use of a benzodiazepine such as lorazepam or clonazepam, while also obtaining laboratory tests and initiating lithium or divalproex.

Lithium in Acute Mania

Many controlled studies have demonstrated that at a serum level of approximately 1 mEq/L, lithium is effective treatment of manic episodes in approximately 70% to 80% of cases. Lithium also has been shown to be more effective overall than antipsychotic drugs used as single agents in treating acute mania. Onset of improvement with lithium usually takes at least 10 to 14 days, and full improvement may take 4 weeks or more. When manic symptoms are not so severe as to require immediate control of abnormal behavior, lithium may be used alone. However, when mania is severe, especially in settings where hospitalization time is limited, the onset of the therapeutic response to lithium is impracticably slow. Thus, early in the treatment of acute mania, antipsychotic drugs are often used as adjuncts to lithium or divalproex therapy. They are effective when administered at full antipsychotic doses (e.g., 8 to 10 mg of haloperidol). With the introduction of relatively less toxic second-generation antipsychotic medications, the clinician can more easily add these drugs with less concern for the EPS, danger of NMS, or incidence of dystonia that attended the use of older antipsychotics. Nonetheless, to minimize undesirable side effects at higher doses of antipsychotic drugs (see Chapter 2), benzodiazepines are often used if temporary additional sedation is required during the early treatment of acute mania (e.g., lorazepam 1 to 2 mg or clonazepam 0.5 mg every 2 hours as needed), either in addition to lithium alone or with an antipsychotic drug. Similarly, lithium can be used in conjunction with antiseizure medications such as divalproex or carbamazepine for refractory manic episodes (see later section on treatment-refractory mania). Other anticonvulsants, such as gabapentin, lamotrigine, and topiramate, unfortunately have been shown ineffective in randomized, placebo-controlled trials for the treatment of acute mania. Milder cases of mania can be treated with lithium alone. However, even mild episodes that occur in the context of lithium prophylaxis generally require the temporary addition of other compounds. If, at the time of a hypomanic or manic breakthrough, the patient's lithium level has been maintained at 0.8 mM or less, the lithium dose can be increased to achieve a level of 0.8 to 1.2 mEq/L (as side effects allow) and an antipsychotic drug added until the symptoms are well controlled. The treating physician must then weigh the frequency of relapses against side effects experienced by the individual patient and decide whether to attempt future prophylaxis with a higher serum level of lithium.

In treating any acutely manic patient, a low-stimulation environment should be provided. Limits should be set clearly and firmly, and provocative interactions avoided. If hospitalized patients attempt to feign compliance with medication, mouth checks and use of liquid preparations, such as lithium citrate, may be necessary. When patients refuse treatment because their judgment is impaired by mental illness, a mechanism of substituted judgment is required. Most states require evidence that there is a high risk of serious harm if the patient remains untreated, leading to a judicial process for establishing substituted judgment.

Valproate in Acute Mania

Several studies have shown that valproate, as either divalproex or divalproex extended-release formulation, is effective for acute mania. It is as effective as lithium, and somewhat better tolerated. There have not been comparison studies with second-generation antipsychotics, though the time course for improvement with divalproex seems somewhat slower than that for the second-generation antipsychotics. The **loading dose method** (20 to 30 mg per kilogram per day) appears to improve the onset of benefit, though the higher starting doses may prove toxic for some patients. Lower doses (10 to 15 mg per kilogram per day) are generally better tolerated. Initial dosing is best done as twice daily dosing, but divalproex can generally be given as a single bedtime dose later in treatment. Plasma concentrations of valproate can be determined several days after starting treatment, though dose adjustments are generally driven by response and tolerability. In acute mania, a target concentration of 100 to 125 μg/mL is reasonable. Antipsychotics or benzodiazepines can be added to divalproex for further therapeutic benefit in acute mania, though combination treatment may lead to greater toxicity. Once mania is controlled, benzodiazepines can be withdrawn and the valproate dose may need to be reduced somewhat.

Carbamazepine in Acute Mania

Although carbamazepine was the first anticonvulsant found effective in acute mania, it was only recently FAD approved, largely because its extended-release formulation was studied in a large sample of patients with acute mania. Carbamazepine ER is better tolerated than carbamazepine and is the preferable formulation for acute mania because higher initial doses can be used. Patients can generally tolerated carbamazepine ER at 200 mg twice daily, and the dose can be gradually increased over 4 to 5 days to 800 to 1,200 mg per day. As noted before, its propensity to induce cytochrome enzymes that reduce its and other drug concentrations make it less desirable than other antimanic drugs. For patients with past traumatic brain injury or aggression, carbamazepine may be a logical first choice.

Antipsychotics in Acute Mania

All of the second-generation antipsychotics are effective in acute mania. They are first-line agents for acute mania, either alone or in combination with lithium or divalproex. There are no convincing studies finding one antipsychotic superior to another for acute mania. The older antipsychotics, other than haloperidol, are not well studied in acute mania. Haloperidol, at approximately 10 mg per day, is also effective as monotherapy in acute mania. The second-generation antipsychotics are generally well tolerated in clinical practice, although for reasons of toxicity and lack of efficacy there are high dropout rates in short-term monotherapy studies. Patients with acute mania may tolerate higher doses than patients with schizophrenia, at least in the short term. Rapid dose increases of the antipsychotics in clinical practice, however, are often associated with **EPS for bipolar disorder patients,** even with the second-generation antipsychotics. On the other hand, using the antipsychotics in combination with lithium or divalproex often reduces the need for high-dose antipsychotics. As in schizophrenia, the antipsychotics take time to achieve significant therapeutic effects in acute mania, often several weeks. Patients may show some benefits within a few days, but core manic symptoms take longer.

Many clinicians start with the antipsychotics alone, though using them in combination with lithium or divalproex is not uncommon. Starting with one drug alone followed by adding another helps to identify toxicity origins and make adjustments accordingly. Quetiapine and olanzapine are often preferred by clinicians because of their sedating qualities in acute mania, though this property may be problematic for longer-term treatment. Olanzapine can generally be started at 10 to 15 mg at bedtime, and increased to 20 to 30 mg per day as tolerated over several days. Some patients may tolerate up to 50 mg per day. Weight gain and effects on lipids may be problematic with continued use of olanzapine. Quetiapine, particularly in its extended-release formulation, can be started at 200 to 300 mg at bedtime and increased to 500 to 800 mg per day over several days, though some patients may tolerate even higher doses. For both olanzapine and quetiapine, patients must be monitored closely for **orthostatic hypotension** during dose escalation. Aripiprazole is less sedating than the others are but may cause gastrointestinal distress or akathisia when given at high doses at first. An aripiprazole starting dose of 15 mg per day is often better tolerated than 30 mg per day, though most patients eventually tolerate 30 mg per day. Risperidone has been well studied in acute mania. It can generally be started at 2 mg at night and increased over several days to 4 to 6 mg as single bedtime dose. Patients treated with risperidone should be monitored for orthostasis and EPS, both of which are common. Dose can be modified according to sedation. Ziprasidone is less well studied than the other second-generation antipsychotics, though it is also effective for acute mania. It has been studied at starting doses of at 40 to 80 mg twice daily, though many clinicians give it as single bedtime dose, starting at 80 mg and increase to 120 to 160 mg over several days. Akathisia and EPS are sometimes problematic. Asenapine, an unapproved antipsychotic similar to the other second-generation antipsychotics has also been shown effective in placebo-controlled trials for acute mania. Its place in the treatment of acute mania remains to be determined. Dissolvable forms of olanzapine and risperidone may be useful for patients with limited insight, and the long-acting form of risperidone may be useful for severe bipolar patients who will not take oral mood stabilizers.

The newer antipsychotics are unfortunately quite expensive, and some patients may be unable to afford the second-generation antipsychotics. Risperidone, however, is recently available in generic form and is more affordable. These older drugs, such as haloperidol and fluphenazine, however, are generally more problematic for inducing EPS or TD in bipolar patients. Loxapine, however, has pharmacologic profile reasonably similar to the newer antipsychotic drugs, and has been a clinical favorite for acute mania because of its salutary effects on sleep and low rates of EPS. Loxapine can be used as an adjunctive treatment, given at bedtime, with a starting dose of 25 mg. and can be increased as tolerated to 100 mg at bedtime. Sedation and orthostasis are the most common dose-related adverse effects.

Treatment-Refractory Mania

In clinical practice a number of patients do not respond well to a single agent or even two agents. This patient group, unfortunately, has not been well studied. Reported predictors of poorer response to lithium or divalproex in acute mania include a prior history of response, rapid cycling, psychotic symptoms, mixed symptoms of depression and mania, psychiatric comorbidity (including personality disorders and substance abuse), and medical comorbidity. However, the presence of one of these features of illness does not necessarily mean that a patient should not have a lithium trial; for example, some studies suggest patients with rapid cycling nonetheless respond to lithium and more recent data suggest that lithium may be as effective as valproic acid for long-term management of rapid cycling, though both drugs were associated with high rates of relapse. Medical illnesses may complicate attempts to achieve adequate lithium levels. For example, the presence of renal disease alters lithium excretion and therefore requires careful monitoring of both lithium levels and salt balance. The presence of sinoatrial node dysfunction raises the question of whether it is safe to use lithium in the absence of a cardiac pacemaker. The presence of even mild dementia complicates the use of lithium (as well as all other psychotropic drugs) by increasing the risk of drug-induced cognitive impairment. Comorbidity of mania with either a medical disorder or a nonaffective psychiatric disorder decreases the likelihood that patients will receive adequate lithium doses or respond well if they do.

For patients who have not shown significant response to their initial mood stabilization treatment after 2 to 3 weeks at therapeutic levels, reconsider the possibility of an undetected complicating medical, psychiatric, or drug abuse disorder. Patients who do not respond to the combination of lithium or divalproex and an antipsychotic drug may respond to treatment with the combination of lithium and valproate and an antipsychotic, or to treatment with another antipsychotic.

There is reasonable evidence to suggest that some patients who do not respond to lithium alone or an anticonvulsant alone respond to combination therapy. There are literally dozens of ways to mix and match the anticonvulsants divalproex or carbamazepine, or antipsychotics, to reduce symptomatology in treatment-resistant patients. However, combined therapy does increase the risk of central nervous system side effects, especially in elderly patients. There have been reports of success with a divalproex-carbamazepine combination in lithium-refractory or lithium-intolerant patients. Because of pharmacokinetic interactions, the dose of divalproex will usually have to be increased and the dose of carbamazepine decreased if this combination is used. Carbamazepine also may speed the metabolism of concomitantly administered antipsychotic and benzodiazepine drugs that are metabolized by cytochrome P450 3A4. Very severe episodes of mania that do not respond satisfactorily to first-line treatments may respond to ECT. ECT has the advantage of rapidity, with remission often occurring after six treatments (with treatments given three times weekly). ECT is not a first-line treatment, in part because the treatment of bipolar disorder requires long-term prophylaxis, which is not provided by ECT. Thus, even after successful ECT treatment, it is still necessary to find an effective prophylactic regimen. Relapse of depression is common after ECT, and aggressive treatments such as maintenance ECT or maintenance ECT with lithium may be needed. Maintenance ECT has not been studied in bipolar patients, though in unipolar patients, even the combination of lithium and nortriptyline provides modest prophylaxis against depressive relapse. ECT is safe and effective in patients receiving lithium or antipsychotic drugs; use of divalproex or carbamazepine will elevate the seizure threshold, requiring some adjustments in treatment.

Patients with **refractory mania** with psychosis should be considered for a trial with **clozapine**. Clozapine can be added to other anticonvulsants or lithium, but not to carbamazepine. Some clinicians will continue with an antipsychotic that is being used, and others will switch to clozapine. As in schizophrenia treatment, the dose escalation should be slow, starting at 25 mg per day and increasing by 25 mg every couple of days, as tolerated, to reach a tolerable dose, usually between 200 and 400 mg per day, depending on the concomitant medications. In our experience, some patients rapidly respond to clozapine. Benzodiazepines should generally be avoided in combination with clozapine because of excessive sedation and effects on ventilation. The usual weekly blood monitoring of the white blood cell count complicates long-term treatment with clozapine. In some cases, the clozapine may be useful in the short term and other treatments used for prophylaxis, though this method has not been carefully studied.

Mixed Episodes

When an episode is characterized by mixed symptoms of mania and depression, the episode is best treated like acute mania, that is, with a mood-stabilizing drug (lithium, divalproex, carbamazepine, or a second-generation antipsychotic) or a combination. As in acute mania, ECT is generally reserved for patients who are refractory to initial drug treatments and who are so severely ill that rapid treatment is required. Patients who respond to ECT will still need subsequent pharmacologic prophylaxis. In mixed episodes, as in acute mania, adjunctive antipsychotic drugs are frequently employed. Benzodiazepines may also be used for adjunctive sedation. Antidepressants are to be avoided because they are likely to worsen the overall course of the episode.

Acute Bipolar Depression

The treatment of bipolar depression is much less satisfactory than the treatment of acute mania. Very few treatments are clearly effective. Although antidepressants have been historical mainstays in combination with lithium or divalproex, more recent evidence is disappointing. Lamotrigine as well as the second-generation antipsychotics, quetiapine and olanzapine/fluoxetine combinations, may be the best treatments for bipolar depression. In all of the studies, however, **remission rates for bipolar depression are relatively low.**

In the long-term course of bipolar disorder, the role of antidepressant therapy remains controversial, and a recent multicenter study found that neither bupropion nor paroxetine provided benefit compared with placebo for acute bipolar depression when added to a mood stabilizer at therapeutic concentrations. This National Institute of Mental Health funded study questions what role, if any, antidepressants should play in acute bipolar depression, although the study also found that there was no higher rate of switch to mania or hypomania overall for the antidepressant group. Antidepressants may be problematic for depressed bipolar patients who have concurrent mild manic symptoms, by either inducing mania or worsening the course of the illness. In addition, it is generally accepted that antidepressant treatment in bipolar patients, particularly using TCAs, poses a risk of triggering a switch into mania or hypomania or of inducing rapid cycling or cycle acceleration. Switch into mania has been observed with virtually every antidepressant class, but the tricyclics and venlafaxine appear most problematic for manic switches. Thus, the central rule in treatment of bipolar depression is that, if antidepressants are used, they should be used together with a mood stabilizer and that antidepressants should be used for the briefest time possible, quite a different approach than in unipolar patients (see Chapter 3).

If psychosis is present during a depressive episode, an antipsychotic drug should be added or ECT should be considered. Two of the second-generation antipsychotics, quetiapine and the olanzapine-fluoxetine combination drug, show clear benefit for bipolar depression, with or without psychosis. Both of these studies were also notable for the rapid onset of efficacy, which has generally not been observed with other agents, although some of this benefit may be a result of side effects such as sedation being reflected in depressive rating scales. Interestingly, the antipsychotic studies were not being conducted in conjunction with lithium or divalproex, though there is nothing to suggest that adding the second-generation antipsychotics would detract from their benefit. **Quetiapine** at doses of 300 and 600 mg per day have proven effective for bipolar depression, though many patients cannot tolerate the higher dose. The quetiapine is best titrated slowly and then given all at bedtime. The studies were short term, and it is therefore unknown if long-term treatment is useful for prophylaxis. It is, however, reasonable to continue the treatment if it is effective, because it may also prevent manic recurrence. Quetiapine may be sedating or contribute to weight gain when used in combination with lithium or valproate. Use with lamotrigine may be better tolerated. The combination of quetiapine with lamotrigine may be better for patients with primarily depressive recurrence. Other second-generation antipsychotics, particularly aripiprazole, which has shown benefit for treatment resistant depression, may also prove useful for bipolar depression.

The **olanzapine-fluoxetine combination** treatment, like quetiapine, has been studied without the benefit of a concurrent mood stabilizer. Although the combination drug has been FDA approved for bipolar depression, it is not clear if the olanzapine fluoxetine combination is any more effective than fluoxetine alone, for the pivotal trial did not include a fluoxetine monotherapy group. The rationale that the olanzapine addition to fluoxetine would prevent mania is reasonable, though it remains unclear if fluoxetine alone, perhaps in combination with lithium or divalproex would prove as useful as the olanzapine/fluoxetine combination. The olanzapine/fluoxetine combination has also proved useful for continuation treatment, though weight gain and lipid changes may be problematic.

Lamotrigine may also be helpful in the treatment of acute bipolar depression, with one controlled trial suggesting some benefit, particularly when used at a daily dose of 200 mg. The down side of lamotrigine for acute bipolar depression is that the drug must be titrated very slowly to prevent rash. Its benefit is better established in the prevention of depressive episodes (see later). Lithium is not as well established for acute bipolar depression, and valproate and carbamazepine appear to have very little benefit for acute bipolar depression. Lithium, valproate, and carbamazepine are more effective as antimanic agents than as antidepressants.

ECT is effective in all phases of bipolar disorder, including depression, and should be considered when medications are unsuccessful or in the presence of psychosis, catatonia, active suicidal plans, and pregnancy.

In summary, if a depression occurs in a bipolar patient who is not currently on lithium or another mood stabilizer, there are several options: (a) treatment should be started with lithium or lamotrigine; (b) quetiapine monotherapy may be begun; or (c) olanzapine/fluoxetine combination can be started. Although the antipsychotics have not been studied in combination with other mood stabilizers, their combined use is common in clinical practice. Adjunctive lamotrigine to lithium or adjunctive antidepressants to lithium or divalproex should be second-line treatments for bipolar depression. A structured psychotherapy such as cognitive-behavioral therapy may also be initiated. The choice will depend on the patient's prior history of responsiveness and the severity of the episode. When depression occurs in bipolar patients on long-term lithium therapy, the clinician is cautioned that lithium may cause hypothyroidism, which may masquerade as or exacerbate depression. It is prudent to withdraw the antidepressant, if possible, in bipolar patients after acute depressive episodes have passed and then to maintain the patients on a mood stabilizer alone.

Should manic symptoms emerge during treatment of a depressive episode, the antidepressant should be discontinued and therapy continued with a mood-stabilizing agent (lithium, divalproex, carbamazepine, or an atypical antipsychotic). Antidepressant-precipitated mania often continues, however, after the antidepressant is stopped, requiring institution of full antimanic treatment, which may include adjunctive use of antipsychotic or benzodiazepine drugs as well as the mood stabilizer. Some patients may require the addition of a second mood stabilizer in these cases (Table 4.15).

TABLE 4.15   Suggested Pharmacologic Treatments for Bipolar Depression

First Line	Second Line	Third line
Lithium	Lithium + divalproex	Lithium + lamotrigine + SSRI
Quetiapine	Lithium or divalproex + olanzapine	Lithium + second-generation antipsychotic
Olanzapine/ fluoxetine	Lithium or valproate + lamotrigine	Lithium + TCA
Lamotrigine	Lithium or valproate + SSRI	Lithium or divalproex + pramipexole
	Quetiapine + SSRI	
	Lithium or divalproex + bupropion	

SSRIs, selective serotonin reuptake inhibitors; TCA, tricyclic antidepressant.

Prophylaxis in Bipolar Disorder

Bipolar disorder must be treated with a longitudinal view of the illness because essentially all patients will suffer recurrences. Several treatments are proven effective for long-term treatments of bipolar disorder, though all treatments, except lamotrigine, are better for preventing manic than depressive relapse. Indeed, lithium, aripiprazole, and olanzapine are approved for long-term treatment of bipolar disorder, but only olanzapine and lithium have not been found to prevent depressive relapse compared with placebo. Interestingly, despite its common use in bipolar prophylaxis, there are no studies confirming that valproate prevents mood recurrence. The best evidence remains for lithium, though the other drugs also have several studies proving efficacy. **None of the drugs completely prevents recurrence of mania or depression.** Overall, experience suggests that lithium and olanzapine are somewhat more effective in preventing manic than depressive recurrences. Episodes of mild depression are reported by many patients despite treatment. Lithium appears to be less effective for patients with a history of frequent recurrences, especially if they are rapid cyclers (more than three cycles per year). Rapid withdrawal of lithium from previously stable patients, or rapid change in lithium levels, appears to predispose to early manic relapses, suggestive of a rebound phenomenon (see later section on discontinuation of lithium therapy).

If the most recent episode was a mania, prophylaxis should generally be undertaken with a continuation of the mood-stabilizing drug or drugs that were effective for that episode. In the past, guidelines suggested that any adjunctive antipsychotic drugs used during the acute episode should generally be tapered and discontinued, but in some cases second-generation antipsychotics may be used as maintenance medications because at least two drugs (olanzapine and aripiprazole) have shown efficacy in preventing recurrence. When possible, second-generation antipsychotics are preferred to minimize the risk of side effects, including TD, though weight gain and lipid rises may limit olanzapine use. For some treatment-refractory patients, clozapine has proven particularly efficacious.

If the most recent episode was depressive, recently added antidepressants should be tapered and discontinued, if possible, and prophylaxis continued with mood stabilizers alone. Lithium and lamotrigine have the most data to support their use for patients with predominate depressive episodes. There are conflicting data on optimal lithium serum levels for prophylaxis. Although effective prophylaxis has been reported with serum levels of lithium as low as 0.4 mM, a randomized double-blind prospective study of 94 patients found levels of 0.8 to 1.0 mM clearly superior to levels of 0.4 to 0.6 mM. (However, that study was confounded by rapid change in lithium levels in some patients, so the superiority of higher doses is unclear.) The main cost of higher levels is worsened side effects, which affect quality of life. It is prudent to start prophylaxis with a target level of 0.8 mM and to educate and reassure patients about side effects.

For patients who cannot tolerate lithium, lamotrigine is an obvious second choice. Doses of lamotrigine are not well established, though most studies have found doses of 200 mg more effective than lower doses. Evidence from two, randomized, lithium-comparator trials shows that lamotrigine is efficacious in the prevention of depressive episodes. Similarly, olanzapine has shown efficacy for the prevention of both depressive and manic episodes, although weight gain and lipid changes often limit its long-term use, and aripiprazole was effective for up to 26 weeks in preventing recurrence compared with placebo in recently manic subjects. Despite the burden of side effects of prophylaxis, given morbidity and life disruption caused by manic and depressive recurrences, **prophylaxis is the rule.** Some patients are resistant to the idea of long-term prophylaxis (this is particularly true in adolescent populations) and insist on a trial of cessation of medication despite an awareness of the substantial risk of recurrence.

Although previously antipsychotics were tapered once there was marked symptomatic improvement, because of the evidence that olanzapine and aripiprazole prevent manic relapse, it is common and reasonable practice that if patients tolerate lithium or divalproex along with the antipsychotic, then **maintenance treatment,** including the antipsychotic, often follows. Indeed, there is one placebo-controlled study that found olanzapine added to lithium or divalproex prolonged time to symptomatic relapse. This may well be true for the other second-generation antipsychotics. Olanzapine in combination with divalproex, however, may lead to significant weight gain, though in this study, patients gained approximately 15 pounds over 18 months. Long-term use of older antipsychotic drugs for prophylaxis of bipolar illness has generally not been recommended because patients with mood disorders appear to have heightened susceptibility to TD. Bipolar patients, however, clearly benefit from antipsychotic drugs when breakthrough symptoms of mania emerge despite prophylaxis with mood stabilizers, and patients with unremitting or rapidly cycling manic symptoms (despite other treatments) have stabilized with antipsychotic medication. Given the lower risk of EPS and the possibility that the second-generation antipsychotic drugs may cause less TD the potential role of newer antipsychotics in the long-term treatment of bipolar illness is being redefined.

Several studies have suggested that carbamazepine may be effective for prophylaxis against recurrences in bipolar disorder, but there is a paucity of placebo-controlled or double-blind studies supporting this. Studies also suggest that carbamazepine may be more effective for prophylaxis in patients with bipolar II disorder than classical mania. Taken together, the published studies and clinical experience underscore the point that long-term prophylactic use of carbamazepine in bipolar disorder is much less well established than its use in acute mania. Clearly more research is necessary, but for the present, it may be reasonable to use carbamazepine for long-term prophylaxis either singly or with lithium in patients who have been treated with that regimen for their acute mania. The effectiveness of carbamazepine or any other prophylactic agent can only be judged after a sufficiently long period to compare the patient's rate of cycling on carbamazepine with the patient's prior rate of cycling. This will vary depending on the patient's base rate. Dosage for prophylaxis is not established; it is reasonable to use the same dosage that is effective for the patient during acute manic episodes and to decrease the dosage only if side effects may limit therapy. The current evidence suggests that carbamazepine may be more effective in prophylaxis against manic than against depressive recurrences.

The efficacy and safety of newer antidepressants for maintenance use in bipolar disorder are not established by placebo-controlled clinical trials, and few comparative data exist to choose between the newer antidepressants. In one small study, over the course of 1 year, bupropion had a lower likelihood of initiating a switch into mania than the tricyclic desipramine, but it is not free of risk. Similarly, in a controlled trial, imipramine yielded greater risk than paroxetine for inducing mania when added to lithium. Of note, in the same trial, neither antidepressant was superior to placebo in bipolar depression. As noted before, venlafaxine appears the most problematic of the newer antidepressants for inducing mania in depressed patients, so other agents are preferable in prophylaxis treatment of bipolar depression.

Prophylaxis for Rapid-Cycling Bipolar Disorder
A minority of bipolar patients has four or more recurrences in a year and is considered to have a rapid cycling course. Rapid cycling is more common in women. It occurs in pedigrees along with classic bipolar disorder, suggesting that it does not have a different genetic basis. Some patients have onset of rapid cycling while

being treated with antidepressants. All classes of antidepressants and even ECT have been implicated in initiating rapid cycling in some cases. It also has been reported that thyroid abnormalities may predispose to rapid cycling, although this finding has not always been replicated.

In general, patients with rapid cycling are less responsive to long-term treatment than patients with infrequent cycles. Although lithium had been thought to be less effective than valproate for rapid cycling, more recent studies suggest no difference. Hence, lithium as well as valproate should be considered for patients with rapid cycling. Lamotrigine, on the other hand, does not appear effective in preventing relapse in rapid cycling patients with bipolar I disorder, though it may be helpful in bipolar II patients. In either case, lamotrigine's role appears primarily for preventing depressive relapse. The second-generation antipsychotics are effective for acute mania for patients with or without rapid cycling. Evidence for long-term prophylaxis is less established, though one post-hoc analysis of a long-term study comparing divalproex with olanzapine found that in rapid-cycling patients, olanzapine was as effective as divalproex for preventing manic relapse. Hence, olanzapine, and perhaps the other second-generation antipsychotics, should be considered for prophylaxis of rapid cycling if more simple regimens are ineffective.

In managing rapidly cycling patients, it is useful to have the patient graphically chart mood state and medications. Thyroid abnormalities should be vigorously sought and treated. Many clinicians advocate administration of T_4 for TSH elevations even in the absence of abnormalities in free T_4 levels, although this has not been systematically studied. Trials of lithium or divalproex should not be terminated too quickly because some rapid cyclers will only begin to show improvement after a year of treatment, especially if antidepressants can be avoided. Clozapine, which is relatively free of EPS, has also shown promise in the treatment of rapidly cycling individuals.

Antidepressant drugs should be avoided if possible in rapid cyclers. Although the utility of discontinuing antidepressants as an intervention for the treatment of rapid cycling has never been studied systematically, it remains a prudent first-line intervention—especially given the lack of data supporting standard antidepressant use in bipolar depression—to discontinue antidepressants in rapid cycling. When used, however, antidepressants should be used for the shortest time possible. Venlafaxine appears more likely than the SSRIs or bupropion to induce mania and should be avoided in rapid cyclers. ECT may be the best antidepressant modality in some rapidly cycling patients, although it too may precipitate switches into mania.

Bibliography

Lithium

Pharmacology
Hardy BG, Shulman KI, Mackenzie SE, et al. Pharmacokinetics of lithium in the elderly. *J Clin Psychopharmacol* 1987;7:153.
Vitiello B, Behar D, Malone R, et al. Pharmacokinetics of lithium carbonate in children. *J Clin Psychopharmacol* 1988;8:355.

Mechanism of Action
Berridge MJ, Downes CP, Hanley MR. Neural and developmental actions of lithium: a unifying hypothesis. *Cell* 1989;59:411.
Klein PS, Melton DA. A molecular mechanism for the effect of lithium on development. *Proc Natl Acad Sci USA* 1996;93:8455.
Lenox RH, Wang L. Molecular basis of lithium action: integration of lithium-responsive signaling and gene expression networks. *Mol Psychiatry* 2003;8:135–144.

Indications

Mood Disorders
Black DW, Winokur G, Bell S, et al. Complicated mania. *Arch Gen Psychiatry* 1988;45:232.

Bowden CL, Brugger AM, Swann AC, et al. Efficacy of divalproex vs. lithium and placebo in the treatment of mania. *JAMA* 1994;271:918.

Calabrese JR, Goldberg JF, Ketter TA, et al. Recurrence in bipolar I disorder: a post hoc analysis excluding relapses in two double-blind maintenance studies. *Biol Psychiatry* 2006;59:1061–1064.

Calabrese JR, Shelton MD, Rapport DJ, et al. A 20-month, double-blind, maintenance trial of lithium versus divalproex in rapid-cycling bipolar disorder. *Am J Psychiatry* 2005;162(11):2152–2161.

Faedda GL, Tondo L, Baldessarini RJ, et al. Outcome after rapid vs. gradual discontinuation of lithium treatment in bipolar patients. *Arch Gen Psychiatry* 1993;50:448.

Gelenberg AJ, Kane JM, Keller MB, et al. Comparison of standard and low serum levels of lithium for maintenance treatment of bipolar disorder. *N Engl J Med* 1989;321:1489.

Hartong EG, Moleman P, Hoogduin CA, et al. LitCarGroup. Prophylactic efficacy of lithium versus carbamazepine in treatment-naive bipolar patients. *J Clin Psychiatry* 2003;64:144.

Price LH, Heninger GR. Lithium in the treatment of mood disorders. *N Engl J Med* 1994;331:591.

Prien RF, Kupfer DJ, Mansky PA, et al. Drug therapy in the prevention of recurrences in unipolar and bipolar affective disorders. *Arch Gen Psychiatry* 1984;41:1096.

Shapiro DR, Quitkin FM, Fleiss JL. Response to maintenance therapy in bipolar illness: effect of an index episode. *Arch Gen Psychiatry* 1989;46:401.

Suppes T, Baldessarini RJ, Faedda GL, et al. Risk of recurrence following discontinuation of lithium treatment in bipolar disorder. *Arch Gen Psychiatry* 1991;48:1082.

Method of Use
Cooper TB, Simpson GM. The 24-hour lithium level as a prognosticator of dosage requirements: a two-year follow-up study. *Am J Psychiatry* 1976;133:440.

Jefferson JW, Greist JH, Clagnaz PJ, et al. Effect of strenuous exercise on serum lithium level in man. *Am J Psychiatry* 1982;139:1593.

Perry PJ, Dunner FJ, Hahn RL, et al. Lithium kinetics in single daily dosing. *Acta Psychiatr Scand* 1981;64:281.

Side Effects and Toxicity

Acute Lithium Intoxication
Sadosty AT, Groleau GA, Atcherson MM. The use of lithium levels in the emergency department. *J Emerg Med* 1999;17:887–891.

Schou M. The recognition and management of lithium intoxication. In: Johnson FN, ed. *Handbook of lithium therapy*. Lancaster, England: MTP Press, 1980.

Lithium and the Kidney
Battle DC, von Riotte AB, Gavira M, et al. Amelioration of polyuria by amiloride in patients receiving long-term lithium therapy. *N Engl J Med* 1985;312:408.

Bowen RC, Grof P, Grof E. Less frequent lithium administration and lower urine volume. *Am J Psychiatry* 1991;148:189.

Raedler TJ, Wiedemann K. Lithium-induced nephropathies. *Psychopharmacol Bull* 2007;40:134–149.

Schou M. Forty years of lithium treatment. *Arch Gen Psychiatry* 1997;54:9.

Thomsen K, Schou M. Avoidance of lithium intoxication: advice based on knowledge about the renal lithium clearance under various circumstances. *Pharmacopsychiatry* 1999;32:83.

Neurologic Toxicities
Apte SN, Langston JW. Permanent neurological deficits due to lithium toxicity. *Ann Neurol* 1983;13:452.

Engelsmann F, Katz J, Ghadirian AM, et al. Lithium and memory: a long-term follow-up study. *J Clin Psychopharmacol* 1988;8:207.

Joffe RT, MacDonald C, Kutcher SP. Lack of differential cognitive effects of lithium and carbamazepine in bipolar affective disorder. *J Clin Psychopharmacol* 1988;8:425.

Kores B, Lader MH. Irreversible lithium neurotoxicity: an overview. *Clin Neuropharmacol* 1997;20:283–299.

Saul RF, Hamberger HA, Selhorst JB. Pseudotumor cerebri secondary to lithium carbonate. *JAMA* 1985;253:2869.

Other Toxicities

Bowden CL, Calabrese JR, Ketter TA, et al. Impact of lamotrigine and lithium on weight in obese and nonobese patients with bipolar I disorder. *Am J Psychiatry* 2006;163:1199–1201.

Deandrea D, Walker N, Mehlmauer M, et al. Dermatological reactions to lithium: a critical review of the literature. *J Clin Psychopharmacol* 1982;2:199.

Franks RD, Dubovsky SL, Lifshitz M, et al. Long-term lithium carbonate therapy causes hyperparathyroidism. *Arch Gen Psychiatry* 1982;39:1074.

Garland EJ, Remick RA, Zis AP. Weight gain with antidepressants and lithium. *J Clin Psychopharmacol* 1988;8:323.

Mitchell JE, Mackenzie TB. Cardiac effects of lithium therapy in man: a review. *J Clin Psychiatry* 1982;43:47.

Yassa R, Saunders A, Nastase C, et al. Lithium-induced thyroid disorders: a prevalence study. *J Clin Psychiatry* 1988;48:14.

Drug Interactions

Miller F, Meninger J. Lithium-neuroleptic neurotoxicity is dose dependent. *J Clin Psychopharmacol* 1987;7:89.

Phelan KM, Mosholder AD, Lu S. Lithium interaction with the cyclooxygenase 2 inhibitors rofecoxib and celecoxib and other nonsteroidal anti-inflammatory drugs. *J Clin Psychiatry* 2003;64(11):1328–1334.

Use in Pregnancy

Cohen LS, Friedman JM, Jefferson JW, et al. A reevaluation of risk of in utero exposure to lithium. *JAMA* 1994;271:146.

Licht RW, Vestergaard P, Kessing LV, et al. Psychopharmacological treatment with lithium and antiepileptic drugs: suggested guidelines from the Danish Psychiatric Association and the Child and Adolescent Psychiatric Association in Denmark. *Acta Psychiatr Scand Suppl* 2003;(419):1.

Newport DJ, Viguera AC, Beach AJ, et al. Lithium placental passage and obstetrical outcome: implications for clinical management during late pregnancy. *Am J Psychiatry* 2005;162:2162–2170.

Viguera AC, Whitfield T, Baldessarini RJ, et al. Risk of recurrence in women with bipolar disorder during pregnancy: prospective study of mood stabilizer discontinuation. *Am J Psychiatry* 2007;164(12):1817–1824.

Viguera AC, Newport DJ, Ritchie J, et al. Lithium in breast milk and nursing infants: clinical implications. *Am J Psychiatry* 2007;164:342–345.

Valproic Acid

Use in Bipolar Disorder

Bowden CL, Brugger AM, Swann AC, et al. Efficacy of divalproex vs lithium and placebo in the treatment of mania. The Depakote Mania Study Group. *JAMA* 1994;271:918.

Bowden CL, Swann AC, Calabrese JR, et al. A randomized, placebo-controlled, multicenter study of divalproex sodium extended release in the treatment of acute mania. *J Clin Psychiatry* 2006;67:1501–1510.

Calabrese JR, Shelton MD, Rapport DJ, et al. A 20-month, double-blind, maintenance trial of lithium versus divalproex in rapid-cycling bipolar disorder. *Am J Psychiatry* 2005;162:2152–2161.

Swann AC, Bowden CL, Morris D, et al. Depression during mania. Treatment response to lithium or divalproex. *Arch Gen Psychiatry* 1997;54:37.

Side Effects and Toxicity

Bryant AE III, Dreifuss FE. Valproic acid hepatic fatalities. III. U.S. experience since 1986. *Neurology* 1996;46:465–469.

Joffe H, Cohen LS, Suppes T, et al. Longitudinal follow-up of reproductive and metabolic features of valproate-associated polycystic ovarian syndrome features: A preliminary report. *Biol Psychiatry* 2006;60(12):1378–1381.

Smith MC, Black TP. Convulsive disorders: toxicity of anti-convulsants. *Clin Pharmacol* 1991;14:97.

Wisner KL, Perel JM. Serum levels of valproate and carbamazepine in breastfeeding mother-infant pairs. *J Clin Psychopharmacol* 1998;18:167.

Carbamazepine

Use in Bipolar Disorder

Greil W, Kleindienst N, Erazo N, et al. Differential response to lithium and carbamazepine in the prophylaxis of bipolar disorder. *J Clin Psychopharmacol* 1998;18:455.

Hartong EG, Moleman P, Hoogduin CA, et al. Prophylactic efficacy of lithium versus carbamazepine in treatment-naive bipolar patients. *J Clin Psychiatry* 2003;64:144.

Weisler RH, Kalali AH, Ketter TA; SPD417 Study Group. A multicenter, randomized, double-blind, placebo-controlled trial of extended-release carbamazepine capsules as monotherapy for bipolar disorder patients with manic or mixed episodes. *J Clin Psychiatry* 2004;65:478.

Weisler RH, Keck PE Jr, Swann AC, et al. Extended-release carbamazepine capsules as monotherapy for acute mania in bipolar disorder: a multicenter, randomized, double-blind, placebo-controlled trial. *J Clin Psychiatry* 2005;66:323–330.

Side Effects and Toxicity

Hart RG, Easton JD. Carbamazepine and hematological monitoring. *Ann Neurol* 1982;11:309.

Heh CW, Sramek J, Herrera J, et al. Exacerbation of psychosis after discontinuation of carbamazepine treatment. *Am J Psychiatry* 1988;145:878.

Joffe RT, Post RM, Roy-Byrne PP, et al. Hematological effects of carbamazepine in patients with affective illness. *Am J Psychiatry* 1985;142:1196.

Drug Interactions

Ketter TA, Post RM, Worthington K. Principles of clinically important drug interactions with carbamazepine: parts I and II. *J Clin Psychopharmacol* 1991;11:198.

Perucca E. Clinically relevant drug interactions with antiepileptic drugs. *Br J Clin Pharmacol* 2006;61:246–255.

Use in Pregnancy

Altshuler LL, Cohen L, Szuba MP, et al. Pharmacologic management of psychiatric illness during pregnancy: dilemmas and guidelines. *Am J Psychiatry* 1996;152:592.

Jones KL, Johnson KA, Adams J. Pattern of malformations in children of women treated with carbamazepine during pregnancy. *N Engl J Med* 1989;320:1661.

Meador KJ, Baker GA, Finnell RH, et al. In utero antiepileptic drug exposure: fetal death and malformations. *Neurology* 2006;67(3):407–412.

Rosa FW. Spina bifida in infants of women treated with carbamazepine during pregnancy. *N Engl J Med* 1991;324:674.

Lamotrigine

Aldenkamp AP, Arends J, Bootsma HP, et al. Randomized double-blind parallel-group study comparing cognitive effects of a low-dose lamotrigine with valproateand placebo in healthy volunteers. *Epilepsia* 2002;43:19.

Bowden CL, Calabrese JR, Sachs G, et al. A placebo-controlled 18-month trial of lamotrigine and lithium maintenance treatment in recently manic or hypomanic patients with bipolar I disorder. *Arch Gen Psychiatry* 2003;60:392.

Calabrese JR, Bowden CL, Sachs GS, et al. A double-blind placebo-controlled study of lamotrigine monotherapy in outpatients with bipolar I depression. Lamictal 602 Study Group. *J Clin Psychiatry* 1999;60:79.

Chen C, Veronese L, Yin Y. The effects of lamotrigine on the pharmacokinetics of lithium. *Br J Clin Pharmacol* 2000;50:193.

Goodwin GM, Bowden CL, Calabrese JR, et al. A pooled analysis of 2 placebo-controlled 18-month trials of lamotrigine and lithium maintenance in bipolar I disorder. *J Clin Psychiatry* 2004;65:432–441.

Gabapentin

Obrocea GV, Dunn RM, Frye MA, et al. Clinical predictors of response to lamotrigine and gabapentin monotherapy in refractory affective disorders. *Biol Psychiatry* 2002;51:253.

Vieta E, Manuel Goikolea J, Martínez-Arán A, et al. A double-blind, randomized, placebo-controlled, prophylaxis study of adjunctive gabapentin for bipolar disorder. *J Clin Psychiatry* 2006;67(3):473–477.

Topiramate

Evins AE. Efficacy of newer anticonvulsant medications in bipolar spectrum mood disorders. *J Clin Psychiatry* 2003;64(suppl 8):9.

Marcotte D. Use of topiramate, a new anti-epileptic as a mood stabilizer. *Affect Disord* 1998;50:245.

McElroy SL, Frye MA, Altshuler LL, et al. A 24-week, randomized, controlled trial of adjunctive sibutramine versus topiramate in the treatment of weight gain in overweight or obese patients with bipolar disorders. *Bipolar Disord* 2007;9:426–434.

McIntyre RS, Mancini DA, McCann S, et al. Topiramate versus bupropion SR when added to mood stabilizer therapy for the depressive phase of bipolar disorder: a preliminary single-blind study. *Bipolar Disord* 2002;4:207.

Antipsychotics and Other Agents

Ghaemi SN, Hsu DJ, Rosenquist KJ. Extrapyramidal side effects with atypical neuroleptics in bipolar disorder. *Prog Neuropsychopharmacol Biol Psychiatry* 2006;30(2):209–213.

Khanna S, Vieta E, Lyons B, et al. Risperidone in the treatment of acute mania: double-blind, placebo-controlled study. *Br J Psychiatry* 2005;187:229–234.

Keck PE Jr, Versiani M, Potkin S, et al. Ziprasidone in the treatment of acute bipolar mania: a three-week, placebo-controlled, double-blind, randomized trial. *Am J Psychiatry* 2003;160:741.

Keck PE Jr, Mintz J, McElroy SL, et al. Double-blind, randomized, placebo-controlled trials of ethyl-eicosapentanoate in the treatment of bipolar depression and rapid cycling bipolar disorder. *Biol Psychiatry* 2006;60(9):1020–1022.

Keck PE Jr, Calabrese JR, McIntyre RS, et al. Aripiprazole monotherapy for maintenance therapy in bipolar I disorder: a 100-week, double-blind study versus placebo. *J Clin Psychiatry* 2007;68:1480–1491.

Sachs G, Sanchez R, Marcus R, et al. Aripiprazole in the treatment of acute manic or mixed episodes in patients with bipolar I disorder: a 3-week placebo-controlled study. *J Psychopharmacol* 2006;20(4):536–546.

Stoll AL, Severus WE, Freeman MP, et al. Omega 3 fatty acids in bipolar disorder: a preliminary double-blind, placebo-controlled trial. *Arch Gen Psychiatry* 1999;56:407.

Suppes T, Webb A, Paul B, et al. Clinical outcome in a randomized 1-year trial of clozapine versus treatment as usual for patients with treatment-resistant illness and a history of mania. *Am J Psychiatry* 1999;156:1164.

Thase ME, Macfadden W, Weisler RH, et al. Efficacy of quetiapine monotherapy in bipolar I and II depression: a double-blind, placebo-controlled study (the BOLDER II study). *J Clin Psychopharmacol* 2006;26:600–609.

Tohen M, Ketter TA, Zarate CA, et al. Olanzapine versus divalproex sodium for the treatment of acute mania and maintenance of remission: a 47-week study. *Am J Psychiatry* 2003;160:1263.

Tohen M, Sanger TM, McElroy SL, et al. Olanzapine versus placebo in the treatment of acute mania. *Am J Psychiatry* 1999;156:702.

Tohen M, Vieta E, Calabrese J, et al. Efficacy of olanzapine and olanzapine-fluoxetine combination in the treatment of bipolar I depression. *Arch Gen Psychiatry* 2003;60:1079.

Yatham LN, Grossman F, Augustyns I, et al. Mood stabilisers plus risperidone or placebo in the treatment of acute mania. International, double-blind, randomised controlled trial. *Br J Psychiatry* 2003;182:141–147.

Zarate CA, Tohen M, Baldessarini RJ. Clozapine in severe mood disorders. *J Clin Psychiatry* 1995;56:411.

Bipolar Depression

Frank E, Kupfer DJ, Thase ME, et al. Two-year outcomes for interpersonal and social rhythm therapy in individuals with bipolar I disorder. *Arch Gen Psychiatry* 2005;62(9):996–1004.

Goldberg JF, Perlis RH, Ghaemi SN, et al. Adjunctive antidepressant use and symptomatic recovery among bipolar depressed patients with concomitant manic symptoms: findings from the STEP-BD. *Am J Psychiatry* 2007;164:1348–1355.

Leverich GS, Altshuler LL, Frye MA, et al. Risk of switch in mood polarity to hypomania or mania in patients with bipolar depression during acute and continuation trials of venlafaxine, sertraline, and bupropion as adjuncts to mood stabilizers. *Am J Psychiatry* 2006;163(2):232–239.

Miklowitz DJ, Otto MW. Psychosocial interventions for bipolar disorder: a review of literature and introduction of the systematic treatment enhancement program. *Psychopharmacol Bull* 2007;40:116–131.

Post RM, Altshuler LL, Leverich GS, et al. Mood switch in bipolar depression: comparison of adjunctive venlafaxine, bupropion and sertraline. *Br J Psychiatry* 2006;189:124–131.

Sachs GS, Nierenberg AA, Calabrese JR, et al. Effectiveness of adjunctive antidepressant treatment for bipolar depression. *N Engl J Med* 2007;356:1711–1722.

Yatham LN, Kennedy SH, O'Donovan C, et al. Canadian Network for Mood and Anxiety Treatments (CANMAT) guidelines for the management of patients with bipolar disorder: update 2007. *Bipolar Disord* 2006;8(6):721–739.

Zarate CA Jr, Payne JL, Singh J. Pramipexole for bipolar II depression: a placebo-controlled proof of concept study. *Biol Psychiatry* 2004;56:54–60.

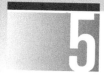

Drugs for the Treatment of Anxiety Disorders

Anxiety is a ubiquitous human emotion. Most instances of anxiety do not call for medical treatment. However, anxiety can become severe enough to cause severe distress and produce disability; in such circumstances, treatment is warranted. Anxiety may be (a) a normal response to stressful life events, (b) a symptom of an anxiety disorder, (c) a symptom of another psychiatric disorder such as depression, or (d) a symptom of a medical illness, such as hyperthyroidism.

GENERALIZED ANXIETY DISORDER

Generalized anxiety disorder (GAD) is characterized by unrealistic and excessive worry and anxiety (occurring more days than not for at least 6 months), accompanied by three or more of specific anxiety symptoms such as restlessness (or feeling keyed up), being easily fatigued, difficulty concentrating, irritability, muscle tension, and difficulty falling asleep or staying asleep. Although the focus of the worry may shift, it is present even in the absence of a clear stressor, with excessive concern about minor day-to-day matters. For this diagnosis, the symptoms must cause substantial distress and psychosocial impairment and cannot be the result of another psychiatric or medical disorder. The lifetime prevalence of GAD is estimated to range between 4.1% and 6.6% in the general population, with a point prevalence of 1.2% to 1.6%. As with many anxiety disorders, women are twice as likely to suffer from GAD as men. Although the age of onset is typically before 25 years, GAD may present at any age. The lifetime psychiatric comorbidity of GAD is about 90%. Between 40% and 50% of GAD patients have comorbid major depressive disorder (MDD), and panic disorder and substance abuse/dependence also commonly co-occur with GAD. Risk factors for GAD include a family history of GAD, an increase in psychosocial stressors, and a history of physical or emotional trauma. Family and genetic studies and the high likelihood of comorbidity suggest that GAD may share risk factors with MDD. A recent study reported that a genetic variant of the serotonin transporter gene may predispose individuals to both GAD and MDD. GAD is highly persistent, with only one third of the patients having spontaneous remissions. It is important to carefully consider the differential diagnosis prior to diagnosing GAD because even when presented by the patient as the chief complaint, **generalized anxiety symptoms are often features of other major psychiatric disorders** or medical disorders or may be secondary to medications or drugs (secondary anxiety). Anxiety symptoms often accompany depression, manic or mixed affective states, psychoses, obsessive-compulsive disorder (OCD), and other psychiatric disorders. They also may be the manifestation of medical illnesses such as angina, congestive heart failure, arrhythmias, asthma and other obstructive pulmonary diseases, and hyperthyroidism, or they may result from overuse of drugs to treat asthma, stimulants, thyroid supplements, caffeine, or over-the-counter decongestants or appetite suppressants. **Secondary anxiety** also may be the result of withdrawal from alcohol or other central nervous system (CNS) depressants or abuse of psychostimulants such as cocaine. Secondary generalized anxiety is best approached in the long term by treatment of the underlying disorder. However, in many situations, short-term or intermittent use of adjunctive benzodiazepines or selective serotonin reuptake inhibitors (SSRIs) may be helpful, whereas in situations resulting in agitation or psychosis, antipsychotic drugs may provide a preferable form of anxiolysis. In medically ill patients with delirium, dementia, or decreased respiratory drive, a benzodiazepine may prove harmful.

Diagnosis

1. Unrealistic and excessive ongoing worry and anxiety (occurring more days than not for at least 6 months) about a number of events or activities.
2. Three or more specific anxiety symptoms such as restlessness (or feeling keyed up), being easily fatigued, difficulty concentrating, irritability, muscle tension, and difficulty falling asleep or restless sleep.
3. A careful medical and psychiatric history should be obtained to rule out medical and psychiatric disorders that may cause significant anxiety.

Laboratory testing is warranted if a medical diagnosis, such as hyperthyroidism, is suspected.

Pharmacologic Treatment

Antidepressants

The Food and Drug Administration (FDA) approval of duloxetine, venlafaxine, paroxetine, and escitalopram for the treatment of GAD underscores the safety and efficacy of antidepressants for this disorder. Indeed, when studied in the past, even tricyclics proved to be as efficacious as the benzodiazepines. The choice of drug class can thus be made on the basis of side-effect profile, comorbidity, and the patient's ability to tolerate the delayed onset of antidepressant effects. Specifically, antidepressants would be favored when depression is also present, and they may be better tolerated in the long term, which is particularly relevant to chronic anxiety disorders such as GAD. SSRIs are often used in the treatment of GAD. Only two of the SSRIs (paroxetine and escitalopram) are FDA approved for the treatment of GAD, but this is likely to represent selective research and marketing. Other SSRIs are often used off-label, partly because of positive placebo-controlled studies, as in the case of sertraline and fluvoxamine, and because of a lack of data demonstrating superior efficacy for any one SSRI compared with another. (See Chapter 3 for a description of the pharmacology of SSRIs.) The **dosing of the SSRIs used in the treatment of GAD is similar to that used in the treatment of depression** (e.g., paroxetine dosages range from 20 to 50 mg per day), although higher dosages may be clinically indicated for refractory patients. Studies have suggested that the benefit of SSRI pharmacotherapy persists over the long term, with significantly lower recurrences of GAD among those continuing SSRI treatment for 6 months compared with a switch to placebo. Recent studies have shown that the addition of nonbenzodiazepine hypnotics such as eszopiclone and sustained-release zolpidem can augment the efficacy of SSRIs in the treatment of sleep disturbances among patients with GAD and insomnia, and another nonbenzodiazepine hypnotic agent eszopiclone can be used in the treatment of anxiety symptoms as well.

Serotonin-norepinephrine reuptake inhibitors (SNRIs), such as venlafaxine and duloxetine, are also good options for the treatment of GAD, and have been approved by the FDA for the treatment of this disorder. The recently approved desvenlafaxine is not approved for the treatment of GAD but is at times used off-label. (See Chapter 3 for a description of the pharmacology of SNRIs.) The dosing of venlafaxine and duloxetine used in the treatment of GAD is similar to that used in the treatment of depression (e.g., dosages ranging from 75 to 225 mg per day for venlafaxine and from 60 to 120 mg per day for duloxetine), although clinically higher dosages, at least for venlafaxine, may be of benefit for some treatment-refractory patients.

Tricyclic antidepressants (TCAs) such as imipramine and nortriptyline are also used off-label in the treatment of GAD, although typically only after other pharmacologic treatments have failed. They are second-line treatments because of

TABLE 5.1 Available Benzodiazepine Preparations for Anxiety			
Preparations	**Regular Oral Dose Forms (mg)**	**Slow-Release Forms (mg)**	**Available Parenteral Forms**
Alprazolam (Xanax)	0.25, 0.5, 1.0, 2.0 (tablet)	0.5, 1.0, 2.0, 3.0 (tablet XR)	
Chlordiazepoxide (Librium)[a]	5, 10, 25 (capsule)		100 mg/2 mL (ampule)
Clonazepam (Klonopin)	0.5, 1.0, 2.0 (tablet) 0.125, 0.25, 0.5, 1.0, 2.0 (wafer)		
Clorazepate (Tranxene)	3.75, 7.5, 15.0 (tablet)	11.25, 22.5	
Diazepam (Valium)	2, 5, 10 (tablet)	15	10 mg/2 mL (ampule or syringe) 50 mg/10 mL (vial)
Lorazepam (Ativan)	0.5, 1.0, 2.0 (tablet)		20 mg/10 mL; 40 mg/10 mL (vial) 2 mg/mL; 4 mg/mL (syringe)
Oxazepam (Serax)	10, 15, 30 (capsule)		

[a]Available with clidinium bromide (Librax, Clipoxide) and amitriptyline (Limbitrol).

their side-effect profile; indeed, anxious patients may be particularly intolerant of the side effects of tricyclics. (See Chapter 3 for a description of the pharmacology of TCAs.) The typical dosing of TCAs used in the treatment of GAD appears to be somewhat lower than that used in the treatment of depression (e.g., imipramine dosage ranging from 50 to 200 mg per day).

Benzodiazepines

Benzodiazepines are efficacious for treatment of GAD. Several benzodiazepines (see Table 5.1 for a list of benzodiazepines with an anxiety or anxiety disorder indication) have demonstrated efficacy in the treatment of GAD compared to placebo. Generally, low-potency, long-acting benzodiazepines are considered to be safe and effective. High-potency, short-acting compounds, such as the immediate-release formulation of alprazolam, although effective as well, carry a higher risk of dependence and interdose rebound symptoms, unless an extended-release formulation is used. Typically, dosages of 15 to 30 mg per day of diazepam or the equivalent are effective, but occasional patients have required the equivalent of 40 to 60 mg per day of diazepam. Similarly, daily doses of clonazepam between 0.5 and 2 mg, alprazolam (in its sustained-release formulation) doses between 1.0 and 4 mg, and lorazepam doses between 2 and 8 mg are typically used in the treatment of GAD. Some patients with generalized anxiety improve with short-term treatment (2 to 6 weeks), but the majority will have recurrences if treatment is stopped at that time. **Long-term treatment appears to be safe and effective for many patients,** who may continue their medication for years; nonetheless, it is worth trying to taper the medication slowly and periodically to see if the underlying condition

| | | **TABLE** 5.2 | Pharmacologic Characteristics of Available Benzodiazepines for Anxiety | | |

Preparations	Oral Dose Elimination Equivalency (mg)	Onset After Oral Dose	Distribution Half-life	Half-life (h)[a]
Alprazolam (Xanax)	0.5	Intermediate	Intermediate	6–20
Chlordiazepoxide (Librium)	10.0	Intermediate	Slow	30–100
Clonazepam (Klonopin)	0.25	Intermediate	Intermediate	18–40
Clorazepate[b] (Tranxene)	7.5	Rapid	Rapid	30–100
Diazepam (Valium)	5.0	Rapid	Rapid	30–100
Lorazepam (Ativan)	1.0	Intermediate	Intermediate	10–20
Oxazepam (Serax)	15.0	Intermediate–slow	Intermediate	8–12

[a]The elimination half-life represents the total for all active metabolites; elderly patients tend to have the longer half-lives in the range reported. Chlordiazepoxide, clorazepate, and diazepam have desmethyldiazepam as a long-acting active metabolite. With chronic dosing, these active metabolites represent most of the pharmacodynamic effect of these drugs.
[b]Clorazepate is an inactive prodrug for desmethyldiazepam, which is the active compound in the blood.

has remitted. When tapering medication, it is important to distinguish recurrence of the original symptoms from **transient rebound or withdrawal symptoms.**

The benzodiazepines are a group of closely related compounds. The name benzodiazepine is derived from the fact that the structures are composed of a benzene ring fused to a seven-member diazepine ring. A large number of benzodiazepines (Table 5.1) are currently available. The benzodiazepines are rarely associated with death from overdose in the absence of other drugs. The effectiveness and relative safety of the benzodiazepines have led to their extensive use in the treatment of GAD. Benzodiazepines should be **avoided in patients with a history of alcohol or drug abuse unless there is a compelling indication,** no good alternative, and close follow-up. Most benzodiazepines are well absorbed when given orally on an empty stomach; many achieve peak plasma levels within 1 to 3 hours, although there is a wide range among the benzodiazepine drugs approved for anxiety or anxiety disorders (Table 5.2). Antacids seriously interfere with benzodiazepine absorption; thus, benzodiazepines should be taken well ahead of any antacid dose. The rate of onset of action after an orally administered benzodiazepine (Table 5.2) is not an important variable in choosing a drug for the treatment of GAD, as the symptoms are chronic in nature. The available benzodiazepines differ markedly in the rate of onset of their therapeutic effect (Table 5.2), offering a wide choice of drugs to fit the patient's needs. For benzodiazepines, simple half-life data are potentially misleading regarding duration of clinical effect. Clinical efficacy depends on the presence of at least a minimum effective concentration in the blood, which is reflected by levels in well-perfused tissues such as those in the brain. After a single dose, the levels may decrease to ineffective concentrations, either by being distributed into peripheral tissues, such as fat (α-phase), or by metabolic inactivation or elimination from the body altogether (β-phase). The volume of distribution represents the size of the pool of tissues into which the drug may be drawn; this is determined by the drug's lipid solubility and tissue-binding properties. With repeated drug dosing, its volume of distribution becomes saturated, and the elimination half-life becomes the more important parameter in describing its behavior. Benzodiazepines differ markedly in their half-lives of distribution and elimination, producing varying clinical effects. For example, the distribution half-life (α-phase) of oral diazepam is 2.5 hours, whereas the elimination half-life (β-phase) is more than 30 hours. Desmethyldiazepam, diazepam's major active metabolite, extends the overall elimination half-life to 60 to 100 hours (up to 200 hours in elderly patients). This means that a single dose of diazepam will be active for a relatively short period based on the rapid distribution of the drug, whereas with repeated administration, **elimination half-life becomes the important parameter to consider,** making diazepam a very long-acting drug (i.e., one that will accumulate in the body to high levels). Conversely, despite the relatively short elimination half-life of lorazepam (10 hours) and its lack of active metabolites, it has a smaller volume of distribution than diazepam and therefore a longer action when given as a single dose. Another important clinical issue related to duration of effect applies to the use of the high-potency, short-acting benzodiazepines, immediate-release alprazolam and, to a lesser extent, lorazepam. Such drugs pose a potential clinical problem because their high potency may make them more liable to cause dependence and their rapid termination of effect unmasks any dependence that develops. Patients may therefore experience rebound symptoms. Such problems can be addressed by switching to longer-acting drugs when indicated (e.g., replacing alprazolam with clonazepam).

Metabolism. Except for lorazepam and oxazepam, the commonly used benzodiazepines in the treatment of GAD are metabolized by hepatic microsomal enzymes to form demethylated, hydroxylated, and other oxidized products that are pharmacologically active. Most of the benzodiazepines are substrates of the cytochrome P450 3A4; therefore, they tend to accumulate when coadministered with inhibitors of such pathways. The active metabolites of benzodiazepines are, in turn, conjugated with glucuronic acid; the resulting glucuronides are inactive, and, because they are more water soluble than the parent compounds, they are readily excreted in the urine. Some of the active metabolites of benzodiazepines, such as desmethyldiazepam, have extremely long half-lives and with repeat dosing may come to represent most of the pharmacologically active compound in serum. In contrast, under normal circumstances (e.g., excluding cirrhosis) the active metabolic products of alprazolam are of little clinical importance. **Lorazepam and oxazepam are metabolized only by conjugation** with glucuronic acid with no intermediate steps, and they have no active metabolites. Unlike the pathways involved in the initial metabolism of other benzodiazepines, glucuronidation is less affected by aging and liver disease; thus, if benzodiazepines are to be used in elderly patients or those with cirrhosis, lorazepam and oxazepam are the drugs of choice. In liver cirrhosis, the elimination of benzodiazepines metabolized by oxidation and demethylation may be reduced by as much as fivefold; thus, routine doses could lead to toxicity. In cirrhosis, even alprazolam may accumulate to dangerous levels.

Mechanism of Action. Acting through its γ-aminobutyric acid A (GABA$_A$) receptor, the amino acid neurotransmitter GABA is the major inhibitory neurotransmitter in the brain. GABA$_A$ receptors are ligand-gated channels, meaning that the neurotransmitter-binding site and an effector ion channel are part of the same macromolecular complex. Because GABA$_A$ receptor channels selectively admit the anion chloride into neurons, activation of GABA$_A$ receptors hyperpolarizes neurons and thus is inhibitory on neuronal firing. **Benzodiazepines produce their effects by binding to a specific site on the GABA$_A$ receptor.** The pharmacology of GABA$_A$ receptors is complex; GABA$_A$ receptors are the primary site of action not only of benzodiazepines but also of barbiturates and of some of the intoxicating effects of ethanol. GABA$_A$ receptors comprise multiple subunits. GABA$_A$/benzodiazepine receptors have a pentameric structure made up of a coassembly of subunits. There are six known α, four β, three γ, two p, and one δ subunits. GABA$_A$ receptors in the brain are most commonly composed of different subtypes of α, β, and γ subunits, with different subunit composition in different brain regions. Series of transgenic mice have been constructed in which each α-subunit was genetically disrupted by a point mutation. This selective inactivation strategy revealed that GABA$_A$ receptors containing the α1 subunit mediate sedation, anterograde amnesia, and part of the seizure protection, whereas GABA$_A$ receptors containing α2 subunits are thought to mediate the anxiolytic effects of benzodiazepines. This finding has led to attempts to develop drugs that selectively interact with different GABA$_A$ receptor subtypes. Benzodiazepines, barbiturates, and alcohol allosterically regulate the GABA$_A$ receptor (changing its conformation) so that it has a greater affinity for its neurotransmitter GABA. At higher doses, barbiturates and ethanol, but not benzodiazepines, can also open the chloride channel within the receptor independent of GABA. The fact that benzodiazepines, barbiturates, and ethanol all have related actions on a common receptor explains their pharmacologic synergy (and therefore the dangers of combined overdose) and their cross-tolerance. Their cross-tolerance is exploited in detoxification of alcoholics with benzodiazepines.

Clinical Uses of Benzodiazepines in GAD. Most patients do not misuse or become addicted to benzodiazepines, though a prior history of alcohol or other substance abuse is a relative contraindication to the use of benzodiazepines. Patients with a history of substance abuse or dependence may become addicted to benzodiazepines. Clinically, the major pharmacologic problem with benzodiazepines is their tendency to cause physiologic dependence, that is, a risk of significant discontinuation symptoms, especially with long-term use. Discontinuation symptoms may pose a serious clinical problem in some patients, causing worsening of (rebound) insomnia, distress, or inability to discontinue treatment. Prior to starting a benzodiazepine, patients should be cautioned about possible sedation and warned not to drive vehicles or operate dangerous machinery until it is determined that the dose does not affect performance. Patients should be instructed to take their medication on an empty stomach and not concomitantly with antacids because meals and antacids may decrease absorption.

When starting benzodiazepines for the treatment of GAD, lower doses (e.g., diazepam, 2 to 5 mg three times daily) should be used initially to **assess patient sensitivity to the drug and to avoid initial oversedation.** The dosage can be slowly increased until a therapeutic effect occurs. Dosage titration with long-acting drugs (e.g., diazepam, chlordiazepoxide, or clorazepate) should proceed more slowly because the drugs reach steady-state levels over a period of several days. Dosages of short-acting drugs (e.g., lorazepam or alprazolam) can be increased more rapidly (e.g., after 2 days).

In follow-up, patients should be asked not only about efficacy but also about side effects. Patients who complain of excessive sedation may do better with a temporary dosage reduction; over time, most individuals develop tolerance to sedative effects. Patients on short-acting compounds such as alprazolam should be questioned about interdose rebound anxiety, which can be addressed by increasing dosing frequency or using the extended-release formulation. Intolerance to or lack of efficacy of a benzodiazepine may result from pharmacokinetic factors, as with sedation or interdose rebound, and thus may improve with the switch to an agent with a different profile (e.g., alprazolam to clonazepam). An alternative approach is the switch to another class of drugs (e.g., an antidepressant).

Tolerance and Discontinuation Symptoms with Benzodiazepines. The benzodiazepines may induce physiologic dependence. Physiologic dependence must be distinguished from addiction, which is defined as compulsive, out of control use of a drug despite negative consequences. Addiction to benzodiazepines in nonsubstance abusers may occur, but is rare. Dependence, which occurs with many classes of both psychotropic and nonpsychotropic medications, represents an adapted state of the body to the drug, such that symptoms emerge on tapering of doses, discontinuation of the drug, or even between doses. Discontinuation symptoms can be conceptually divided into (a) recurrence of the original disorder, (b) rebound (a marked temporary return of original symptoms), and (c) withdrawal (recurrence of the original symptoms plus new symptoms, which for benzodiazepines might include tachycardia or elevations in blood pressure). In clinical practice, these syndromes demonstrate a great deal of overlap and frequently coexist. The nature of the symptoms and their time course may help in making distinctions.

Recurrences reflect the loss of therapeutic benefit and typically do not subside with time; the symptoms are generally indistinguishable from those present prior to treatment. Generally, the response to recurrence of the original disorder is resumption of therapy.

Rebound symptoms occur soon after discontinuation and generally represent a return of original symptoms, such as anxiety or insomnia, but at a greater intensity than the original symptoms. The response to rebound symptoms is to observe whether they resolve quickly or to resume therapy and then taper the benzodiazepine more slowly. For some high-potency compounds with a short half-life, such as alprazolam, rebound symptoms occasionally occur even during maintenance therapy as blood levels between doses reach their nadir. If interdose rebound symptoms or rebound occurring with attempts to decrease the dosage represent a serious clinical problem, a switch to a compound with a longer half-life may prove helpful.

The onset of withdrawal symptoms generally reflects the half-life of the drug used, usually 1 to 2 days after the last dose for short-acting drugs, 2 to 5 days for long-acting drugs (although symptoms beginning as late as 7 to 10 days have been reported). Withdrawal symptoms generally peak days after onset and slowly disappear over 1 to 3 weeks. In contrast to recurrence and rebound, **withdrawal syndromes include symptoms that the patient has not previously experienced.** Benzodiazepine withdrawal symptoms include anxiety, irritability, insomnia, tremulousness, sweating, anorexia, nausea, diarrhea, abdominal discomfort, lethargy, fatigue, tachycardia, systolic hypertension, delirium, and seizures.

The risk of developing dependence and thus rebound and withdrawal symptoms is higher with long-term treatment, higher doses, and higher-potency drugs. The likelihood and severity of rebound and withdrawal symptoms also reflect the half-life of the compound; such symptoms occur more frequently and are generally more severe with compounds with a short half-life.

Although dependence can be induced by any benzodiazepine, rebound and withdrawal symptoms are relatively uncommon with low-potency and long-acting drugs and are typically mild and self-limited when they do occur. Dependence is most likely, and rebound and withdrawal symptoms are most severe with short-acting benzodiazepines, such as alprazolam and lorazepam. These are the compounds that are most likely to produce delirium and seizures after abrupt discontinuation from high doses. In addition to the more common benzodiazepine withdrawal symptoms, severe dysphoria and psychotic-like symptoms have been reported in patients discontinuing alprazolam. Because they are atypical, these symptoms may be extremely confusing on presentation unless a history of alprazolam discontinuation is obtained.

For some patients, discontinuation of alprazolam may be easier via a switch to equipotent doses of a longer-acting, high-potency benzodiazepine such as clonazepam (see next section on switching from alprazolam to clonazepam). A small number of reports also have suggested that anticonvulsants such as carbamazepine, valproic acid, and gabapentin (Neurontin) may be useful adjuncts for alprazolam withdrawal. Although this strategy may aid an individual patient, a large controlled study failed to show evidence of efficacy for carbamazepine.

Switching from Alprazolam to Clonazepam. Despite the apparently equivalent efficacy of alprazolam and clonazepam for anxiety disorders and the recent introduction of the extended-release formulation of alprazolam, which has greatly reduced the need for a switch, there are still clinical circumstances in which it is helpful to switch patients from alprazolam to clonazepam. These circumstances include significant interdose rebound anxiety or difficulty with tapering and discontinuing alprazolam. As described previously, these issues reflect the high potency and short half-life of alprazolam. Switching to clonazepam appears to address these clinical problems because clonazepam is potent enough to replace alprazolam but has a long half-life (1 to 2 days). One method is based on an open study of patients with panic disorder. The switch takes approximately 1 week (the minimum time to reach a steady-state level of clonazepam).

1. Clonazepam is given at half the total daily alprazolam dose, divided into an early morning and a midafternoon dose.
2. Regular alprazolam doses are stopped but, during the first 7 days, alprazolam can be taken as needed up to the full amount taken previously.
3. Alprazolam is stopped entirely after day 7.
4. If more medication is needed after day 7, clonazepam is increased by 0.25 to 0.5 mg every week until efficacy is reestablished.

Benzodiazepine Abuse. In contrast to public impressions, it appears that few patients who have received benzodiazepines for valid indications become abusers (i.e., increase their dosage without medical supervision and take the drugs for nonmedical purposes) or addicted in the sense of using compulsively. **Most abusers of benzodiazepines also have abused other drugs.** Serious abusers of CNS depressants may use the equivalent of hundreds of milligrams of diazepam per day. Serious CNS depressant abusers should be detoxified as inpatients using either phenobarbital or a long-acting benzodiazepine, such as diazepam, as the detoxification agent.

Benzodiazepine Use in Elderly Patients. Slowed hepatic metabolism and increased pharmacodynamic sensitivity mean that great care must be taken when prescribing benzodiazepines in elderly patients. In general, short-acting benzodiazepines are safest, especially those metabolized by glucuronidation alone (lorazepam and oxazepam). In one study of patients older than 65 years, use of benzodiazepines with an elimination half-life of more than 24 hours, but not benzodiazepines with a short half-life, was associated with a 70% increase in the risk of hip fracture due to falls compared with individuals not using any psychotropic drugs. Accumulation of long-acting benzodiazepines must always be considered in the differential diagnosis of delirium or rapid cognitive decline in elderly patients.

Benzodiazepine Use in Pregnancy. Earlier reports associating diazepam with both cleft lip and cleft palate have not been substantiated. A cohort study and some but not all case-control studies suggest that benzodiazepines may be safe during pregnancy. However, it would be wise to avoid benzodiazepines, especially early in pregnancy, unless there are compelling reasons for their use.

Benzodiazepine Side Effects and Toxicity. Fatigue and drowsiness are the most common side effects associated with benzodiazepine treatment. In addition, impairment of memory and other cognitive functions and impairments of motor coordination may occur. The benzodiazepines have little effect on autonomic function.

Thus, adverse effects on blood pressure, pulse, and cardiac rhythm are not typically seen. The development of these side effects depends on dosage used (concomitant use of other medications, especially CNS depressants, and alcohol) and the sensitivity of the individual being treated. With repeated dosing, most patients develop tolerance to sedation. The suggestion that automobile accidents are more likely to occur among benzodiazepine users (assuming tolerance to the early sedative effects) is complicated by the possibility that the condition being treated (e.g., anxiety, insomnia) may be a contributing factor. The interpretation of laboratory studies of attention, cognitive control, and driving ability are difficult to generalize to real-life situations.

Acute dosages of benzodiazepines may produce transient anterograde amnesia. This effect appears to be independent of sedation; acquisition of new information is specifically impaired. The risk of anterograde amnesia appears to be worsened by concomitant ingestion of alcohol.

Uncommon side effects include dysarthria, confusion, abnormal coordination, ataxia, depression or worsening of mood (see below), dry mouth, constipation, nausea, slurred speech, dizziness, and tremor. Side effects due to rapid decrease or abrupt withdrawal from benzodiazepines may include agitation, heightened sensory perception, paresthesias, muscle cramps, muscle twitching, diarrhea, reduced concentration, worsening of mood, anxiety, nervousness, restlessness, sleeping difficulties, insomnia, tremors, and, in rare cases, seizures and hallucinations.

Benzodiazepine-Induced Disinhibition. Reports of paradoxical reactions to benzodiazepines (disinhibition), in particular describing rage outbursts or aggression in patients on chlordiazepoxide, diazepam, alprazolam, or clonazepam, have been published. Disinhibition can probably occur with any benzodiazepine, but the lower potency, slowly absorbed oxazepam may be less likely to trigger this effect. Many clinicians feel that the highest incidence of disinhibition occurs in personality disorder patients with prior histories of dyscontrol. When paradoxical excitement occurs in a patient given a benzodiazepine in an emergency department or inpatient ward, the administration of an antipsychotic drug is often effective in reversing the state.

Benzodiazepine-Induced Depression. All benzodiazepines have been associated with the emergence or worsening of depression; whether they were causative or only failed to prevent the depression is unknown. If the depression occurs during the course of treatment, the benzodiazepine can be combined with or replaced by an antidepressant.

Benzodiazepine Overdose. With respect to lethality, benzodiazepines have proved to be relatively safe in overdose in that benzodiazepines alone have only rarely been implicated in fatal overdoses. However, when combined with other CNS depressants, such as alcohol, barbiturates, or narcotics, benzodiazepines may contribute to the lethality of the overdose.

The treatment of benzodiazepine overdose includes induction of emesis or gastric lavage, when appropriate, and supportive care for patients who are stuporous or comatose. The benzodiazepine antagonist flumazenil is available for the treatment of benzodiazepine overdose. In benzodiazepine-dependent patients, this drug may precipitate withdrawal symptoms in analogy with the actions of naloxone in opiate-dependent individuals.

Benzodiazepine Interactions with Alcohol and Other Drugs. Serious pharmacokinetic drug interactions are rare with benzodiazepines but may occur (Table 5.3). Benzodiazepines can cause a mild to moderate increase in CNS depression caused by

TABLE 5.3	Interactions of Benzodiazepines with Other Drugs
Decrease absorption	Antacids
Increase central nervous system depression	Antihistamines Barbiturates and similarly acting drugs Cyclic antidepressants Ethanol
Increase benzodiazepine levels (compete for microsomal enzymes; probably little or no effect on lorazepam and oxazepam)	Cimetidine Disulfiram Erythromycin Estrogens Isoniazid SSRIs
Decrease benzodiazepine levels	Carbamazepine (possibly other anticonvulsants)

SSRIs, selective serotonin reuptake inhibitors.

coingested alcohol; when taken together in overdose, ethanol and benzodiazepines can result in death.

Buspirone

An alternative to antidepressants or benzodiazepines for GAD is buspirone (BuSpar), a partial agonist of the serotonin 5-HT$_{1A}$ receptor. Buspirone has also slight affinity for the dopamine D$_2$ receptors. Buspirone may be a good initial choice in patients with GAD who are at elevated risk for benzodiazepine abuse, but it is not indicated in GAD with comorbid depression and/or panic disorder, where antidepressant monotherapy is typically the first choice. Buspirone, which has been approved for treatment of GAD, is a member of a chemical group called the azaspirodecanediones. Buspirone has no direct effects on GABA$_A$ receptors, it has no pharmacologic cross-reactivity with benzodiazepines or barbiturates, and it lacks the sedative, anticonvulsant, and muscle relaxant effects of benzodiazepines. A major advantage of buspirone is that it does not produce dependence, and it has no abuse potential.

Buspirone is believed to exert its anxiolytic effect by acting as a partial agonist at 5-HT$_{1A}$ receptors. Because 5-HT$_{1A}$ receptors are autoreceptors, their activation by buspirone decreases serotonin release. Investigations of the role of serotonin in anxiety suggest that there is a complex relationship between the neurotransmitter and anxiety symptoms. This complexity is highlighted by the fact that SSRIs increase synaptic serotonin rather than decrease it. Ultimately because both buspirone and SSRIs produce therapeutic actions only after a latency of days to weeks, it is likely that their beneficial effects reflect adaptations within certain circuits to drug stimulation. Of interest, buspirone has an active metabolite, 1-phenylpiperazine, that acts via α_2-adrenergic receptors initially to increase the rate of firing of locus coeruleus neurons. Because the ratio of the plasma level of this metabolite to the parent compound increases with treatment over time, this stimulation of adrenergic systems may play a key role in the agent's therapeutic as well as adverse effects.

Buspirone is 100% absorbed from the human gastrointestinal tract but undergoes extensive first-pass metabolism by the liver so that only 4% may be bioavailable. Buspirone is metabolized by the liver; the half-life of the parent compound is 2 to 11 hours. Oxidative metabolism of buspirone is carried out through cytochrome P450 3A4. Therefore, inhibitors of 3A4 activity such as grapefruit juice may significantly elevate buspirone blood levels.

When used to treat GAD, buspirone has been found to be as effective as standard benzodiazepine treatments in some but not all studies. Buspirone is most often ineffective as a sole treatment for panic disorder. It appears that patients with GAD who have taken benzodiazepines within 4 weeks prior to taking buspirone may be less likely to benefit from buspirone. Unlike benzodiazepines, buspirone is effective only when taken regularly. It takes 1 to 2 weeks to show its initial effects, and maximal effectiveness may be reached only after 4 to 6 weeks. This must be clearly explained to patients who are accustomed to using benzodiazepines. Because of this time course of effectiveness, buspirone is not useful in emergencies or when rapid onset of anxiolysis is required. The initial dosage of buspirone is 5 mg three times daily; in most trials, 20 to 30 mg per day in two or three divided doses has been effective, but a total dosage of up to 60 mg per day may be required for an optimal response. Buspirone is available in 5-, 10-, 15-, and 30-mg tablets.

Because of its lack of cross-reactivity with benzodiazepines, **buspirone cannot prevent benzodiazepine withdrawal symptoms.** Therefore, when switching patients from a benzodiazepine to buspirone, the benzodiazepine must be slowly tapered as if no new drugs were being introduced. If buspirone is started before the taper has concluded (which should be safe), it is important not to confuse benzodiazepine withdrawal or rebound symptoms with buspirone side effects.

Buspirone does not cause sedation; however, it may occasionally produce restlessness. It does not appear to impair psychomotor performance. The other most common side effects of buspirone are dizziness, headache, light-headedness, gastrointestinal distress, nausea, insomnia, paresthesia, and drowsiness. Buspirone does not appear to be highly toxic in overdose. Buspirone has been somewhat disappointing in general clinical use in that a smaller percentage of anxious patients benefit from buspirone than from benzodiazepines. Whether this reflects inappropriate expectations and inadequate dose and duration of treatment on the part of both physicians and patients who are accustomed to the rapid effects of benzodiazepines is unclear. For patients who respond to buspirone, it has the marked advantages of being free of sedation, lacking any prominent discontinuation symptomatology.

Anticonvulsants

Anticonvulsants are occasionally used off-label in the treatment of GAD when other pharmacologic treatments have failed. In theory, anticonvulsants that enhance GABA transmission in the brain might have useful anxiolytic effects. (See Chapter 4 for a description of the pharmacology of anticonvulsants.) The dosing of anticonvulsants used in the treatment of GAD appears to be similar to that used in the treatment of epilepsy [e.g., tiagabine (Gabitril) dosage ranging from 4 to 16 mg per day]. Although there are currently no anticonvulsants considered first line for GAD owing to limited clinical trials data, agents of emerging clinical and research interest include gabapentin (600 to 3,600 mg per day), tiagabine (4 to 16 mg per day), and levetiracetam (Keppra) (500 to 3,000 mg per day), in part due to their relative tolerability compared with older anticonvulsants (e.g., valproate).

Pregabalin (Lyrica) is an anticonvulsant ligand of the α-2-δ subunit of voltage-gated calcium channels, which was approved by the European Commission in 2006 for the treatment of GAD, with FDA approval for neuropathic pain, postherpetic neuralgia, and epilepsy augmentation. Data from a combination of five placebo-controlled studies led to the approval of European Commission, showing that pregabalin can provide rapid and sustained efficacy for the treatment of GAD. As early as the first week of treatment, pregabalin was shown to be significantly effective in providing relief of both emotional symptoms, such as depressive symptoms and panic, as well as physical symptoms, including headaches and muscle aches. Pregabalin dosages between 150 and 600 mg per day are typically used for the treatment of GAD, in divided doses. Although research is needed in this area to understand the efficacy and tolerability of these agents in GAD, anticonvulsants may have a specific role in the treatment of anxiety disorders in patients who are refractory to initial intervention, have difficulties with substance use disorders, and/or have bipolar disorder comorbid with GAD.

Second-Generation Antipsychotics

Second-generation antipsychotics such as risperidone, olanzapine, aripiprazole, ziprasidone, and quetiapine are typically used off-label as adjuncts in the treatment of GAD only when other pharmacologic treatments have failed or when patients present with disorganized and/or explosive and aggressive behavior. (See Chapter 2 for a description of the pharmacology of second-generation antipsychotics.) The dosing of second-generation antipsychotics used in the treatment of GAD is similar to that used in the treatment of psychotic disorders (e.g., risperidone dosage ranging from 0.5 to 8 mg per day, olanzapine dosage ranging from 5 to 20 mg per day, aripiprazole dosage ranging from 2 to 20 mg per day, ziprasidone dosage ranging from 40 to 160 mg per day, quetiapine dosage ranging from 50 to 300 mg per day). Both open and controlled studies provide evidence in support of the usefulness of second-generation antipsychotics as adjuncts in the treatment of GAD. There are also positive placebo-controlled data on the use of some of these agents (for example, 50 to 150 mg per day of the prolonged-release formulation of quetiapine) as monotherapy for GAD. Although research is needed in this area to understand the efficacy and tolerability of these agents in GAD, second-generation antipsychotics may have a specific role in the treatment of GAD in patients who are refractory to initial interventions and/or have bipolar disorder comorbid with GAD.

Riluzole

Riluzole, an antiglutamatergic agent approved by the FDA for the treatment of amyotrophic lateral sclerosis, is occasionally used as well in patients with drug-resistant GAD. In an 8-week, open-label, fixed-dose study, where 18 patients with GAD received treatment with riluzole (100 mg per day), 12 of the 15 patients who completed the trial responded positively to riluzole. Although these findings are very preliminary and uncontrolled, there is an interest in exploring the efficacy of this compound in resistant GAD.

Psychotherapy

Cognitive-behavioral therapy (CBT) is probably the best evidence-based form of psychotherapy for the treatment of GAD, although not as effective as for the treatment of phobia-based anxiety disorders. Patients are typically taught to record thoughts and feelings in diaries and to replace anxiety-provoking thoughts with positive thoughts. Relaxation therapy, primarily focused on helping patients imagine calming situations to induce muscular and mental retardation, is an alternative to CBT. Both forms of psychotherapy are typically delivered as short-term treatments over 6 to 12 weeks. Many patients do, however, continue to receive more open-ended, supportive, or dynamic psychotherapies with the view that they may be useful in helping patients identify and manage life stressors; however, data supporting their efficacy for the relief of GAD symptoms are limited.

SITUATIONAL OR STRESS-RELATED ANXIETY

This is usually self-limited and rarely calls for medical treatment. When patients complain of anxiety due to a specific life stress, the questions to address include the following:

1. Is the anxiety harmful to the individual? In many situations, anxiety may be helpful in terms of motivation to respond, cope, or adapt, but in other situations, anxiety can lead to maladaptive behavior or severe distress. In such situations, treatment is indicated.
2. Would psychosocial treatment (generally CBT) be effective and acceptable to the patient?
3. What are the risks and benefits of short-term antianxiety treatment? Specifically, the physician must consider side effects, the acceptability of pharmacologic treatment to the individual, possible dependence (if benzodiazepine treatment is contemplated), and possible interactions with other medications or medical disorders.

If drug treatment is indicated, a low-potency benzodiazepine such as diazepam or oxazepam might be prescribed. See the section on GAD treatment for a description of the pharmacology of benzodiazepines. Of the benzodiazepines, compounds such as diazepam or oxazepam have the lowest risk of causing dependence and subsequent rebound or withdrawal symptoms. A typical regimen might be diazepam, 5 mg three times daily or the equivalent. (Diazepam also appears to offer muscle relaxant properties and may therefore provide relief from stress-related muscle tension.) Doses may be increased as needed, but the equivalent of 30 mg of diazepam or less should suffice for almost all cases of situational anxiety. The duration of treatment should be limited, guided by the time course of the stressor that precipitated the anxiety.

Benzodiazepines also can be useful for the **symptomatic treatment of transient anxiety, fear, or tension associated with medical illnesses** (e.g., post–myocardial infarction) and surgical illnesses (e.g., for pre- or postoperative anxiety). The dosage is similar to that for other situational anxieties, usually less than the equivalent of 30 mg per day of diazepam. However, in elderly patients or in patients with compromised hepatic function, lorazepam or oxazepam is clearly superior to diazepam or other long-acting drugs because they will not accumulate (and thus cause somnolence or other toxicities); in such patients, lower doses are also prudent.

SOCIAL ANXIETY DISORDER (SOCIAL PHOBIA)

Social anxiety disorder (or social phobia), as defined by *Diagnostic and Statistical Manual of Mental Disorders*, 4th edition (*DSM-IV*), consists of persistent fears of one or more social situations in which the person is exposed to possible scrutiny by others and fears humiliation. Perhaps the best known example is public speaking anxiety, in which an individual is unable to speak before an audience. Other specific features of social anxiety disorder include being unable to eat in front of others, write or sign one's name under scrutiny, use public urinals, or speak on the telephone. In the generalized form of the condition, the sufferer avoids or experiences intense distress in multiple social situations where the potential exists for scrutiny by others. Many patients with social anxiety disorder experience symptoms of physiologic arousal, including flushing, palpitations, tremulousness, and in some cases even full panic attacks in feared situations. These symptoms may further heighten fear and avoidance of those situations. The focus of concern is embarrassment and performance, which generally differentiates severe social anxiety disorder from panic disorder with agoraphobia. Social anxiety disorder is associated with marked impairment in social and work function. The lifetime prevalence of social anxiety disorder was 13.3% in the National Comorbidity Survey, but prior epidemiologic surveys suggested markedly lower prevalence rates, probably because of differences in the stringency of the definition of this condition. Women are more likely than men to suffer from it, although the ratio (3:2) is not as pronounced as other anxiety disorders. Social anxiety disorder is often comorbid, most frequently with agoraphobia, specific phobia, substance use disorders, and MDD. The onset of social anxiety disorder is typically during childhood and adolescence. Several risk factors have been identified, including family history of social anxiety disorder and the trait of behavioral inhibition. Social anxiety disorder tends to persist over time and, when untreated, it is typically chronic. Treating social anxiety disorder is important, because this condition may interfere with school and work progression given its early age of onset, chronicity, and resultant avoidance of many activities required in our culture for success and may be a risk factor for the development of MDD and/or substance use disorders.

Diagnosis

1. Persistent fears of one or more social situations in which the person is exposed to possible scrutiny by others and fears humiliation.
2. A careful psychiatric history should be obtained to rule out psychiatric disorders that may cause significant social anxiety, such as MDD with atypical features (where the hypersensitivity to rejection may cause significant social anxiety).

Pharmacologic Treatment

Antidepressants

Antidepressants have demonstrated safety and efficacy in the treatment of social anxiety disorder, as demonstrated by the FDA approval of venlafaxine, sertraline, and paroxetine for the treatment of this condition. Antidepressants are also useful in addressing the frequent comorbidity of social anxiety disorder with depression and other anxiety disorders such as panic disorder.

SSRIs are often used in the treatment of social anxiety disorders. Only two of the SSRIs (paroxetine and sertraline) are FDA approved for the treatment of social anxiety disorder, whereas the other SSRIs are typically used off-label, partly because experience to date suggests similar efficacy across the SSRIs as a class for social anxiety disorder. (See Chapter 3 for a description of the pharmacology of SSRIs.) The dosing of the SSRIs used in the treatment of social anxiety disorder appears to be similar to that used in the treatment of depression (e.g., paroxetine dosage ranging from 20 to 50 mg per day and sertraline dosage ranging from 50 to 150 mg per day).

SNRIs such as venlafaxine and duloxetine are also used in the treatment of social anxiety disorder, although only the former has been approved by the FDA for the treatment of social anxiety disorder. (See Chapter 3 for a description of the pharmacology of SNRIs.) The dosing of venlafaxine used in the treatment of social anxiety disorder appears to be similar to that used in the treatment of depression (e.g., dosage ranging from 75 to 225 mg per day).

Monoamine oxidase inhibitors (MAOIs), such as phenelzine and moclobemide, are also used off-label in the treatment of social anxiety disorder, although typically only after other pharmacologic treatments have failed, given the side-effect profile of MAOIs, the risk of drug–drug interactions, and, in the case of the irreversible MAOIs, the need for tyramine-free diet. (See Chapter 3 for a description of the pharmacology of MAOIs.) The dosing of MAOIs used in the treatment of social anxiety disorder appears to be similar to that used in the treatment of depression (e.g., phenelzine dosage ranging from 45 to 90 mg per day, moclobemide dosage ranging from 300 to 900 mg per day).

Although effective for other anxiety disorders, two well-controlled studies have shown that TCAs are not effective for social anxiety disorder. Although the reason for this differential efficacy remains unknown, tricyclics should not be considered in the algorithm of effective pharmacotherapy for social anxiety disorder—unlike the situation for panic disorder or GAD.

It should be noted that longer-term studies (e.g., 6 months) of antidepressants such as venlafaxine suggest that reduction in fear and avoidance symptoms continue over the course of at least 6 months. This may be because of a need for patients to be confronted in their day-to-day lives over time with many of the previously feared or avoided situations and to learn that their prior symptoms are either milder or lacking in these situations before a full remission occurs. Thus, although short-term studies suggest antidepressants result in greater improvement than placebo in 10 to 12 weeks, clinically full response may be delayed, suggesting the need for longer trials before considering a switch or augmentation strategy than typically used in practice for depression or other anxiety disorders. Research is needed to better understand the treatment of refractory social anxiety disorder.

A number of compounds have been used to augment SSRIs and SNRIs in patients who do not respond to these agents alone. Among them, D-cycloserine, a partial agonist at the glycine recognition site of the N-methyl-D-aspartic acid receptor in the amygdala, the serotonin 5-HT$_{1A}$ partial agonists buspirone, the serotonin 5-HT$_{1A}$ antagonist and β-blocker pindolol (Visken), and second-generation antipsychotics, have shown some promise.

Benzodiazepines

Benzodiazepines also have demonstrated efficacy for social anxiety disorder, although data are more limited than for antidepressants. (See section on GAD above for a description of the pharmacologic characteristics of benzodiazepines.) Several benzodiazepines (e.g., clonazepam, alprazolam, and bromazepam) have shown efficacy in the treatment of social anxiety disorder compared to placebo. Generally, high-potency compounds, such as alprazolam and clonazepam, are favored. Typically, dosages of 2 to 6 mg per day of alprazolam (typically in its extended-release formulation), clonazepam 1 to 3 mg per day, or the equivalent are effective, but occasional patients have required higher dosages. Long-term treatment (6 months) appears to be safe and effective for many patients; nonetheless, it is worth trying to taper the medication slowly and periodically to see if the underlying symptoms have improved. When tapering medication, it is important to distinguish recurrence of the original symptoms from transient rebound or withdrawal symptoms. Limitations of benzodiazepines for social anxiety disorder include their lack of antidepressant properties in a disorder with very high lifetime depression comorbidity and, given relatively high rates of self-medication with alcohol in social anxiety disorder, their abuse potential. In addition, **benzodiazepines are generally not useful as-needed (p.r.n.) agents,** particularly for those with the generalized form of the disorder because situations often cannot be predicted ahead of time, and the use of p.r.n. agents may result in a higher level of sedation than daily use, which can impair performance. All patients with social anxiety disorder should be queried about their alcohol use, particularly in social situations, prior to initiating any treatment but especially before initiating benzodiazepine therapy.

β-Blockers

β-Adrenergic blockers have been used off-label to treat performance anxiety. The evidence for the efficacy of β-blockers in the treatment of generalized social anxiety disorder is scant and unconvincing. β-blockers are clinically useful when the disorder is not generalized but **limited to performance anxiety.** Performance anxiety, a well-known example of which is stage fright, is considered a specific form of social anxiety disorder. When severe, performance anxiety can interfere with life activities that are important to many individuals. It may lead to poor performance in or avoidance of such activities as interviews, speaking in class, public speaking, acting, or performing in musical events. Symptoms include dry mouth, hoarse voice, pounding heart, difficulty in breathing, tremor, and, occasionally, weakness and dizziness. The anxiety may feed on itself, creating a vicious cycle of anticipatory anxiety leading up to the activity and worsening anxiety during the activity. When this syndrome interferes with important activities, treatment is indicated.

β-Adrenergic blockers in clinical use are competitive antagonists of norepinephrine and epinephrine at β-adrenergic receptors. Thus, they are peripherally sympatholytic. Their relative lack of sedation compared with benzodiazepines makes their use as p.r.n. agents prior to performance situations a useful option. The β-blockers do not appear to induce tolerance to their psychiatric effects or to have abuse potential.

When β-blockers are used for the treatment of performance anxiety, a single dose of propranolol (Inderal), 10 to 40 mg or its β-blocker equivalent, usually suffices, although higher doses have been used. The dose can be given 30 minutes prior to the anxiogenic event. It is reasonable to administer a **test dose** on some anxiogenic occasion prior to an all-important engagement to ensure that hypotension or other troublesome side effects will not interfere with performance. Because most of the distressing symptoms of performance anxiety are peripheral, less lipophilic agents [e.g., nadolol (Corgard) or atenolol (Tenormin)] are also effective.

β-Adrenergic blockers have a variety of significant side effects (Table 5.4). β-Blockers have no apparent effect on memory. They may actually improve performance of tasks that require a mixture of perceptual motor, learning, and memory skills, perhaps because such tasks are sensitive to even low levels of anxiety. Several drug interactions have been reported, including increased levels of theophylline and thyroxine. β-Blockers, used in optimal doses, have minimal central

 TABLE 5.4 Side Effects and Toxicity of β-blockers

Cardiovascular	Hypotension Bradycardia Dizziness Congestive failure (in patients with compromised myocardial function)
Respiratory	Asthma (less risk with β_1-selective drugs)
Metabolic	Worsened hypoglycemia in diabetics on insulin or oral hypoglycemic agents
Gastrointestinal	Nausea Diarrhea Abdominal pain
Sexual function	Impotence
Neuropsychiatric	Lassitude Fatigue Dysphoria Insomnia Vivid nightmares Depression Psychosis (rare)
Other (rare)	Raynaud's phenomenon Peyronie's disease Withdrawal syndrome Rebound worsening of preexisting angina pectoris when β-blockers are discontinued

side effects and generally improve performance. This is contrary to the benzodiazepines, which may cause some sedation or disinhibition, and are likely to worsen performance. For patients with asthma or other obstructive pulmonary disorders, a relatively selective β-antagonist [metoprolol (Lopressor and Toprol XL) or atenolol] is preferable. However, for such patients, the risk, even with selective agents, probably outweighs their established psychiatric benefits. β-Blockers should be used cautiously in diabetics prone to hypoglycemia, because they may interfere with the normal response to hypoglycemia.

β-Blockers are begun at low doses, and side effects, such as bradycardia, hypotension, or bronchospasm, should be monitored. Doses are typically withheld if blood pressure is less than 90/60 mm Hg or heart rate is less than 55 beats per minute. **Bradycardia or hypotension also precludes dosage increases.** If patients develop asthma symptoms during treatment, the dangers of drug therapy may outweigh the established benefits.

Although not supported by efficacy data, daily use of β-blockers is occasionally used as monotherapy or as an augmentation strategy for social anxiety disorder. Propranolol may be started at dosages of 10 mg three times daily or 10 to 20 mg twice daily and slowly increased (e.g., by no more than 20 to 30 mg per day at first) until therapeutic effects are achieved. It must be given in divided doses because of its short half-life. Metoprolol is usually begun at dosages of 50 mg twice daily. Nadolol (40 or 80 mg) and atenolol (50 or 100 mg) can be given in single daily doses. Patients who have coronary artery disease or hypertension risk rebound worsening when β-blockers are discontinued; in such patients, slow weaning with careful follow-up is the safest course.

The major beneficial effects of β-blockers appear to be peripheral. Possible anxiolytic mechanisms within the CNS are not well understood. Within the brain, norepinephrine is produced by a small number of neurons, all located in the brainstem. The major noradrenergic nucleus is the locus coeruleus, found within the dorsal pons, which projects widely throughout the CNS. Functionally, noradrenergic systems in the brain appear to be involved in modulation of global vigilance, regulation of hormone release, modulation of pain perception, and central regulation of the sympathetic nervous system. It has been hypothesized that noradrenergic systems are involved in important aspects of anxiety and fear. There is evidence that norepinephrine acts in the amygdala to enhance the cognitive component of emotionally charged memories (e.g., most individuals have a very clear memory of where they were when they heard about the attacks of September 11, 2001). This effect has led to clinical trials of β-blockers after trauma to prevent posttraumatic stress disorder (PTSD) (see later in this chapter). Peripherally, norepinephrine is the major transmitter of postganglionic sympathetic neurons. Epinephrine has only a limited role in the CNS; it appears to be involved in blood pressure control. Peripherally, both epinephrine and norepinephrine are released from the adrenal medulla in response to stress.

Four major features differentiate the β-blockers: their relative receptor selectivity, their relative lipophilicity, their route of metabolism, and their half-lives. The advent of relatively selective β-receptor antagonists (metoprolol and atenolol), with less effect at β_2 than β_1 receptors, has decreased the problem of bronchospasm induced by the older nonselective drugs. The selectivity is only relative; however, caution must still be exercised in treating patients with asthma. Both nonselective and β_1-selective compounds have been used for psychiatric disorders.

β-Receptor blockers differ markedly in their lipophilicity. The least lipophilic drugs, nadolol and atenolol, cross the blood–brain barrier poorly and therefore have a higher ratio of peripheral to central effects, whereas the more lipophilic drugs, propranolol and metoprolol, have potent central as well as peripheral

TABLE 5.5	Relevant Pharmacologic Properties of Commonly used β-adrenergic Blockers			
Drug	Selectivity	Lipophilicity	Half-life (h)	Route of Drug Elimination
Propranolol	None	High	3–6	Hepatic
Metoprolol	β	High	3–4	Hepatic
Atenolol	β	Low	6–9	Renal
Nadolol	None	Low	14–24	Renal

effects. Compounds of intermediate lipophilicity include acebutolol (Sectral) and timolol (Blocadren). Pindolol is also of intermediate lipophilicity; however, it differs from the other β-blockers because it also has intrinsic sympathomimetic activity, is a serotonin 5-HT$_{1A}$ receptor antagonist, and has been used to accelerate response to antidepressants and to augment their effects in resistant depression.

The drugs also vary markedly in elimination half-life. Nadolol and atenolol have relatively long half-lives, thus allowing once a day administration. In contrast, propranolol, if used as a standing regimen, requires multiple daily dosing unless a sustained-release form is used. The major features of commonly used β-adrenergic blockers are given in Table 5.5.

Anticonvulsants
Anticonvulsants such as gabapentin, pregabalin, topiramate, and levetiracetam are typically used off-label in the treatment of social anxiety disorder when other pharmacologic treatments have failed, mostly because of some evidence of efficacy in both uncontrolled and placebo-controlled trials and because of their lack of abuse potential. They may also have a role in patients with comorbid bipolar disorder, although data are lacking. (See Chapter 4 for a description of the pharmacology of anticonvulsants.) As with benzodiazepines, **anticonvulsants do not protect against MDD,** which is commonly comorbid with social anxiety disorder. The dosing of the anticonvulsants used in the treatment of social anxiety disorder appears to be similar to that used in the treatment of epilepsy (e.g., gabapentin dosage ranging from 900 to 3,600 mg per day; pregabalin dosage ranging from 300 to 600 mg per day, topiramate dosage ranging from 100 to 400 mg per day; levetiracetam dosage ranging from 500 to 3,000 mg per day; valproic acid dosage ranging from 500 to 2,500 mg per day). It remains unknown whether longer treatment periods, as with antidepressants, may be necessary to see optimal efficacy of anticonvulsants for social anxiety disorder.

Psychotherapy
CBT is the best evidence-based form of psychotherapy in the treatment of social anxiety disorder, whereas the usefulness of interpersonal psychotherapy is supported only by uncontrolled studies. CBT for social anxiety disorder typically includes one or more of the following elements:

1. Exposure, aimed at helping patients face social situations that are anxiety provoking so that habituation and extinction can occur.
2. Cognitive restructuring, with the goal of helping patients challenge maladaptive assumptions and beliefs.
3. Social skills training, with the goal of helping patients acquire the basic component skills required in social situations.

CBT, whether offered in individual or group settings, is a treatment of choice for diminishing distress and avoidance related to performance anxiety and also may be useful in combination with pharmacotherapy, although the optimal ordering and combination of CBT with pharmacotherapy for social anxiety disorder remains unclear.

PANIC DISORDER

The core manifestation of panic disorder is recurrent unexpected panic attacks. In addition, patients with panic disorder develop anticipatory anxiety with concern about the occurrence and/or impact of future attacks. A substantial proportion of patients also develop phobic avoidance, which may prove more disabling than the panic attacks themselves. When severe, phobic avoidance in the form of agoraphobia (fear of situations in which it may be difficult to gain help or escape) may cause patients to become entirely housebound. This combination of symptoms must cause substantial distress and/or psychosocial impairment and cannot be the result of another psychiatric or medical disorder. The lifetime prevalence of panic disorder is estimated to be ranging from 1.5% to 3.5% in the general population. Women are twice as likely as men to suffer from panic disorder, and the age of onset is typically between adolescence and early adulthood. Patients with panic disorder often have comorbid MDD, other anxiety disorders, and substance abuse/dependence. Panic disorder has recently also been identified as common and impairing in patients with bipolar disorder. Panic attacks may be the manifestation of medical illnesses such as asthma and other obstructive pulmonary diseases, inner ear vestibular dysfunction (with vertigo), and hyperthyroidism, or they may result from overuse of some drugs used to treat asthma, thyroid supplements, caffeine, or over-the-counter decongestants or appetite suppressants.

Diagnosis

1. Recurrent unexpected panic attacks.
2. Anticipatory anxiety.
3. Phobic avoidance.
4. A careful medical and psychiatric history should be obtained to rule out medical and psychiatric disorders that may cause panic attacks.

When patients present with panic disorder, the role of laboratory testing is not always straightforward. It is important not to miss underlying medical conditions, but at the same time, panic disorder is common and often has onset in younger patients for whom detailed medical investigations are not likely to be cost-effective. The need for further workup can often be determined from the history, and certainly focused laboratory tests, such as thyroid studies and an electrocardiogram, may well be warranted. A more substantial workup is warranted in older patients, atypical patients, and treatment-refractory patients.

Pharmacologic Treatment

The optimal duration of pharmacotherapy for panic disorder is unknown; however, to reduce risk of relapse it is best to continue medication if tolerated for at least 1 year after being symptom free. For patients with agoraphobic avoidance, it is important to determine that the patient has returned to avoided situations and is not just panic free, because avoidance of panic triggers can masquerade as remission. Many patients with panic disorder have a history of vulnerability to anxiety symptoms across the life cycle, beginning with anxiety difficulties in early childhood, including separation anxiety and school avoidance, followed by social anxiety in adolescence, and panic attacks in early adulthood; these individuals also have family histories of anxiety disorders and more comorbidity with anxiety disorders. It may be unrealistic to expect these patients to continue to feel and function well over time without treatment in contrast to those with a more defined, acute syndrome, which may more often remit with treatment.

Antidepressants

The FDA approval of paroxetine, sertraline, and venlafaxine for the treatment of panic disorder underscores the usefulness of antidepressants for this condition; when studied in the past, both TCAs and MAOIs have shown efficacy. Antidepressants are also useful in addressing the frequent comorbidity of panic disorder with depression and other anxiety disorders such as GAD and social anxiety disorder (with the exception of social anxiety disorder in which TCAs have failed to show efficacy). The typical approach to the treatment of panic disorder with antidepressants involves the "starting low and going slow" strategy, with use of low starting doses and very gradual dosing escalations to avoid initial activation and jitteriness. Patients with panic disorder are highly sensitive to side effects because of the fear of physical sensations that affects many of them. In some cases, titration may need to be further slowed, although educating the patient about the often transitory side effects that may occur will also improve tolerability and treatment adherence.

SSRIs are often used in the treatment of panic disorder. Only two of the SSRIs (paroxetine and sertraline) are FDA approved for the treatment of panic disorder, whereas the other SSRIs (citalopram, escitalopram, fluoxetine, fluvoxamine) are typically used off-label, based on positive placebo-controlled studies. (See Chapter 3 for a description of the pharmacology of SSRIs.) The **dosing of the SSRIs used in the treatment of panic disorder appears to be similar to that used in the treatment of depression** (e.g., paroxetine dosage ranging from 10 to 50 mg per day, sertraline dosage ranging from 50 to 150 mg per day), although higher doses may be needed for refractory patients.

SNRIs such as venlafaxine and duloxetine are also used in the treatment of panic disorder, on-label in the case of venlafaxine and off-label in the case of duloxetine and desvenlafaxine. (See Chapter 3 for a description of the pharmacology of SNRIs.) The dosing of venlafaxine, desvenlafaxine, and duloxetine used in the treatment of panic disorder is similar to that used in the treatment of depression (e.g., venlafaxine 75 to 225 mg per day, duloxetine 60 to 120 mg per day, and desvenlafaxine 50 to 100 mg per day).

Norepinephrine reuptake inhibitors such as reboxetine are also used off-label in the treatment of panic disorder, mostly because of positive, double-blind, placebo-controlled data with reboxetine. (See Chapter 3 for a description of the pharmacology of norepinephrine reuptake inhibitors.) The dosing of reboxetine used in the treatment of panic disorder is similar to that used in the treatment of depression (4 to 6 mg per day).

TCAs such as imipramine, clomipramine, and desipramine are also used off-label in the treatment of panic disorder, although typically only after other pharmacologic treatments have failed, given the less favorable side-effect profile of TCAs. (See Chapter 3 for a description of the pharmacology of TCAs.) The dosing of TCAs used in the treatment of panic disorder is similar to that used in the treatment of depression (e.g., imipramine dosage ranging from 50 to 200 mg per day).

MAOIs such as phenelzine and moclobemide are also used off-label in the treatment of panic disorder, although typically only after many other pharmacologic treatments have failed, given the side-effect profile of MAOIs, the risk of drug–drug interactions, and, in the case of the irreversible MAOIs, the need for tyramine-free diet. (See Chapter 3 for a description of the pharmacology of MAOIs.) The dosing of MAOIs used in the treatment of panic disorder is similar to that used in the treatment of depression (e.g., phenelzine dosage ranging from 45 to 90 mg per day; moclobemide dosage ranging from 300 to 900 mg per day). Despite an initial negative open study with bupropion, a more recent open study raises the possibility that this antidepressant may also have positive effects in panic disorder, although controlled data are lacking at this point.

Benzodiazepines

Two high-potency benzodiazepines, alprazolam and clonazepam, have shown efficacy in the treatment of panic disorder compared with placebo in a number of studies and are FDA approved for the treatment of this condition. Generally, low-potency benzodiazepines are considered to be less effective. If they could be given in adequate doses, it is possible that all benzodiazepines might prove effective in preventing panic attacks; however, the required doses of lower-potency compounds, such as diazepam, would be so high as to produce oversedation. Therefore, the high-potency compounds are the ones most clinically useful for this indication, although there is some evidence to support the clinical utility of lorazepam as well. The high-potency benzodiazepines alprazolam and clonazepam have demonstrated comparable efficacy to the antidepressants for the reduction of panic attacks, anticipatory anxiety, and phobic avoidance. (See above section on GAD for a description of the pharmacologic characteristics of benzodiazepines.) Typically, dosages of 1 to 6 mg per day of alprazolam or 0.5 to 3 mg per day of clonazepam are effective, but occasional patients have required the equivalent of 10 mg per day of alprazolam and 5 mg per day of clonazepam. The extended-release formulation of alprazolam is clearly preferred to the immediate-release formulation, because it minimizes the problem of interdose rebound. Some patients with panic disorder improve with short-term treatment (2 to 6 weeks), but the majority will have recurrences if treatment is stopped at that time. **Long-term treatment (6 months) appears to be safe and effective for many patients,** and, as with antidepressants, if benzodiazepines are used as monotherapy, patients should ideally be free of symptoms for at least 1 year to reduce the likelihood of relapse. At this time, it may be worth trying to taper the medication slowly and periodically to see if the underlying symptoms have improved. When tapering medication, it is important to distinguish recurrence of the original symptoms from transient rebound or withdrawal symptoms. In some cases, the anticonvulsants valproic acid and gabapentin, as well as CBT, have been reported as useful for some patients in helping with benzodiazepine discontinuation.

Benzodiazepines are not considered to be as effective as antidepressants and thus have disadvantages over antidepressants for many patients with depression comorbid with panic disorder. Benzodiazepines have been demonstrated to be useful in combination with antidepressants at treatment initiation to reduce anxiety and improve tolerability of antidepressants during the initial weeks before antipanic efficacy of antidepressants takes effect; when benzodiazepines are used to aid in antidepressant initiation, the benzodiazepine may be tapered after the first few weeks or so of treatment. Finally, although p.r.n. benzodiazepine use remains common in many clinical settings, this may be detrimental for patients with panic disorder and associated avoidance and may paradoxically result in a higher risk of psychological dependence on the benzodiazepine daily dosing for these patients.

Buspirone

There is no good evidence that buspirone, even at higher doses, has significant antipanic effects, as suggested by several inconclusive placebo-controlled trials. Thus, buspirone should not be used as a monotherapy for panic disorder, although it may have a role as an augmentation strategy for patients remaining symptomatic on SSRIs.

Anticonvulsants

Anticonvulsants such as gabapentin, pregabalin, levetiracetam, tiagabine, and valproate are typically used off-label in the treatment of panic disorder when other pharmacologic treatments have failed, partly because of anecdotal reports, open trials, and some positive double-blind, placebo-controlled data. (See Chapter 4 for a description of the pharmacology of anticonvulsants.) The dosing of the anticonvulsants used in the treatment of panic disorder appears to be similar to that used in the treatment of epilepsy (e.g., tiagabine dosage ranging from 4 to 16 mg per day; gabapentin 600 to 3,600 mg per day, pregabalin 150 to 600 mg per day, levitiracetam 500 to 3,000 mg per day).

Second-Generation Antipsychotics

Second-generation antipsychotics such as risperidone, olanzapine, aripiprazole, ziprasidone, and quetiapine are typically used off-label as adjuncts in the treatment of panic disorder only when other pharmacologic treatments have failed. (See Chapter 2 for a description of the pharmacology of second-generation antipsychotics.) The dosing of second-generation antipsychotics used in the treatment of panic disorder is similar to that used in the treatment of psychotic disorders (e.g., risperidone dosage ranging from 0.5 to 8 mg per day, olanzapine dosage ranging from 5 to 20 mg per day, aripiprazole dosage ranging from 2 to 20 mg per day, ziprasidone dosage ranging from 40 to 160 mg per day, quetiapine dosage ranging from 50 to 300 mg per day). Mostly open studies provide some evidence in support of the usefulness of second-generation antipsychotics as adjuncts in the treatment of panic disorder. Although research is needed in this area to understand the efficacy and tolerability of these agents in panic disorder, second-generation antipsychotics may have a specific role in the treatment of panic disorder in patients who are refractory to initial interventions and/or have bipolar disorder comorbid with panic disorder.

Psychotherapy

Nonpharmacologic treatments, especially packaged interventions of CBT techniques (e.g., panic control therapy), are also first-line interventions, demonstrating comparable efficacy and superior durability after treatment is discontinued when compared with pharmacotherapy. Given the high rates of chronic and recurrent distress, many patients require multimodal treatment. **CBT is probably the best studied form of psychotherapy in the treatment of panic disorder,** although interpersonal psychotherapy has shown promise as well. CBT is typically delivered as short-term treatment over approximately 12 weeks. Exposure to feared physical sensations and situations appears to be the most effective component of CBT; p.r.n. benzodiazepines should not be used in combination with CBT, because they may interfere with the effectiveness of this psychosocial intervention.

SIMPLE PHOBIAS

Benzodiazepines are generally not the treatment of choice for simple object phobias, such as fear of bees, dogs, snakes, spiders, or heights. CBTs those emphasize exposure appear to be successful with few contraindications. Nonetheless, if a patient with a simple phobia of a situation that can be anticipated or is likely to endure (e.g., airplanes) must confront the phobic stimulus on particular occasions (e.g., an airplane flight), p.r.n. use of a benzodiazepine (1 to 2 mg of lorazepam or 5 to 10 mg of diazepam) may be helpful. In such circumstances it is important to factor in the possibility of sedation.

OBSESSIVE-COMPULSIVE DISORDER

OCD is a psychiatric disorder characterized by obsessions and/or compulsions, with significant interference in social and occupational functioning. The lifetime prevalence of OCD is between 2% and 3% of the U.S. population. Epidemiologic studies show that by late adolescence OCD has a lifetime prevalence of 2% to 3%. The age of onset tends to be earlier in boys than in girls and has a first peak around puberty and another in early adulthood. The natural course of the disorder is fairly stable, with complete remission rates of 10% to 15%. Comorbid conditions include MDD, movement disorders, and anxiety disorders. In a recent study, in the subgroup of OCD patients younger than 15 years, boys showed a higher incidence of tic disorders, whereas OCD girls showed a tendency toward more frequent comorbid mood and eating disorders. OCD has been shown to be familial disorder, although phenotypic and genetic heterogeneity of OCD makes locating susceptibility genes difficult.

Diagnosis
1. Recurrent obsessive thoughts (obsessions) and/or compulsions.
2. Marked distress and psychosocial impairment.
3. A careful medical psychiatric history should be obtained to rule out medical and psychiatric disorders that are associated with OCD behavior, such as rheumatic fever with and without Sydenham's chorea, hypothyroidism, and tic disorders.

Pharmacologic Treatment

Antidepressants
The FDA approval of clomipramine, fluvoxamine, fluoxetine, paroxetine, and sertraline for the treatment of OCD demonstrates the usefulness of antidepressants for this condition. Antidepressants are also useful in addressing the frequent comorbidity of OCD with MDD and other anxiety disorders such as GAD and panic disorder.

SSRIs are often used in the treatment of OCD. Only four of the SSRIs (fluvoxamine, fluoxetine, paroxetine, and sertraline) are FDA approved for the treatment of OCD, whereas citalopram and escitalopram are typically used in an off-label mode, partly because of positive placebo-controlled studies. (See Chapter 3 for a description of the pharmacology of SSRIs.) The **dosing of the SSRIs used in the treatment of panic disorder is somewhat higher** than that used in the treatment of depression (e.g., fluvoxamine dosage ranging from 200 to 300 mg per day, fluoxetine dosage ranging from 40 to 80 mg per day, paroxetine dosage ranging from 40 to 80 mg per day, sertraline dosage ranging from 100 to 200 mg per day), although even higher doses may be required for resistant cases of this disorder.

Relatively serotonergic TCAs such as clomipramine are also used in the treatment of OCD, although typically only after SSRIs have failed, given the unfavorable side-effect profile of clomipramine and the other TCAs. (See Chapter 3 for a description of the pharmacology of TCAs.) Clomipramine is FDA approved for the treatment of OCD. The dosing of clomipramine used in the treatment of OCD appears to be similar to that used in the treatment of depression (e.g., clomipramine dosage ranging from 100 to 250 mg per day).

SNRIs such as venlafaxine (150 to 300 mg per day), duloxetine (60 to 120 mg per day), and desvenlafaxine (50 to 100 mg per day) are also used off-label in the treatment of OCD, partly because of studies suggesting comparable efficacy of venlafaxine to clomipramine or SSRIs. (See Chapter 3 for a description of the pharmacology of SNRIs.)

Benzodiazepines
Benzodiazepines are not generally as effective as sole treatments in OCD, although case series and one clinical trial indicated efficacy of clonazepam compared with placebo.

Treatment-Resistant OCD: Augmentation Strategies
Because overall response and remission rates to monotherapy with antidepressants tend to be rather low in OCD, augmentation strategies are common:

1. Buspirone (dosing: 10 to 90 mg per day) may have some use as an adjunct to SSRIs in the treatment of OCD, but the support for this recommendation comes from two of four controlled trials.
2. Clonazepam (dosing: 0.5 to 4 mg per day) may augment clomipramine or SSRIs, although the benefit was shown in one of three outcome measures in a placebo-controlled trial.
3. Antipsychotic drugs, both typical (e.g., haloperidol and pimozide at dosages between 2 and 10 mg per day) and atypical (e.g., risperidone at dosages of 2 to 6 mg per day, olanzapine at dosages of 5 to 20 mg per day, aripiprazole 5 to 20 mg per day, and quetiapine at dosages of 50 to 300 mg per day), may boost the efficacy of SSRIs or clomipramine, based on evidence of both open and controlled trials. The presence of comorbid schizotypal personality disorder and/or tic disorders is often considered a positive predictor of the efficacy of antipsychotic drug augmentation in OCD, but the evidence for this association is relatively weak.
4. Lithium (at doses leading to serum levels of 0.4 to 1.0 mmol/L) may be a helpful adjunct, but double-blind studies question its efficacy.
5. Clomipramine (at dosages ranging from 75 to 150 mg per day) may augment SSRIs, but there is a risk of toxicity due to drug–drug interactions, and blood levels of clomipramine and desmethylclomipramine and electrocardiograms need to be monitored.
6. Inositol (at doses of 18 grams per day) may be a helpful adjunct, based on a crossover study.
7. Glutamergic drugs (e.g., memantine at dosages ranging from 10 to 20 mg per day; riluzole 50 mg b.i.d.; lamotrigine 100 to 300 mg per day) may augment SSRIs or SNRIs, based primarily on open trials and anecdotal reports, and on the evidence that glutaminergic hyperactivity is involved in OCD.
8. Anticonvulsants (e.g., gabapentin at dosages ranging from 900 to 2,700 mg per day, phenytoin at dosages ranging from 100 to 200 mg per day) may augment SSRIs and SNRIs, but their evidence is weak.
9. Other agents (e.g., trazodone, naltrexone, tramadol, ondansetron, and pergolide) may augment SSRIs and SNRIs, but their evidence is lacking at this point.

Psychotherapy
Nonpharmacologic treatments, especially behavioral and CBT techniques, are also first-line interventions, demonstrating comparable efficacy and superior durability after treatment is discontinued versus drug therapy. Exposure and response prevention are often key elements of these psychotherapeutic interventions. Given the high rates of chronic and recurrent distress, many patients require multimodal treatment.

POSTTRAUMATIC STRESS DISORDER (PTSD)
Time-limited posttraumatic stress responses that do not persist or affect one's functioning are normal reactions to external threats, analogous to normal grief reactions. PTSD is an anxiety disorder characterized by exposure to a markedly distressing traumatic event followed by at least 1 month of recurrent reexperiencing of the event, persistent avoidance of stimuli associated with the trauma and numbing of general responsiveness, and persistent symptoms of hyperarousal. This is an often chronic and highly disabling condition, with a lifetime prevalence in the community of 1.3% to 7.8% and a greater risk among women than men. The most common comorbid conditions are substance use disorders, MDD, simple phobia, and GAD.

Diagnosis

1. History of exposure to a markedly distressing traumatic event.
2. Recurrent reexperiencing of the event, persistent avoidance of stimuli associated with the trauma, numbing of general responsiveness, and persistent symptoms of hyperarousal.
3. A careful psychiatric history should be obtained to diagnose conditions that are associated with PTSD.

The cost-effectiveness of laboratory testing is unclear, and physical examinations, although potentially useful in ruling out medical conditions with secondary symptoms of hyperarousal, are typically performed only when the clinical presentation is suggestive.

Pharmacologic Treatment

Pharmacologic treatment of PTSD is typically continued over the long term, because there is evidence of significant prophylaxis of relapses and recurrences with continued antidepressant treatment for 9 months. Furthermore, many patients, particularly those with a history of repeated trauma, do not respond to initial intervention and may require more than one medication, along with psychosocial intervention to achieve remission.

Antidepressants

Antidepressants are relatively efficacious in the treatment of PTSD. They are also useful in addressing the frequent comorbidity of MDD, panic disorder, and other anxiety disorders such as GAD.

SSRIs are often used in the treatment of PTSD. Only two of the SSRIs (sertraline and paroxetine) are FDA approved for the treatment of PTSD, whereas the other SSRIs are typically used in an off-label mode, partly because of positive placebo-controlled studies such as in the case of fluoxetine. (See Chapter 3 for a description of the pharmacology of SSRIs.) The dosing of the SSRIs used in the treatment of PTSD appears to be similar to that used in the treatment of depression (e.g., sertraline dosage ranging from 50 to 200 mg per day).

SNRIs such as venlafaxine, duloxetine, and desvenlafaxine are also used off-label in the treatment of PTSD, partly because of promising open trials with venlafaxine. (See Chapter 3 for a description of the pharmacology of SNRIs.) The dosing of venlafaxine, duloxetine, and desvenlafaxine used in the treatment of PTSD is similar to that used in the treatment of depression (e.g., venlafaxine dosages ranging from 75 to 225 mg per day).

The α_2-adrenergic receptor antagonist mirtazapine (dosage 15 to 45 mg per day) has shown efficacy in a small placebo-controlled trial in PTSD, whereas there is no good evidence of efficacy for bupropion and trazodone.

TCAs such as imipramine and amitriptyline are also used off-label in the treatment of PTSD, although typically only after other pharmacologic treatments have failed, given the side-effect profile of TCAs and lethality risk in overdose. (See Chapter 3 for a description of the pharmacology of TCAs.) Their efficacy in the treatment of PTSD appears to be rather modest. The dosing of TCAs used in the treatment of PTSD is similar to that used in the treatment of depression (e.g., imipramine dosage ranging from 100 to 300 mg per day).

MAOIs such as phenelzine are in rare cases used off-label in the treatment of PTSD, although typically only after many other pharmacologic treatments have failed, given the side-effect profile of MAOIs, the risk of drug–drug interactions, and the need for tyramine-free diet for a disorder that may result in impulsivity for some patients. Some researchers have argued that MAOIs may be more effective than TCAs in the treatment of PTSD. (See Chapter 3 for a description of the pharmacology of MAOIs.) The dosing of MAOIs used in the treatment of PTSD is similar to that used in the treatment of depression (e.g., phenelzine dosage ranging from 30 to 90 mg per day).

Benzodiazepines
High-potency benzodiazepines such as alprazolam and clonazepam are most commonly prescribed, but the evidence to support their clinical utility is weak, and the common comorbidity of substance use with PTSD makes the use of benzodiazepines even less attractive for PTSD. Thus, benzodiazepines are not considered first-line pharmacotherapy for PTSD. (See above section on GAD for a description of the pharmacologic characteristics of benzodiazepines.) Typically, dosages of 1 to 6 mg per day of alprazolam and 0.5 to 3 mg per day of clonazepam may be helpful, but occasional patients have required the equivalent of 10 mg per day of alprazolam and 5 mg per day of clonazepam. The extended-release formulation of alprazolam is clearly preferred to the immediate-release formulation, because it minimizes the problem of interdose rebound.

Buspirone
There is very modest evidence that buspirone (at daily doses between 15 and 60 mg) has significant anti-PTSD effects; its use clinically is largely limited to augmentation of antidepressants.

Anticonvulsants
Anticonvulsants such as carbamazepine, oxcarbazepine, gabapentin, tiagabine, lamotrigine, topiramate, and valproic acid are typically used off-label in the treatment of PTSD when other pharmacologic treatments have failed. (See Chapter 4 for a description of the pharmacology of anticonvulsants.) The dosing of the anticonvulsants used in the treatment of PTSD appears to be similar to that used in the treatment of epilepsy (e.g., gabapentin dosage ranging from 300 to 2,400 mg per day, topiramate dosage ranging from 50 to 400 mg per day, lamotrigine dosage ranging from 50 to 400 mg per day, valproic acid dosage ranging from 500 to 2,000 mg per day, tiagabine dosage ranging from 4 to 16 mg per day, and carbamazepine dosage ranging from 400 to 1,000 mg per day). The evidence in support of the usefulness of anticonvulsants in the treatment of PTSD primarily derives from uncontrolled studies (although there is one positive double-blind study), and more research is needed.

β-Blockers, α$_2$-Adrenergic Receptor Agonists, and α$_1$-Adrenergic Receptor Antagonists
Preliminary data suggest that β-blockers such as propranolol administered within a few hours of the traumatic event may reduce the chances of developing PTSD as a complication of the trauma exposure by blocking the enhancement of explicit (conscious) memories that characterizes emotionally charged situations. β-Blockers do not produce amnesia but only block this enhancement. A large clinical trial to study the utility of β-blockers in preventing PTSD is ongoing. β-Blockers (e.g., propranolol 40 to 160 mg per day) have also shown some benefit in the treatment of established PTSD.

The α$_2$-adrenergic receptor agonists [e.g., clonidine (Catapres) 0.2 to 0.6 mg per day; guanfacine (Tenex) 0.5 to 3 mg per day] have shown some possible utility as a treatment of PTSD as either monotherapy or as adjunctive treatment, although a recent study showed no benefit from augmentation with guanfacine. The most common side effects of these agents are dry mouth, dizziness, fatigue, and drowsiness.

The α$_1$-adrenergic receptor antagonist prazosin (Minipress) (2 to 10 mg per day) has shown some efficacy in the treatment of PTSD in a double-blind crossover protocol. Dreams and sleep are improved more than other symptoms of PTSD. The most common side effects of prazosin are dizziness, drowsiness, fatigue, and headache.

Second-Generation Antipsychotics

Second-generation antipsychotics such as risperidone, olanzapine, and quetiapine are typically used off-label as adjuncts in the treatment of PTSD only when other pharmacologic treatments have failed. These agents may also have a role in the reduction of flashbacks and dissociation. (See Chapter 2 for a description of the pharmacology of second-generation antipsychotics.) The dosing of second-generation antipsychotics used in the treatment of PTSD is similar to that used in the treatment of psychotic disorders (e.g., risperidone dosage ranging from 0.5 to 8 mg per day, olanzapine dosage ranging from 5 to 20 mg per day, aripirazole dosage ranging from 5 to 20 mg per day, quetiapine dosage ranging from 50 to 300 mg per day). Both open and controlled studies provide evidence in support of the usefulness of second-generation antipsychotics as adjuncts in the treatment of PTSD.

Psychotherapy

Nonpharmacologic treatments typically include prolonged exposure therapy, CBT techniques, and their combination. Studies support the efficacy of these approaches, which may also be considered a first-line intervention. Eye movement and desensitization reprocessing, involving exposure accompanied by saccadic eye movements, has been found to be less effective than other exposure-based structured psychotherapies.

Bibliography

Generalized Anxiety Disorder (GAD)
Fricchione G. Clinical practice. Generalized anxiety disorder. *N Engl J Med* 2004;351:675.
Pollack MH. Optimizing pharmacotherapy of generalized anxiety disorder to achieve remission. *J Clin Psychiatry* 2001;62(suppl 19):20.

Antidepressants in GAD
Davidson J, Allgulander C, Pollack MH, et al. Efficacy and tolerability of duloxetine in elderly patients with generalized anxiety disorder: a pooled analysis of four randomized, double-blind, placebo-controlled studies. *Hum Psychopharmacol* 2008;23(6):519–526.
Pollack M, Kinrys G, Krystal A, et al. Eszopiclone coadministered with escitalopram in patients with insomnia and comorbid generalized anxiety disorder. *Arch Gen Psychiatry* 2008;65(5):551–562.
Rickels K, Mangano R, Khan A. A double-blind, placebo-controlled study of a flexible dose of venlafaxine ER in adult outpatients with generalized social anxiety disorder. *J Clin Psychopharmacol* 2004;24:488.
Zohar J, Westenberg HG. Anxiety disorders: a review of tricyclic antidepressants and selective serotonin reuptake inhibitors. *Acta Psychiatr Scand Suppl* 2000;403:39–49.

Toxicity of Benzodiazepines
Buffett-Jerrott SE, Stewart SH. Cognitive and sedative effects of benzodiazepine use. *Curr Pharm Des* 2002;8:45.
Isbister GK, O'Regan L, Sibbritt D, et al. Alprazolam is relatively more toxic than other benzodiazepines in overdose. *Br J Clin Pharmacol* 2004;58:88.

Dependence and Abuse with Benzodiazepines
Brunette MF, Noordsy DL, Xie H, et al. Benzodiazepine use and abuse among patients with severe mental illness and co-occurring substance use disorders. *Psychiatr Serv* 2003;54:1395.
de las Cuevas C, Sanz E, de la Fuente J. Benzodiazepines: more "behavioural" addiction than dependence. *Psychopharmacology (Berl)* 2003;167:297.

Kan CC, Hilberink SR, Breteler MH. Determination of the main risk factors for benzodiazepine dependence using a multivariate and multidimensional approach. *Compr Psychiatry* 2004;45:88.

Sellers EM, Schneiderman JF, Romach MK, et al. Comparative drug effects and abuse liability of lorazepam, buspirone, and secobarbital in nondependent subjects. *J Clin Psychopharmacol* 1992;12:79.

van Broekhoven F, Kan CC, Zitman FG. Dependence potential of antidepressants compared to benzodiazepines. *Prog Neuropsychopharmacol Biol Psychiatry* 2002;26:939.

Discontinuation of Benzodiazepines

Morin CM, Bastien C, Guay B, et al. Randomized clinical trial of supervised tapering and cognitive behavior therapy to facilitate benzodiazepine discontinuation in older adults with chronic insomnia. *Am J Psychiatry* 2004;161:332.

Otto MW, Hong JJ, Safren SA. Benzodiazepine discontinuation difficulties in panic disorder: conceptual model and outcome for cognitive-behavior therapy. *Curr Pharm Des* 2002;8:75.

Rynn M, Garcia-Espana F, Greenblatt DJ, et al. Imipramine and buspirone in patients with panic disorder who are discontinuing long-term benzodiazepine therapy. *J Clin Psychopharmacol* 2003;23:505.

Voshaar RC, Gorgels WJ, Mol AJ, et al. Tapering off long-term benzodiazepine use with or without group cognitive-behavioural therapy: three-condition, randomised controlled trial. *Br J Psychiatry* 2003;182:498.

Benzodiazepine Use in the Elderly

Madhusoodanan S, Bogunovic OJ. Safety of benzodiazepines in the geriatric population. *Expert Opin Drug Saf* 2004;3:485.

Wagner AK, Zhang F, Soumerai SB, et al. Benzodiazepine use and hip fractures in the elderly: who is at greatest risk? *Arch Intern Med* 2004;164:1567.

Benzodiazepine Use in Pregnancy

Eros E, Czeizel AE, Rockenbauer M, et al. A population-based case-control teratologic study of nitrazepam, medazepam, tofisopam, alprazolam and clonazepam treatment during pregnancy. *Eur J Obstet Gynecol Reprod Biol* 2002;101:147.

Lin AE, Peller AJ, Westgate MN, et al. Clonazepam use in pregnancy and the risk of malformations. *Birth Defects Res A Clin Mol Teratol* 2004;70:534.

Anticonvulsants in GAD

Bech P. Dose-response relationship of pregabalin in patients with generalized anxiety disorder. A pooled analysis of four placebo-controlled trials. *Pharmacopsychiatry* 2007;40(4):163–168.

Mula M, Pini S, Cassano GB. The role of anticonvulsant drugs in anxiety disorders: a critical review of the evidence. *J Clin Psychopharmacol* 2007;27(3):263–272.

Antipsychotics in GAD

Hoge EA, Worthington JJ III, Kaufman RE, et al. Aripiprazole as augmentation treatment of refractory generalized anxiety disorder and panic disorder. *CNS Spectr* 2008;13(6): 522–527.

Katzman MA, Vermani M, Jacobs L, et al. Quetiapine as an adjunctive pharmacotherapy for the treatment of non-remitting generalized anxiety disorder: a flexible-dose, open-label pilot trial. *J Anxiety Disord* 2008;22(8):1480–1486.

Pollack MH, Simon NM, Zalta AK, et al. Olanzapine augmentation of fluoxetine for refractory generalized anxiety disorder: a placebo controlled study. *Biol Psychiatry* 2006;59(3): 211–215.

Riluzole in GAD

Mathew SJ, Amiel JM, Coplan JD, et al. Open-label trial of riluzole in generalized anxiety disorder. *Am J Psychiatry* 2005;162(12):2379–2381.

Psychotherapy in GAD

Hofmann SG, Smits JA. Cognitive-behavioral therapy for adult anxiety disorders: a meta-analysis of randomized placebo-controlled trials. *J Clin Psychiatry* 2008;69(4):621–632.

Social Anxiety Disorder

Davidson JR. Use of benzodiazepines in social anxiety disorder, generalized anxiety disorder, and posttraumatic stress disorder. *J Clin Psychiatry* 2004;65(suppl 5):29.

Davidson JR. Pharmacotherapy of social anxiety disorder: what does the evidence tell us? *J Clin Psychiatry* 2006;67(suppl 12):20–26.

Hofmann SG, Pollack MH, Otto MW. Augmentation treatment of psychotherapy for anxiety disorders with D-cycloserine. *CNS Drug Rev* 2006;12(3/4):208–217.

Otto MW, Pollack MH, Gould RA, et al. A comparison of the efficacy of clonazepam and cognitive-behavioral group therapy for the treatment of social phobia. *J Anxiety Disord* 2000;14:345.

Pande AC, Feltner DE, Jefferson JW, et al. Efficacy of the novel anxiolytic pregabalin in social anxiety disorder: a placebo-controlled, multicenter study. *J Clin Psychopharmacol* 2004;24:141.

Rodebaugh TL, Holaway RM, Heimberg RG. The treatment of social anxiety disorder. *Clin Psychol Rev* 2004;24:883.

Seedat S, Stein MB. Double-blind, placebo-controlled assessment of combined clonazepam with paroxetine compared with paroxetine monotherapy for generalized social anxiety disorder. *J Clin Psychiatry* 2004;65:244.

Simon NM, Worthington JJ, Doyle AC, et al. An open-label study of levetiracetam for the treatment of social anxiety disorder. *J Clin Psychiatry* 2004;65:1219.

Stein DJ, Ipser J, Balkom A. Pharmacotherapy for social phobia. *Cochrane Database Syst Rev* 2004:CD001206.

Stein MB, Fyer AJ, Davidson JR, et al. Fluvoxamine treatment of social phobia (social anxiety disorder): a double-blind, placebo-controlled study. *Am J Psychiatry* 1999;156:756.

Stein MB, Sareen J, Hami S, et al. Pindolol potentiation of paroxetine for generalized social phobia: a double-blind, placebo-controlled, crossover study. *Am J Psychiatry* 2001;158(10):1725–1727.

Van Ameringen M, Mancini C, Pipe B, et al. An open trial of topiramate in the treatment of generalized social phobia. *J Clin Psychiatry* 2004;65(12):1674–1678.

Zhang W, Connor KM, Davidson JR. Levetiracetam in social phobia: a placebo controlled pilot study. *J Psychopharmacol* 2005;19(5):551–553.

Panic Disorder

Asnis GM, Hameedi FA, Goddard AW, et al. Fluvoxamine in the treatment of panic disorder: a multi-center, double-blind, placebo-controlled study in outpatients. *Psychiatry Res.* 2001;103(1):1–14.

Bandelow B, Stein DJ, Dolberg OT, et al. Improvement of quality of life in panic disorder with escitalopram, citalopram, or placebo. *Pharmacopsychiatry* 2007;40(4):152–156.

Hoge EA, Worthington JJ 3rd, Kaufman RE, et al. Aripiprazole as augmentation treatment of refractory generalized anxiety disorder and panic disorder. *CNS Spectr* 2008;13(6):522–527.

Kampman M, Keijsers GP, Hoogduin CA, et al. A randomized, double-blind, placebo-controlled study of the effects of adjunctive paroxetine in panic disorder patients unsuccessfully treated with cognitive-behavioral therapy alone. *J Clin Psychiatry* 2002;63:772.

Mavissakalian MR, Guo S. Early detection of relapse in panic disorder. *Acta Psychiatr Scand* 2004;110:393.

Michelson D, Allgulander C, Dantendorfer K, et al. Efficacy of usual antidepressant dosing regimens of fluoxetine in panic disorder: randomised, placebo-controlled trial. *Br J Psychiatry* 2001;179:514–518.

Pande AC, Pollack MH, Crockatt J, et al. Placebo-controlled study of gabapentin treatment of panic disorder. *J Clin Psychopharmacol* 2000;20:467.

Papp LA. Safety and efficacy of levetiracetam for patients with panic disorder: results of an open-label, fixed-flexible dose study. *J Clin Psychiatry* 2006;67(10):1573–1576.

Pollack MH, Otto MW, Worthington JJ, et al. Sertraline in the treatment of panic disorder: a flexible-dose multicenter trial. *Arch Gen Psychiatry* 1998;55:1010.

Rosenbaum JF, Moroz G, Bowden CL. Clonazepam in the treatment of panic disorder with or without agoraphobia: a dose-response study of efficacy, safety, and discontinuance. *J Clin Psychopharmacol* 1997;17:390.

Sepede G, De Berardis D, Gambi F, et al. Olanzapine augmentation in treatment-resistant panic disorder: a 12-week, fixed-dose, open-label trial. *J Clin Psychopharmacol* 2006;26(1):45–49.

Simon NM, Safren SA, Otto MW, et al. Longitudinal outcome with pharmacotherapy in a naturalistic study of panic disorder. *J Affect Disord* 2002;69:201.

Stahl SM, Gergel I, Li D. Escitalopram in the treatment of panic disorder: a randomized, double-blind, placebo-controlled trial. *J Clin Psychiatry* 2003;64:1322.

Buspirone

Davidson JR, DuPont RL, Hedges D, et al. Efficacy, safety, and tolerability of venlafaxine extended release and buspirone in outpatients with generalized anxiety disorder. *J Clin Psychiatry* 1999;60:528.

DeMartinis N, Rynn M, Rickels K, et al. Prior benzodiazepine use and buspirone response in the treatment of generalized anxiety disorder. *J Clin Psychiatry* 2000;61:91.

Grady TA, Pigott TA, L'Heureux F, et al. Double-blind study of adjuvant buspirone for fluoxetine-treated patients with obsessive-compulsive disorder. *Am J Psychiatry* 1993;150:819.

Laakmann G, Schule C, Lorkowski G, et al. Buspirone and lorazepam in the treatment of generalized anxiety disorder in outpatients. *Psychopharmacology (Berl)* 1998;136:357.

Obsessive-Compulsive Disorder (OCD)

Bystritsky A, Ackerman DL, Rosen RM, et al. Augmentation of serotonin reuptake inhibitors in refractory obsessive-compulsive disorder using adjunctive olanzapine: a placebo-controlled trial. *J Clin Psychiatry* 2004;65:565.

Dell'Osso B, Nestadt G, Allen A, et al. Serotonin-norepinephrine reuptake inhibitors in the treatment of obsessive-compulsive disorder: a critical review. *J Clin Psychiatry* 2006;67(4): 600–610.

Denys D, de Geus F, van Megen HJ, et al. A double-blind, randomized, placebo-controlled trial of quetiapine addition in patients with obsessive-compulsive disorder refractory to serotonin reuptake inhibitors. *J Clin Psychiatry* 2004;65:1040.

Denys D. Pharmacotherapy of obsessive-compulsive disorder and obsessive-compulsive spectrum disorders. *Psychiatr Clin North Am* 2006;29(2):553–584, xi.

Dougherty DD, Rauch SL, Jenike MA. Pharmacotherapy for obsessive-compulsive disorder. *J Clin Psychol* 2004;60:1195.

Geller DA, Wagner KD, Emslie G, et al. Paroxetine treatment in children and adolescents with obsessive-compulsive disorder: a randomized, multicenter, double-blind, placebo-controlled trial. *J Am Acad Child Adolesc Psychiatry* 2004;43:1387.

Hollander E, Allen A, Steiner M, et al. Paroxetine OCD Study Group. Acute and long-term treatment and prevention of relapse of obsessive-compulsive disorder with paroxetine. *J Clin Psychiatry* 2003;64:1113.

Hollander E, Baldini Rossi N, Sood E, et al. Risperidone augmentation in treatment-resistant obsessive-compulsive disorder: a double-blind, placebo-controlled study. *Int J Neuropsychopharmacol* 2003;6:397.

Onder E, Tural U, Gökbakan M. Does gabapentin lead to early symptom improvement in obsessive-compulsive disorder? *Eur Arch Psychiatry Clin Neurosci* 2008;258(6):319–323. Epub 2008 Feb 23.

Pasquini M, Biondi M. Memantine augmentation for refractory obsessive-compulsive disorder. *Prog Neuropsychopharmacol Biol Psychiatry* 2006;30(6):1173-1175. Epub 2006 May 30.

Sareen J, Kirshner A, Lander M, et al. Do antipsychotics ameliorate or exacerbate obsessive compulsive disorder symptoms? A systematic review. *J Affect Disord* 2004;82:167.

Posttraumatic Stress Disorder (PTSD)

Davidson J, Pearlstein T, Londborg P, et al. Efficacy of sertraline in preventing relapse of posttraumatic stress disorder: results of a 28-week double-blind, placebo-controlled study. *Am J Psychiatry* 2001;158:1974.

Davidson JR, Stein DJ, Shalev AY, et al. Posttraumatic stress disorder: acquisition, recognition, course, and treatment. *J Neuropsychiatry Clin Neurosci* 2004;16:135.

McNally RJ. Panic and posttraumatic stress disorder: implications for culture, risk, and treatment. *Cogn Behav Ther* 2008;37(2):131–134.

Miller LJ. Prazosin for the treatment of posttraumatic stress disorder sleep disturbances. *Pharmacotherapy* 2008;28(5):656–666.

Penava SJ, Otto MW, Pollack MH, et al. Current status of pharmacotherapy for PTSD: an effect size analysis of controlled studies. *Depress Anxiety* 1996–1997;4:240.

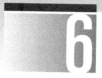

6

Drugs for the Treatment of Substance Use and Addictive Disorders

GENERAL PRINCIPLES

Substance use disorders are extremely common and frequently comorbid with other mental disorders. Treating mental disorders without treating comorbid substance use disorders frequently leads to poor outcomes.

Alcohol and drug addiction may mimic a wide range of mental disorders and lead to misdiagnosis or misguided treatment. For example, covert cocaine use may lead to symptoms of anxiety or mania in toxicity or depression on withdrawal. Alcoholism frequently complicates unipolar depression, bipolar disorder, and anxiety disorders, creating a picture in which the proximate cause of symptoms is muddied. Because patients are often not forthcoming about substance use, the unsuspecting clinician may target the psychiatric symptoms of these **covert disorders** and fail to treat a substance use disorder that is adding complexity to the clinical picture. Moreover, a subset of patients have more than one addiction (e.g., those with opiates dependence frequently also use alcohol or cocaine), and treatment must address each substance.

Substance use may produce a variety of mental and behavioral symptoms even in the absence of dependence. For example, the intermittent binge drinker or cocaine user may exhibit a range of problems from mood lability to risk of accidents. With repetitive use of drugs comes physiologic dependence, an adapted state of brain and other organ systems in which withdrawal symptoms complicate attempts to abstain from drug use. The withdrawal syndrome is substance specific. Alcohol and opiates produce physical withdrawal symptoms that can be severe (agitation, tachycardia, insomnia, seizures in the case of the former, severe abdominal cramps, flulike symptoms in the case of the latter). The withdrawal syndrome of nicotine and cocaine, highly addictive drugs, is dominated by mood and cognitive effects such as irritability and difficulty concentrating and also include prominent insomnia and increased appetite. Addiction is the end stage of substance abuse, defined as a compulsive behavior, usually drug use, that is continued despite negative consequences. The results for the person, family, and society may be severe. Addiction is a chronic and relapsing disorder for which effective treatments exist. Most patients require **multiple treatment** trials before they can sustain abstinence. Individuals with addiction are at high risk of relapse even after extended periods of abstinence, indeed long after withdrawal symptoms other than intense craving to use the drug have subsided.

Treatment of substance use disorders too often ends with detoxification and management of withdrawal symptoms. Because we now know that addiction is a chronic, relapsing disorder that results in brain changes, and because powerful craving to use substances can persist or recur at times of stress or exposure to the drug or drug cues, detoxification and resolution of withdrawal symptoms is really the area at which ongoing outpatient treatment should begin rather than end. The aim of successful treatment is to minimize late relapse (such treatments are often aimed at managing craving elicited by drug-related cues and by stress) and to treat co-occurring mental disorders. In general, extensive (the number of reinforcing sessions and duration of the treatment) rather than intensive (e.g., inpatient rehabilitation, etc.) predict better outcomes.

A number of effective pharmacologic treatments are available for the treatment of addictive disorders. All pharmacologic treatments are recommended to be delivered in combination with psychosocial treatments. Recent studies have examined patients with multiple drug addictions. In some combinations of addiction, medication treatment benefits at least a facet of the addiction. Pharmacologic treatments alone have low long-term success rates and may mislead the patients with substance use disorders, especially addiction, into believing that psychosocial treatments and personal struggles will be less important. Pharmacologic detoxification treatments are more successful than treatments to promote long-term abstinence, although the former treatment must be seen as a prelude to the long-term treatment of persons with addictions. This chapter focuses on the major drugs of abuse and details the pharmacologic treatment of substance abuse disorders.

OPIOID DEPENDENCE

Opioid dependence is associated with severe medical and psychosocial consequences, including violent crimes and spread of HIV infection through unprotected sex or sharing needles used for intravenous injections. Because abused opioids are generally expensive and short acting, persons using these drugs frequently suffer withdrawal symptoms and may go to great extremes such as burglary, prostitution, or drug dealing to prevent withdrawal, although a substantial number finance their addiction through conventional employment. **Antisocial personality disorder** is often seen in men with heroin dependence, and it is not uncommon to see heroin-dependent women present with mood and anxiety disorders. Those with heroin dependence also commonly misuse alcohol and psychostimulants.

OPIOID WITHDRAWAL

Acute cessation of opioids following chronic use leads to nausea and vomiting, sweating, piloerection ("goose flesh"), hypertension, enlarged pupils, tachycardia, muscle and bone pain, anxiety, and insomnia. Hallucinations and confusion are rare; however, they may be precipitated by use of an opioid antagonist such as naltrexone or naloxone. Treatment is supportive. Opioid withdrawal is extremely uncomfortable but generally not dangerous; however, the intense craving that follows acute abstinence often leads to nonadherence with recommended treatments and relapse to drug use.

DRUGS USED IN THE TREATMENT OF OPIOID WITHDRAWAL

Clonidine

Clonidine is an α_2-adrenergic receptor agonist used in the treatment of hypertension that also is useful in the treatment of opioid withdrawal. Because the predominant role of central α_2 receptors is to act as autoreceptors with a negative feedback function, the major effect of clonidine is to decrease the activity of central noradrenergic neurons. It is particularly effective in suppressing autonomic symptoms, having proved more effective than morphine or placebo. Several controlled trials have demonstrated that clonidine suppresses many of the signs and symptoms commonly seen in patients withdrawing from narcotics and thereby contributes significantly to patient comfort and compliance. Although a very useful compound to manage the autonomic symptoms of withdrawal, its sedative and hypotensive effects limit its outpatient use and it is clearly less effective than morphine in reducing drug-craving symptoms.

Pharmacology

Clonidine is almost completely absorbed after oral administration, achieving peak plasma concentrations in 1 to 3 hours. Approximately half of the drug is metabolized in the liver, the rest is excreted unchanged by the kidney, and it has no known active metabolites. It has an elimination half-life of 9 hours; thus, it is usually given in two daily doses. Because clonidine is very lipophilic, it easily penetrates the blood–brain barrier, where it has its principal effects as outlined previously.

Side Effects and Toxicity
Although most of our clinical experience with clonidine comes from its use for hypertension, the side-effects profiles for both medical and psychiatric patients are similar. About 50% of patients report dry mouth and some degree of sedation during the first 2 to 4 weeks of therapy with gradual improvement of these side effects over that period. An estimated 10% of patients discontinue this agent because of persistent side effects, including sedation, **postural dizziness**, dry mouth and/or dry eyes, nausea, impotence, and fluid retention (which may be managed with diuretics).

The similarity between central nervous system (CNS) side effects of these drugs and the disorder for which the drugs are used is a significant complication of treatment and management of these patients, demanding that the clinician pay careful attention to mental status and neurologic examination findings. Therefore, sedation, drowsiness, vivid dreams or nightmares, insomnia, restlessness, anxiety, depression, visual or auditory hallucinations (rare), or erectile dysfunction need to be assessed as possible side effects versus symptoms of the illness being treated. Rare idiosyncratic side effects include rash, pruritus, alopecia, hyperglycemia, gynecomastia, and increased sensitivity to alcohol.

Drug interactions are uncommon, but concurrent use with a tricyclic antidepressant may reduce the antihypertensive effect of clonidine. Use with other agents that cause orthostasis (e.g., trazodone or risperidone) may lead to hypotension.

Overdoses may result in decreased blood pressure, heart rate, and respiratory rate. Patients who have overdosed on these agents may be stuporous or comatose with small pupils, their condition mimicking an opioid overdose. Treatment consists of ventilatory support, intravenous fluids or pressors for hypotension, and atropine for bradycardia.

Dose Forms Available
Clonidine is available for oral use only under the trade name Catapres. Tablets are available in 0.1-, 0.2-, and 0.3-mg strengths. Clonidine is available as a long-acting skin patch, providing the equivalent of 0.1 mg three times a day (t.i.d.), 0.2 mg t.i.d., and 0.3 mg t.i.d.

Method of Use
If patients are being withdrawn from opioids and not placed on methadone, then clonidine may be administered beginning at low dosages, such as 0.1 mg twice a day (b.i.d.) or t.i.d. and increased as needed and tolerated. Blood pressure and symptoms of orthostasis should be monitored every 4 hours. Dosage can be gradually increased over the first few days, rarely to exceed 0.3 mg t.i.d. Clonidine best treats adrenergic signs and symptoms (e.g., hypertension, piloerection) and is not particularly effective for the treatment of gastrointestinal symptoms and drug craving. Bone and muscle pain responds well to nonsteroidal antiinflammatory agents (e.g., ibuprofen 400 to 600 mg t.i.d.), and gastrointestinal symptoms may be treated symptomatically with one or a combination of the following: sucralfate 1 g four times a day (q.i.d.), loperamide 2 mg t.i.d., or dicyclomine 10 to 20 mg t.i.d. Successful treatment of acute withdrawal as outlined previously rarely exceeds a few days, allowing for a rapid taper of clonidine when deemed appropriate. In the absence of replacement therapy with opioid agonists, however, the drug craving may be so strong that many opioid addicts relapse following clonidine detoxification, and because of opioid craving they may leave the hospital prematurely to continue using it.

PHARMACOLOGIC TREATMENT OF CHRONIC OPIOID DEPENDENCE

Opioid dependence is a chronic and frequently relapsing condition. Although treatment of opioid withdrawal is generally straightforward, combined pharmacologic and behavioral treatment of long-term sobriety are somewhat less successful. Some reasons for relapse to drug use include strong cravings associated with stress or environmental cues, treatment onset late in the course of the addiction, and co-occurring addictive, psychiatric, or medical disorders. The mainstay of outpatient relapse prevention treatment is **opioid replacement pharmacotherapy** [i.e., methadone, or buprenorphine]. Antagonist treatment (i.e., naltrexone) alone is generally less effective, except in highly motivated patients with excellent social supports. Patients should be involved in some form of **psychosocial therapy** addressing abstinence to maintain long-term sobriety and addressing any co-occurring illnesses, for example, HIV infection, posttraumatic stress disorder, or alcohol dependence. Contingency management techniques, such as providing vouchers or the ability to take a dose of methadone home in return for urine, saliva, or expired air screens that are negative for substances, are also useful aids to pharmacotherapy. It is the norm for patients to require multiple courses of treatment before sustained abstinence is attained.

Methadone

Methadone is a long-acting synthetic opioid also used in the treatment of chronic pain. It is commonly used to aid long-term abstinence from opiate use as it blocks access of heroin to the μ-opiate receptor, blocking euphoric effects of heroin. Methadone also ameliorates craving, prevents withdrawal symptoms, and has minimal euphoric effects. Thus, someone who has taken an adequate dose of methadone will not gain a desired hedonic effect from heroin. Of course, methadone does not block the target receptors for nonopiate drugs; therefore, other drugs can produce euphoria in the presence of methadone.

The use of methadone has often proved controversial to those who believe that the goals of treatment should be abstinence. A large body of data, however, suggests that **termination of methadone often leads to relapse** to heroin and that from a medical and harm avoidance point of view (taking into account the risks of shared needles among heroin users, the possibility of rehabilitation, and reduction in crime), long-term methadone maintenance and perhaps other opioid replacement therapies are the most effective existing treatments for heroin addiction. Use of methadone for opioid replacement, formerly overseen by the Drug Enforcement Administration, is currently under the auspices of the Substance Abuse and Mental Health Services Administration, leading to less stringent practice requirements. More take-home doses are allowed, and after a period of stability, take-home doses of up to 1 month are permissible, though not all states allow this. Well rehabilitated patients often do well with this extended regimen.

Pharmacokinetics

Methadone is rapidly absorbed and highly plasma protein bound; oral absorption is approximately 50% of subcutaneous absorption. It has a steady-state elimination half-life of 25 hours, allowing for once-a-day dosing; it is N-demethylated and conjugated by the liver with modest first-pass effects. Significant reduction in plasma concentration of methadone may occur with coadministration of drugs that induce hepatic enzymes such as carbamazepine, phenobarbital, nevirapine, or other protease inhibitors used in the treatment of HIV infection. Conversely, plasma concentration may be increased when methadone is coadministered with ketoconazole or fluvoxamine.

Pharmacologic Effects

Methadone has pharmacologic effects similar to those of morphine. The drug is an agonist at opioid receptors, particularly at μ-receptors. Opioid receptors are found in various organs and tissues throughout the body, including the brain, where they inhibit the release of acetylcholine, norepinephrine, and substance P and alter the release of dopamine. Methadone's effects are dose dependent, acting primarily as a CNS, respiratory, and gastrointestinal depressant inducing analgesia without loss of consciousness. Systemic effects are dose dependent and apply to various organ systems. With increasing doses, the following effects may be seen:

CNS: euphoria, sedation, confusion, coma
Cardiovascular: bradycardia, hypotension, shock
Gastrointestinal: nausea and vomiting, constipation, bowel obstruction
Pulmonary: decreased ventilation, pulmonary edema, hypoxia, respiratory arrest
Genital/sexual: decreased libido, impotence, delayed orgasm
Endocrine: hyperprolactinemia and gynecomastia may result with chronic use

Methadone should be used with caution in patients with the following problems:

1. Asthma, chronic obstructive pulmonary disease, preexisting respiratory depression, hypoxia, hypercapnia
2. Volume depletion or drugs with significant α-1 blockade
3. Traumatic brain injury
4. Coadministration of other CNS depressants
5. Acute abdominal pain
6. Alcohol intoxication

Dose Forms Available

The trade name for methadone is Dolophine. Methadone is available as a solution, 120 mg/mL. This may also be available in a cherry-flavored elixir. Tablet forms of 5 or 10 mg are also available. (Tables 6.1 and 6.2).

Method of Use for Withdrawal from Opioids

The mainstay of opiate detoxification is the long-acting opiate methadone. In typical detoxification protocols, the requirement for methadone is determined using objective criteria (hypertension or tachycardia above baseline, dilated pupils, sweating, gooseflesh, rhinorrhea, or lacrimation) rather than subjective complaints. Methadone is administered in dosages of 10 mg orally every 4 hours when at least two objective criteria for withdrawal are met. The total dose of methadone given on day 1 is given the next day in two divided doses. Methadone is then withdrawn by 5 mg per day. The use of methadone for the management of withdrawal in neonates with narcotic abstinence syndrome is best accomplished with dosages of 3 to 4 mg per kilogram per day; reports in the literature find this to be a dose range that optimizes efficacy while minimizing toxicity.

Method of Use for Abstinence from Opioids

When the patient is clinically stable, he or she can be started on a relatively low dosage of methadone, 20 to 40 mg per day. The dosage can be gradually titrated by 5 mg every 3 to 5 days as tolerated to higher dosages, usually reaching a **final dosage of 60 to 120 mg per day,** although some patients may need higher dosages to maintain abstinence from illicit opioids, especially from heroin. Low doses of

Disorder	Drug	Trade Name	Dose Forms
Opioid withdrawal	Clonidine	Catapres	0.1-, 0.2-, 0.3-mg tablets
	Dicyclomine	Bentyl	10-mg capsules, 20-mg tablet
	Sucralfate	Carafate	1-g tablet
Opioid abstinence	Methadone	Dolophine	5-, 10-mg tablets; 5 mg/5 mL, 5 mg/10 mL
	Levomethadyl acetate (LAAM)	Orlaam	5-, 10-mg tablets
	Buprenorphine	Buprenex	2-, 8-mg sublingual tablets
	Buprenorphine/ naloxone	Suboxone	2-mg/0.5-mg sublingual 8-mg/2-mg sublingual
Nicotine dependence	Nicotine	Nicoderm	7-, 14-, 21-mg transdermal
		Habitrol	7-, 14-, 21-mg transdermal
		Commit	2-, 4-mg disintegrating tablets
		Nicorette gum	2-, 4-mg gum
		Nicotrol inhaler	4-mg cartridge
		Habitrol inhaler	4-mg cartridge
		Nicotrol nasal spray	4-mg cartridge
	Bupropion SR	Zyban	100-, 150-mg tablets
	Varenicline	Chantix	0.5-, 1-mg tablets
Cocaine dependence	Modafinil	Provigil	200-, 400-mg tablets
	Disulfiram	Antabuse	250-, 500-mg tablets
	Topiramate	Topamax	25-, 50-, 100-, 200-mg tablets

TABLE 6.1 Drugs Used in the Treatment of Substance Use Disorders

methadone (e.g., 30 to 40 mg) are rarely helpful in maintaining abstinence. The methadone dose should be adjusted to control cravings to prevent relapse, but the clinician is cautioned to monitor the patient carefully to avoid excessive sedation or respiratory depression. Objective observations or information from other sources is sometimes better than relying on patients who may underreport the sedating effects of methadone. Methadone is often dispensed from specialized treatment centers in a liquid form, requiring patients to initially attend the treatment center five times per week. After patients proved themselves reliable by negative urine drug screens, they may begin take-home drug doses.

Levomethadyl Acetate
Levomethadyl acetate, also known as LAAM, is a long-acting congener of methadone. LAAM is a μ-opioid receptor agonist and has pharmacologic properties similar to those of methadone, with a longer half-life. Similarly, LAAM does not have a "rush" or "high" associated with its use. The advantages of LAAM over methadone is that it may be better tolerated, induces less withdrawal, and requires to use only 3 days per week, reducing the need to attend an opioid replacement

TABLE 6.2 Dose Range for Drugs Used in the Treatment of Substance Use Disorders

	Usual Dose	Extreme Dose Range
Opioid Withdrawal		
Clonidine	0.1–0.2 mg t.i.d.	0.1–0.3 mg t.i.d.
Dicyclomine	5–30 mg	5–60 mg
Sucralfate	2–4 g	1–6 g
Nicotine Abstinence		
Nicotine transdermal	7–21 mg	7–28 mg
Nicotine gum/tablet	18–40 mg	10–48 mg
Nicotine inhaler	6–10 cartridges	4–16 cartridges
Nicotine nasal spray	3–4 cartridges	2–5 cartridges
Bupropion SR	150–300 mg	100–450 mg
Varenicline	1–2 mg	0.5–2 mg
Cocaine Abstinence		
Topiramate	100–200 mg	50–400 mg
Disulfiram	250 mg	250–500 mg
Topiramate	100–200 mg	50–400 mg

t.i.d., three times a day.

clinic daily. Some patients will prefer methadone to LAAM and vice versa, but there are no clear predictors of which patients will do better on which drug.

Although LAMM may be better tolerated than methadone, it is similarly effective as methadone at reducing opioid use. Like methadone, LAAM is controlled under the Substance Abuse and Mental Health Administration and Drug Enforcement Agency regulations and requires specialized treatment centers for administration. These special treatment settings, unfortunately, isolate opioid treatment from mainstream medical treatment.

Occasional cases of torsades de pointes, a rare cardiac arrhythmia, are reported with LAAM use, suggesting that electrocardiogram monitoring should be a regular part of LAAM treatment. Because LAAM is proarrhythmic, **it is indicated only for those patients for whom other pharmacologic treatments for opioid dependence have failed;** it is not available in Europe because of this cardiac complication. Because of its toxicity, it is not a first-line agent for opioid dependence.

Pharmacology

LAAM is nearly completely absorbed from the gastrointestinal tract and reaches peak concentration within 2 to 4 hours. It is metabolized extensively by the liver, via cytochrome P450 CYP3A4 enzymes, and there are several active metabolites, including nor-LAAM, that are more potent at μ-opioid receptors than LAAM. The drug and its metabolites are excreted through the kidney and bile. The drug should be used cautiously in patients with liver disease because of the potential drug accumulation. LAAM and its active metabolites have long-lasting effects, with an elimination half-life more than 48 hours.

Like methadone and other opioids, LAAM may cause respiratory depression, nausea and vomiting, constipation, as well as a range of CNS effects including sedation, confusion, abnormal dreams, amnesia, sexual dysfunction, or ataxia. LAAM appears to increase QTc on echocardiograms and should be used with great caution in any patient with cardiac disease or taking a drug known to prolong the Q-T interval (e.g., calcium channel blockers, antimalarials, adenosine, Class II antiarrhythmics, tricyclic antidepressants, chlorpromazine, thioridazine, droperidol).

LAAM is contraindicated for use in patients with the following clinical conditions:

QTc prolongation (QTc greater than 450 milliseconds)
Treatment with monoamine oxidase inhibitors (MAOIs)
Bradycardia or significant heart disease
Treatment with Class I and Class III antiarrhythmics
Treatment with CYP3A4 inducers (e.g., rifampin, phenobarbital, phenytoin) or inhibitors (e.g., ketoconazole, erythromycin, HIV protease inhibitors)
Hypokalemia or hypomagnesemia

LAAM, like other opioids, should be used with caution in patients with heart disease, pulmonary disease, increased intracranial pressure, brain injury, hypothyroidism, or prostatic hypertrophy or in patients concomitantly treated with other CNS depressants. The dose should be carefully titrated in patients with renal or hepatic disease.

Dose Forms Available
LAAM is available as an oral solution, 10 mg/mL. The trade name is Orlaam.

Method of Use
Following detoxification and a careful cardiac history and evaluation, patients can be started on doses of 30 to 40 mg. Subsequent doses are given every other day, and dose increases can be made by 5- to 10-mg intervals. Within 2 weeks, doses can be given 3 days per week on Monday, Wednesday, and Friday, although some patients may not tolerate the 72-hour weekend intervals. Some patients may need a higher dose on Fridays to limit opioid craving or use over the weekend. Patients, at least initially, should be regularly involved in psychosocial treatment aimed at reducing drug and alcohol use.

The target dosage for most patients is between 60 and 100 mg three times per week. Caution should be taken with rapid dose increase because the long half-life may lead to accumulation and delayed sedative effects. The maximum recommended dosage is 140 mg three times per week. For patients being converted from methadone to LAAM, the dose should be approximately 1.2 times higher (e.g., 80 mg of methadone is replaced by 100 mg of LAAM). If a patient misses a few doses, renewed treatment should be restarted at a slightly lower dose. If the patient misses more than a week of treatment, dose titration should start from the beginning.

Buprenorphine
Buprenorphine is a novel synthetic opioid with mixed agonist and antagonist effects at opioid receptors. It is used in the treatment of pain and for abstinence from illicit opioids. It is a schedule III narcotic under the Controlled Substance Act. Unlike methadone, it may be prescribed outside of the usual specialized opioid treatment centers. Buprenorphine is thus an advance over previous treatments because it can be prescribed in **office-based settings**. Buprenorphine, however, is limited for prescribing only by physicians who meet qualifying requirements, and physicians can treat 30 patients for opioid addiction, though they can apply for a waiver to treat up to 100 patients.

Like other opioids, buprenorphine is a useful replacement agent for persons addicted to heroin or other illicit opioids, although it appears to have no advantage over methadone for maintaining long-term sobriety. Buprenorphine, like the other opioid replacement treatments, has modest benefits, leading to long-term abstinence in perhaps one third of those with opioid addiction. Many patients drop out of clinical trials. As with the other opioid replacement treatments, buprenorphine should be prescribed in conjunction with psychosocial therapies aimed at preventing relapse. The intensity of required psychosocial intervention is unclear. A recent study found that once-weekly brief visits with a nurse combined with once-weekly prescriptions was just as effective than thrice weekly prescriptions with more intense psychological interventions. Because of its **long half-life,** buprenorphine may be dosed every other day in some patients.

    Buprenorphine has also been studied in combination with naloxone for the treatment of opioid dependence. The rationale for this treatment is that patients taking the combined agonist and antagonist treatment will experience reduced pleasure if they inject the combination pill. Taken orally, naloxone is not absorbed, but if the combination pill is injected, the naloxone enters the brain and potentially antagonizes the effects of the buprenorphine. This deterrent strategy, however, has not been carefully studied in humans, though anecdotal reports suggest that many patients report an unpleasant experience injecting the buprenorphine-naloxone combination pill. For other patients, the low dose of naltrexone may be inadequate for blocking euphoric effects. For unclear reasons, buprenorphine has a ceiling effect in producing euphoric or analgesic effects, and may even have opioid antagonist effects at high doses. For these reasons, buprenorphine is less prone than other opioid for abuse or to cause respiratory depression.

    Buprenorphine is as effective as moderate doses of methadone, but may be less effective than high-dose methadone (>80 mg per day) for preventing relapse. Opioid addicts with more severe addictions may do better with methadone than buprenorphine. Abstinence rates from illicit drugs generally range between 20% and 40% in short-term buprenorphine trials. Although buprenorphine may be of benefit in the treatment of opioid addiction, it is not a panacea. An advantage of buprenorphine is that it may be initiated early in the course, within 1 year, of opiate dependence, whereas methadone is limited to those with 1 year or more of opiate dependence.

Pharmacology and Mechanism of Action
Buprenorphine is a potent partial opioid agonist with agonist effects at the μ-receptors and antagonist effects at κ-receptors. These properties are different from other opioid agonists and may contribute to buprenorphine's limited potential for abuse and opioid antagonist effects at high doses. Because it tightly binds opioid receptors, it may precipitate opioid withdrawal in patients taking less tightly binding opioids such as methadone or heroin. It is only available in sublingual and injectable forms. Like other opioids, buprenorphine causes CNS, gastrointestinal, respiratory, and cardiovascular depression.

    Buprenorphine is only moderately absorbed (30% bioavailability) when taken sublingually with a time-to-peak concentration at approximately 2 hours. It is highly protein bound and has a terminal half-life of approximately 37 hours. Buprenorphine is metabolized by the liver via the 3A4 cytochrome via *N*-dealkylation and glucuronide addition. Drugs that inhibit 3A4 enzymes (ketoconazole, fluvoxamine, HIV protease inhibitors) may increase buprenorphine plasma concentration and lead to unexpected sedation.

    Buprenorphine may cause **significant sedation,** ataxia, or respiratory compromise when used in combination with other sedative drugs, **especially benzodiazepines or alcohol.** Patients with significant hepatic disease may have concentrations of buprenorphine higher than expected. Buprenorphine should be used with extreme caution in patients with the following clinical conditions or disorders: traumatic brain injury with increased intracranial pressure, chronic obstructive pulmonary disease, asthma, symptomatic hypothyroidism, prostatic hypertrophy, biliary disease, hepatic dysfunction, congestive heart failure, and respiratory depression. Taken in overdose, buprenorphine requires naloxone in a continuous infusion because of its tight binding to opioid receptors.

Adverse Effects
Common adverse effects include dizziness, sedation, constipation, respiratory depression, vertigo, nausea, and vomiting. Buprenorphine has fewer cognitive or sedating effects compared with methadone and is preferred by many opioid addicts as a replacement treatment.

Method of Use
Once the patient has mild withdrawal symptoms, he or she can be started treatment with sublingual buprenorphine up to 8 mg on the first day (held under the tongue for 5 to 10 minutes) and then increased to 16 mg as tolerated over the next few days. If the patient is taking a full opioid agonist (e.g., methadone or heroin) and not yet in withdrawal, buprenorphine may induce acute opioid withdrawal. The patient should be observed daily for the first few days to assess tolerance and craving and gradually less often until stabilized. A dose of **16 mg once daily is the usual maintenance dose.** Alternatively, because of the drug's long half-life, dosing may be spread out during the week (i.e., 32 mg three times per week). Patients also should be involved in a psychosocial program such as Narcotics Anonymous with regular, random urine drug screens to evaluate use of other illicit drugs such as cocaine. After the patient has been abstinent and engaged in treatment, usually for several months, the physician may prescribe buprenorphine-naloxone combination tablet for up to 30 days.

Switching from Methadone to Buprenorphine
Patients with less severe addictions and taking moderate doses of methadone (40 to 80 mg per day) are good candidates for switching to buprenorphine. Patients taking higher doses have more difficulty because of difficulty withdrawing down to a dose of 30 mg per day or lower. **Switching to buprenorphine at higher doses of methadone often leads to problematic withdrawal symptoms.** Ideally patients should be in methadone withdrawal before starting buprenorphine. Methadone's long half-life requires several days' wait to be sure that the drug is eliminated from the body. On the other hand, drugs with shorter half-lives such as oxycodone or heroin require brief periods of sobriety before withdrawal ensues and buprenorphine starts. An intermediate switch from methadone to morphine may be a reasonable way for transition to buprenorphine.

Dose Forms Available
Buprenorphine is available as 2- and 8-mg sublingual tablets. The trade name is Subutex. Buprenorphine is also available in a combination tablet with naloxone, each sublingual tablet containing 2 mg of buprenorphine and 0.5 mg of naloxone or 8 mg buprenorphine with 2 mg naloxone. The trade name of the combination tablet is Suboxone. Buprenorphine is available in an injectable form, 0.3 mg/mL. Trade name of the injectable form is Buprenex.

Naltrexone for Opioid Dependence
Use of naltrexone for the treatment of opioid dependence is not as well established as it is for alcohol dependence. Most reports are open label, and earlier controlled studies were confounded by the bitter taste of the oral solution. Moreover, compliance with naltrexone is notoriously poor, especially among newly detoxified heroin addicts. The overall evidence is that naltrexone provides some benefit for opioid addiction, although the benefits are modest and compliance is often poor

because craving is not treated by naltrexone. Naltrexone may be beneficial in highly motivated patients with good social supports. Naltrexone may also be useful for patients with long-term sobriety from illicit opioids after they have been weaned from methadone treatment.

Pharmacology
The pharmacology is detailed in the section on alcohol dependence.

Method of Use
To ensure that the patient is free of opioids and to prevent a severe withdrawal state related to naltrexone use, a **naloxone challenge** is best performed first. The clinician should give the patient 0.2 mg of naloxone intravenously and observe for signs or symptoms of opioid withdrawal for several minutes. If there is no evidence of withdrawal, another 0.6 mg can be injected and the patient observed for an additional 15 to 20 minutes. If there are no signs of withdrawal, then the patient can be safely started on naltrexone. Alternatively, the patient can be given naloxone, 0.8 mg subcutaneously, and observed for signs and symptoms of withdrawal for 15 to 20 minutes.

Once the patient is suitable for naltrexone treatment, he or she can be started at 25 mg per day for several days to reduce gastrointestinal distress; the dosage can subsequently be increased to 50 mg daily as tolerated by the patient. Dosages may need to be higher than those for the treatment of alcoholism, and many patients will require 100 mg daily to block the euphoric effects of opioids. A common final dosage regimen is 50 to 100 mg per day on weekdays and 150 mg on weekends. Some patients may be given 150 mg three times per week. These dosage patterns, however, are not well established in clinical trials. Liver function tests should be monitored during the course of naltrexone treatment because of its infrequent propensity to elevate transaminase levels. Patients should be monitored with urine drug screens and be involved in a psychosocial treatment aimed at preventing relapse.

DRUGS USED IN THE TREATMENT OF ALCOHOLISM
Alcohol is ubiquitous across the globe. Most individuals use it safely, but due to its broad availability and the apparently high rates of vulnerability to abuse, alcohol dependence and addiction (alcoholism) are enormous health and social problems worldwide. Alcohol abuse leads to a wide range of medical (e.g., gastrointestinal diseases and traumatic brain injury) and psychosocial consequences (e.g., divorce and legal problems), although often these costs are not readily obvious until the person has been drinking regularly for a decade or more. According to epidemiologic studies, 15% of men have a lifetime history of alcohol dependence, and the World Health Organization lists alcohol dependence among the top 10 diseases afflicting all parts of the world.

Acute or chronic use of alcohol often worsens comorbid mental illnesses, especially mood and anxiety disorders. Although drug treatment is useful in limiting the symptoms of alcohol withdrawal, pharmacologic treatments play a limited role in providing abstinence from alcohol; however, a number of agents have shown benefit in clinical trials.

ALCOHOL WITHDRAWAL TREATMENT
Alcohol has a diversity of effects on cells throughout the brain and the rest of the body. This lack of specificity reflects the general membrane effects that alcohol exerts (in addition to any specific effects on receptors or ion channels) at the very high concentrations that people use to achieve psychotropic effects. A major effect of alcohol is to facilitate some actions of γ-aminobutyric acid (GABA), the major

inhibitory neurotransmitter in the brain (acting via the $GABA_A$ receptor) and to inhibit the N-methyl-D-aspartate glutamate receptor, an important excitatory neurotransmitter receptor involved in memory (among other things). With chronic alcohol use, the **brain adapts homeostatically to these effects by upregulating excitatory neurotransmission and reducing inhibitory transmission,** creating an overall bias toward excitation that is balanced by ongoing alcohol use. With cessation of alcohol, the intrinsic overbalancing toward excitation in many brain circuits leads to withdrawal symptoms. Withdrawal seizures reflect this imbalance in the cerebral cortex. Many patients who drink alcohol on a regular basis have very mild symptoms and rarely come for clinical care. Patients who have withdrawal symptoms often do not come to the attention of physicians until withdrawal symptoms are severe. Early on, mild symptoms may include hypertension, anxiety, tremor, sweating, nausea, and vomiting, although over time, as the condition worsens, withdrawal may include seizures, hallucinations, delirium, cardiac arrhythmias, or even death.

Time Course of Alcohol Withdrawal

Although alcohol withdrawal signs and symptoms generally begin after complete metabolism of alcohol, in more severe alcoholism, the withdrawal syndrome may begin when the plasma concentration drops below a certain threshold. During the first day of alcohol withdrawal, typical signs include tremor, tachycardia, sweating, hypertension, mild fever, anxiety, and gastrointestinal distress. For patients with mild withdrawal, these symptoms **generally resolve within 2 days.** Mild withdrawal generally occurs in younger patients and those who are medically stable.

Patients with a longer history of alcoholism or unstable medical conditions are more likely to develop complicated withdrawal as evidenced by profound changes in blood pressure, severe tremulousness, ataxic gait, and seizures that may occur within the first 36 hours of withdrawal. Patients having a seizure after 36 hours should be evaluated for other causes of seizure (i.e., subdural hematoma, meningitis). An agitated delirium may develop 2 to 4 days after the start of the withdrawal syndrome. The delirium often includes **profound sleep-wake cycle disruption, visual or auditory hallucinations, and marked cognitive impairment** including the inability to make new memories or complete simple tasks such as clock drawing. More severe withdrawal syndromes may take a week or more to improve, and subtle cognitive impairment may persist for some time, although the chronic alcohol effects are difficult to distinguish from withdrawal effects. Infrequently, patients whose delirium was accompanied by thiamine deficiency may go on to have a profound amnestic disorder (Korsakoff's syndrome).

General Principles

There are several purposes of pharmacologic treatment of alcohol withdrawal: (a) allow relatively comfortable detoxification such that the patient can move forward with controlled drinking or abstinence, (b) reduce severe symptoms such as seizure or cardiac arrest, and (c) potentially prevent the progression of severity of the withdrawal syndrome over time. A number of medications may be used, often in combination, including drugs that are cross-tolerant with alcohol (i.e., benzodiazepines), drugs used to control adrenergic overactivity (i.e., clonidine or atenolol), drugs used to treat delirium (i.e., haloperidol or risperidone), and drugs used to prevent amnestic syndromes (i.e., thiamine).

Benzodiazepines

The benzodiazepines are the mainstay of the treatment of alcohol withdrawal due to their cross-tolerance with alcohol and their shared agonist effects on $GABA_A$ receptors. As described previously, during alcohol withdrawal there is an excess of excitatory (e.g., glutamate) versus inhibitory (e.g., GABA) neurotransmission. This leads to symptoms such as anxiety, tachycardia, and sweating or, in more severe cases, seizures, arrhythmias, hallucinations, and delirium. The pharmacology of benzodiazepines is described in Chapter 5. The best-studied benzodiazepines for the treatment of alcohol withdrawal are chlordiazepoxide, diazepam, and lorazepam.

Method of Use—Outpatient Detoxification

The first decision is whether the patient will be treated as an outpatient or an inpatient. Persons younger than 45 years or those generally in good health can be managed as outpatients. Older persons with complicated medical conditions, especially symptomatic cardiac disease or pulmonary disease, or those with a history of severe withdrawal in the past are best treated in the hospital. Occasionally, young persons with severe alcoholism may require hospitalization. To reduce the variation in benzodiazepine plasma concentration, a drug with a long elimination half-life, such as chlordiazepoxide or diazepam, is preferred.

For motivated outpatients, lorazepam or diazepam may be used to control withdrawal symptoms. Patients should be evaluated daily for 2 or 3 days and started on a modest dosage of oral lorazepam (1 to 2 mg t.i.d.) or diazepam (5 to 10 mg t.i.d.) and thiamine 100 mg daily. Alternatively, a loading dose of 20 to 30 mg of diazepam may be administered to the patient in the evening on the first day. Patients should also be encouraged to avoid driving and to maintain fluid intake. If signs and symptoms worsen, the patient should be hospitalized. Once withdrawal is completed, the patient should be enrolled in a psychosocial treatment to maintain abstinence.

Method of Use—Inpatient Detoxification

For patients at risk for more severe withdrawal, treatment is more complex and often requires frequent readjustments depending on the clinical progress over several days. Although many patients will have a benign course, the lethality (15% to 30%) of untreated delirium tremens and other complications of acute alcohol intoxication make it imperative that the high-risk patients be monitored closely. Patients most at risk for severe withdrawal and potentially poor outcome include those with past alcohol withdrawal delirium or withdrawal seizure, recent cardiac or hip surgery, unstable cardiac disease, pneumonia, or other unstable systemic illness.

The clinician must decide whether to start medication immediately or to treat following signs of withdrawal. We recommend waiting for withdrawal signs to develop. The principal advantage of waiting for symptom development is that a lower total dose of benzodiazepine is generally needed.

On admission, physical examination, particularly of the heart, lungs, and neurologic systems, must be performed and then reevaluated daily. Patients also should be thoroughly evaluated for alcohol withdrawal progression every few hours by nursing or physician staff, preferably by use of a standard rating instrument such as the Clinical Institute Withdrawal Assessment-Revised. Key clinical items to be evaluated for alcohol withdrawal include the following: vital signs, other manifestations of autonomic excitation (tremor, sweating), cognitive impairment, sleep-wake disruption, gait abnormality, complaints of chest pain, and presence of hallucinations or confusion.

Benzodiazepines are the mainstay of alcohol withdrawal treatment. Treatment sometimes needs to be aggressive at the beginning to control symptoms; however, dosing must be carefully titrated to limit the sedating effects of these compounds. In general, patients with severe alcohol withdrawal will require significant amounts of benzodiazepine (e.g., 100 mg of diazepam or more) to reduce symptoms. Sometimes, however, aggressive treatment may lead to **excessive sedation and respiratory compromise, particularly in smokers with chronic obstructive pulmonary disease** or aspiration pneumonia in patients who have recently eaten or consumed fluids.

Once the patient begins to show signs of withdrawal, treatment should begin. Diazepam, 10 mg t.i.d. or q.i.d., or lorazepam, 2 mg t.i.d. or q.i.d., is a reasonable initial regimen, although individual requirements to control symptoms are variable. Similarly, oxazepam or chlordiazepoxide may be used. Chlordiazepoxide or oxazepam, 15 mg, is approximately equivalent to diazepam, 5 mg, or lorazepam, 1 mg. Patients should be evaluated frequently, every 1 to 2 hours, on the first day to assess drug needs. If signs and symptoms persist despite a typical starting dosage (i.e., diazepam 10 mg t.i.d. or q.i.d.), then the dosage can be titrated upward as needed to control symptoms. If the patient becomes lethargic after the first few doses, then the dose can be reduced; however, most patients with significant alcohol withdrawal symptoms will require at least 30 to 40 mg of diazepam or an equivalent dose of another benzodiazepine. In general, because sleep is disrupted during alcohol withdrawal, a benzodiazepine (e.g., lorazepam, 2 mg, or diazepam, 10 mg) should be given before bedtime.

Many patients will continue to require benzodiazepines on the second and third days of treatment or beyond, with dose and duration of treatment dictated by severity of symptoms. If the patient continues to show signs of withdrawal (i.e., sweating, tremor, tachycardia), benzodiazepine dosing should continue every 4 to 6 hours until signs abate. Mild symptoms generally need not be treated with benzodiazepines. If more severe symptoms, such as hallucinations and delirium, develop after the start of withdrawal, then antipsychotic medications should be started as outlined later.

Diazepam Loading Method
Another method to manage alcohol withdrawal with benzodiazepines is termed "the loading method," capitalizing on the prolonged elimination half-life of diazepam and its principal metabolites. Patients in whom respiratory compromise is not a concern, can be given diazepam, 15 to 20 mg, every 2 hours until sedated. A minimum of 60 mg of diazepam is typically required. After the loading dose, the patient should continue to be monitored, and in many cases, further dosing with diazepam is not required. If the patient becomes sedated before reaching 60 mg, then severe withdrawal is unlikely. Some highly tolerant patients may need very high doses of diazepam (i.e., up to 200 mg of diazepam or even higher).

Lorazepam Versus Diazepam for Withdrawal Treatment
The relative benefit of using lorazepam versus diazepam for acute withdrawal is dictated primarily by pharmacokinetic differences between these two compounds. Lorazepam offers a relatively short elimination half-life, no active metabolites, a catabolic pathway that is maintained even in hepatic disease (lorazepam only requires glucuronidation for elimination), and a readily absorbed intramuscular form. The advantages of these properties allow for the use of lorazepam in ill patients when finer control is required. On the other hand, fluctuation in lorazepam plasma concentration may lead to a more varied symptom presentation, with reemergence of symptoms as plasma concentration drops below therapeutic concentrations.

Diazepam, on the other hand, has a long elimination half-life and an active metabolite, desmethyldiazepam, has an even longer half-life. Diazepam therefore provides a **longer, slower taper with little fluctuation in plasma concentration** and may therefore be somewhat smoother and more predictable in its effects once a therapeutic concentration is achieved. On the other hand, if dosing is too aggressive, diazepam and its metabolite may accumulate and lead to toxicity including excessive sedation, ataxia, and cognitive impairment. In some cases, it is difficult to distinguish the cognitive toxicity of diazepam from subtle delirium. In these cases, alteration of the sleep-wake cycle or presence of hallucinations is a clinical marker to help identify delirium. Hence, diazepam dosing needs to be carefully determined to balance the benefits of controlling symptoms and limiting toxicity. In the course of treating alcohol withdrawal with benzodiazepines, most patients will experience some adverse effects, but the adverse effects generally resolve quickly with relatively low risk of morbidity. The aim is to prevent serious complications such as cardiac ischemia, delirium, or seizures.

Thiamine

Thiamine (vitamin B_1) deficiency is not uncommon in alcoholics experiencing withdrawal symptoms due to their poor dietary practices. Although the development of Wernicke's encephalopathy is uncommon, this severe condition can be avoided by treatment with thiamine. Patients should receive thiamine, 100 mg daily, at the start of treatment. If there is any concern about absorption (poor intake or vomiting), thiamine should be given parenterally daily for several days.

Antipsychotic Drugs

If the person undergoing withdrawal experiences hallucinations or delirium, antipsychotic drugs should be considered. Symptoms may be subtle at first and include illusions (mistaking spots on the ceiling for insects); however, symptoms may progress to florid visual or auditory hallucinations that accompany a confusional state. Although mild illusions may be treated with benzodiazepines, these subtle symptoms are often the harbinger of more serious withdrawal that will follow. The onset of cognitive impairment and delirium can sometimes be subtle, making daily, careful assessments for these conditions essential in the optimal management of these patients. Simple bedside tests such as clock drawing or reciting the months of the year backwards are useful for identifying the onset of confusion. Haloperidol, 2 to 5 mg once or twice daily, or risperidone, 1 to 3 mg daily, often suffices to reduce delirium symptoms. Patients in withdrawal delirium following surgery, however, may require higher doses of haloperidol. The advantage of haloperidol over risperidone or other second-generation antipsychotics is that haloperidol does not cause orthostasis. Patients already taking benzodiazepines generally do not experience akathisia or extrapyramidal signs. Antipsychotics can be withdrawn once the hallucinations or delirium resolves, usually within several days of onset.

Atenolol and Clonidine

Although most patients will not require antihypertensive agents during treatment of acute withdrawal, hypertension accompanying alcohol withdrawal may be augmented with atenolol or clonidine for systolic blood pressure greater than 180 mm Hg or diastolic blood pressure greater than 110 mm Hg. These agents may be particularly useful in patients with coronary artery disease and those at risk for angina or cardiac arrhythmias. Dosing should be cautious and gradually titrated to prevent hypotension. In general, daily doses of atenolol, 25 to 50 mg, may be helpful, although some patients require up to 100 mg per day. Atenolol can be stopped after several days of treatment.

Clonidine may be started at 0.1 mg b.i.d. or t.i.d. and gradually titrated to control hypertension. Again, blood pressure should be frequently monitored to guard against hypotension.

Anticonvulsants in Alcohol Withdrawal

Carbamazepine, valproic acid, and gabapentin have been used in the treatment of alcohol withdrawal. None of these are established for the treatment of withdrawal; however, limited clinical investigation suggests that they may have a role in outpatient detoxification. These drugs have not been well studied in most ill patients, nor are significant placebo-controlled data available. As with all treatments of alcohol withdrawal, which is a self-limited phenomenon that resolves in several days, anecdotal reports of efficacy can often be misleading.

Carbamazepine

Carbamazepine is an anticonvulsant with antikindling properties that may reduce alcohol withdrawal symptoms and potentially limit drinking following detoxification. The advantage of carbamazepine is for outpatients in whom there is some concern about abuse of benzodiazepines. The disadvantages are that it may cause hepatic toxicity or bone marrow suppression. Carbamazepine should not be used in patients with granulocytopenia, thrombocytopenia, or significant liver disease. Pharmacology of carbamazepine is discussed in Chapter 4.

Method of Use. For patients with mild to moderate withdrawal, carbamazepine may be started at 200 mg t.i.d. to q.i.d. If the initial dose is too sedating or causes significant ataxia, the dose can be reduced. The first 2 days of treatment with carbamazepine should use the same daily dose; thereafter, the dose can be tapered over the next 3 or 4 days. If symptoms are not controlled with carbamazepine, a benzodiazepine should be added. Ataxia, visual problems, and sedation are the most common side effects.

Divalproex Sodium

Divalproex sodium is an anticonvulsant with antikindling properties that enhances GABA neurotransmission. Limited data suggest that it may reduce withdrawal symptoms and reduce the need for benzodiazepines, particularly in outpatients with mild to moderate symptoms. Divalproex is preferred over valproic acid because divalproex has much less gastrointestinal toxicity. Like carbamazepine, it may cause hepatic toxicity and its use should be limited in patients with significant hepatic disease.

Method of Use. Divalproex sodium should be started after symptoms begin. The starting dosage is 500 mg b.i.d., although some patients may require 500 mg t.i.d. The second-day dose should be the same as the first or slightly higher if symptoms progress. Dosing thereafter is dictated largely by clinical course with gradual tapering for the patient whose symptoms abate or continued higher dosing for the more refractory patients. Most patients can be detoxified over 4 to 7 days.

Gabapentin

Gabapentin is an anticonvulsant approved for use as an adjunct to standard anticonvulsants. Its principal advantage is that it is well tolerated and, other than sedation or ataxia, causes little toxicity. It does not cause hepatic or bone marrow toxicity and is excreted unchanged by the kidney. Several open-label reports suggest that it may have a role in detoxification; however, in one placebo-controlled study, it did not reduce the need for treatment with a standard agent (clomethiazole). Gabapentin's current role should be limited to mild alcohol withdrawal.

Method of Use. After the onset of withdrawal symptoms, gabapentin should be started at 400 mg t.i.d. to q.i.d. The dosage may need to be slightly adjusted depending on severity of symptoms or toxicity. The second-day dose should be equal to the dose needed on the first day. Thereafter, the dose can be gradually tapered over the next 3 or 4 days.

PHARMACOLOGIC TREATMENT OF CHRONIC ALCOHOLISM

Naltrexone

Naltrexone is a semisynthetic opiate antagonist similar to naloxone, approved in the early 1990s by the Food and Drug Administration for the treatment of alcohol dependence in the United States. Although naltrexone was originally used to aid recovering opioid-dependent patients, it has become more widely used in the treatment of chronic alcohol dependence. Recently, a long-acting, injectable preparation of naltrexone, Vivitrol, became available for alcohol dependence. The rationale for using an opioid antagonist in alcohol dependence is that alcohol enhances the release of endogenous opioids in the brain, and when opioid receptors are blocked in alcohol-preferring rodents, this alcohol preference is diminished. The reduction of alcohol consumption in humans, however, appears to be less robust than in rodents. Moreover, severe alcoholics may not benefit from naltrexone treatment.

When used in combination with group therapy, naltrexone has consistently been shown to be superior to placebo in sustaining alcohol abstinence and reducing alcohol craving; however, the benefits are often modest and much of the improvement appears related to the benefits of psychosocial treatments. Importantly, naltrexone may limit the severity of the relapse once drinking occurs because naltrexone reduces craving. The benefits of using naltrexone are also most evident with highly motivated patients.

A 1-year study suggested that naltrexone may be superior to acamprosate. In this study, patients who were actively involved in psychosocial weekly therapy for the first 3 months were randomized to acamprosate or naltrexone. The patients treated with naltrexone were twice as likely to maintain sobriety as the patients treated with acamprosate (41% vs 17%). Patients treated with naltrexone also had more total days of sobriety (243 vs 180 days) and perhaps more importantly, when patients did relapse, naltrexone patients had fewer drinks than acamprosate-treated patients (4 vs 9).

In a large study ($N = 627$) of patients with severe alcohol dependence treated in Veteran's Administration hospitals, however, naltrexone did not appear to be effective. Patients in this study had intensive behavioral treatment. They were engaged in weekly 12-step individual counseling and were encouraged to attend Alcoholics Anonymous meetings, the rate of relapse was not different between placebo-treated and naltrexone-treated patients after 3 months (38% vs 44%). Moreover, after 1 year, the percentage of days drinking or the number of drinks taken at any given binge was not different between naltrexone- and placebo-treated patients. This may be due to a ceiling effect with intensive behavioral treatment. This study suggests that, although naltrexone may play a role in some patients, it does not appear to be useful in the more severe chronic alcoholics. This study has been criticized because many of the patients were homeless and had minimal psychosocial support. In studies in which patients had better support, outcomes were more favorable. Indeed, in a large, multicenter study ($N = 1,383$) comparing naltrexone with placebo and acamprosate, with or without behavioral therapy, naltrexone fared better than placebo or acamprosate regarding the number of days abstinent and the return to heavy drinking. Interestingly, this advantage held when patients were treated with "medical management" but not with behavior therapy. Also, the combination of naltrexone with acamprosate did no better than naltrexone alone. Of note, the risk reduction for heavy drinking was relatively low, 28%. Naltrexone is not a panacea for alcoholism.

The most recent formulation of naltrexone, a long-acting injection, uses the same technology employed in long-acting risperidone, dissolvable microspheres. The preparation is not effective in patients who are currently drinking alcohol. In recently abstinent drinkers, however, it appears to be effective. In a 6-month registration trial, patients were given injections of naltrexone, 190 or 380 mg, or placebo every 4 weeks. Overall, the study was negative, but the data were analyzed for patients who were abstinent for at least 4 days before starting the treatment. For these recently abstinent patients, the median time to first drink was 12 days for placebo-treated patients and 41 days for naltrexone-treated patients (380 mg). Thirty-two percentage of patients assigned to injectable naltrexone and 11%

assigned to placebo attained continuous abstinence. Hence, a subset of patients may be helped by naltrexone injections.

Pharmacokinetics

Naltrexone is rapidly absorbed with peak concentrations achieved within 2 hours. The drug undergoes extensive first-pass hepatic metabolism with the majority of drug and metabolites excreted in the urine. Naltrexone has a half-life of approximately 4 hours; however, much of the drug is distributed into the tissues and elimination is biphasic with a secondary redistribution resulting in a much longer duration of action. The first metabolite of naltrexone, β-naltrexol, is a weaker antagonist of opioid receptors but has a half-life of approximately 12 hours, which contributes to the long duration of opioid blockade. The drug is conjugated in the liver and excreted by glomerular filtration through the kidney. Naltrexone variably inhibits microsomal enzymes, although there are no established clinical implications. Naltrexone used in combination with yohimbine may lead to increased anxiety or panic, perhaps related to increased noradrenergic sensitivity.

With the injectable formulation, following intramuscular injection there is some absorption in the first few hours with a gradual rise over several days and a peak reached at 2 weeks. Total drug exposure (as measured by area under the curve of concentration over time) is several times higher for the intramuscular dose of 380 mg compared with a daily oral dose of 50 mg.

Pharmacodynamics

Naltrexone is a pure opioid antagonist at μ-opioid receptors without partial agonist effects. Naltrexone initially increases the secretion of the luteinizing hormone, follicle-stimulating hormone, adrenocorticotropin, and cortisol, although these hormones return to normal level with chronic treatment. There are generally no clinical implications of these hormonal changes. Naltrexone may also decrease total cholesterol and triglycerides, but the mechanism of this effect is unknown.

Adverse Effects

Naltrexone side effects include gastrointestinal complaints, including nausea, abdominal pain, and diarrhea ($>15\%$), but generally these symptoms are time limited. A small number of patients may develop transaminasemia; however, this is generally found at higher doses than used for alcoholism. In higher doses, naltrexone may cause hepatocellular injury. Anorexia is uncommon with some patients reporting insomnia, anxiety, fatigue, or irritability. Although joint and muscle pain is a common complaint, rhabdomyolysis appears to be a rare complication. There are no known pulmonary or cardiovascular adverse effects.

For the injectable formulation, injection site reactions are common. Approximately 30% to 40% patients experience pain or swelling, though this adverse effect rarely leads to discontinuation.

The following are contraindications for a patient's use of naltrexone:

1. Use of opioids
2. Opioid withdrawal
3. Hepatitis or significant hepatic impairment

Use of Naltrexone with Opioids

If naltrexone is given to a patient addicted to opioids, a severe withdrawal state may result, including delirium, stupor, hallucinations, nausea, and vomiting. Supportive care, including fluid replacement and treatment of delirium with antipsychotics such as haloperidol, may be needed. Low-dose lorazepam may also be useful. The withdrawal may last several days, and the naltrexone must be stopped immediately.

Dose Forms Available

Naltrexone is available as a 50-mg tablet. The trade name is ReVia. It is also available as an injection of 380 mg suspended in 4 cc saline diluent.

Method of Use

Liver function tests should be done at the start of therapy to ensure that the patient does not have hepatitis or significant hepatic impairment. Avoid naltrexone use in patients with hepatitis. Following detoxification from alcohol, as long as the patient has been free of opioids for a week, he or she may be started on 25 mg per day. Abstinence from opioids may be monitored using urine drug testing, if needed. Patients dependent on opioids should not be given naltrexone until they are sober for at least a week. Nausea is reduced if the medication is taken with food and generally resolves over 1 week. After a week on naltrexone, the dose can be increased to 50 mg.

The injectable formulation is given every 4 weeks in the posterior, lateral aspect of the gluteus muscle. The medication comes in a prepared package with a syringe. The dry drug-microsphere combination must be thoroughly mixed with the diluent. This takes several minutes of vigorous shaking once the diluent is mixed with the drug. The suspension becomes milky white in the vial, and once the entire drug is suspended it can be drawn into the syringe in total. The entire 4 cc can then be injected. The drug must be refrigerated until time of use. Unrefrigerated, the drug retains its long-acting properties only for 7 days. The drug must not get warmer than 77°F.

The patient should be encouraged to attend Alcoholics Anonymous meetings or be enrolled in some form of psychosocial rehabilitation. Duration of treatment is not well established, but 3 to 6 months is reasonable for motivated patients. Longer durations have not been studied, but longer use is reasonable for motivated patients. Liver function tests should be obtained every 3 to 6 months (Tables 6.3 and 6.4).

TABLE 6.3 Drugs Used in the Treatment of Alcohol Dependence

	Drug	Trade Name	Dose Forms
Alcohol withdrawal	Diazepam	Valium	5-, 10-mg tablets
	Lorazepam	Ativan	0.5-, 1-, 2-mg tablets
	Chlordiazepoxide	Librium	5-, 10-, 25-mg capsules
	Oxazepam	Serax	15-, 30-mg capsules
	Gabapentin	Neurontin	100-, 300-mg capsules
	Carbamazepine	Tegretol	100-, 200-mg capsules
	Divalproex	Depakote	500-mg tablet
Alcohol abstinence	Disulfiram	Antabuse	250-mg tablets
	Naltrexone	ReVia	50-mg tablets
		Vivitrol	380-mg microspheres in 4 cc diluent
	Acamprosate	Campral	333-mg tablets
	Ondansetron	Zofran	4-, 8-, 24-mg tablets; 4-, 8-mg disintegrating tablets
	Topiramate	Topamax	25-, 50-, 100-, 200-mg tablets; 15-, 25-mg sprinkle capsules

	Usual Dose (mg)	Extreme Dose Range (mg)
Alcohol Withdrawal		
Diazepam	30–60	10–200
Chlordiazepoxide	45–75	20–200
Lorazepam	6–12	2–24
Oxazepam	45–90	15–225
Gabapentin	900–1,500	600–2,400
Carbamazepine	600–800	400–1,200
Divalproex	500–1,000	500–2,000
Alcohol Abstinence		
Disulfiram	250	125–500
Naltrexone	50	25–150
Acamprosate	999–1,666	333–1,666
Ondansetron	2–4	2–8
Topiramate	100–300	50–400
Baclofen	15–30	5–80

TABLE 6.4 — Dose Range for Drugs Used in the Treatment of Alcohol Dependence

Acamprosate

Although acamprosate is used in more than 20 countries worldwide, it has not yet been approved by the Food and Drug Administration for use in the United States. Acamprosate may be used to maintain abstinence or limit drinking following alcohol detoxification. The rationale for use is that acamprosate, like alcohol, affects GABA and glutamate neurons, and in animal models it limits alcohol drinking. Acamprosate also appears to attenuate withdrawal symptoms and early abstinence craving. Unlike alcohol, it does not cause euphoria or intoxication and it is not prone to habitual use. In controlled trials, however, acamprosate has shown modest benefits in reducing drinking in alcoholics. Many clinical trials have examined the time to relapse as well as the amount of drinking following relapse. Studies generally follow detoxification and are in conjunction with psychosocial therapy, often including weekly cognitive therapy or participation in Alcoholics Anonymous meetings. Although acamprosate increases sobriety periods, the abstinence rates generally decline over the course of time following drug treatment. The amount of heavy drinking may also be decreased; however, in general, the aim for alcoholism treatment is abstinence. Approximately 20% of acamprosate-treated patients remain abstinent over the course of 1 year compared with 10% of placebo-treated patients. Because there is a decline in rates of abstinence following acamprosate treatment, it is difficult to make any recommendations about discontinuation of the medicine.

Acamprosate is superior at maintaining alcohol abstinence during drug treatment; however, the benefits compared with placebo are modest, and there was significant drop-out rate in most studies. In the study with the best outcomes (Sass et al., 1996), 43% of acamprosate-treated patients were alcohol abstinent at the end of 48 treatment weeks compared with 21% of placebo-treated patients. Furthermore, approximately 1 year following treatment cessation, more patients who had taken acamprosate remained abstinent compared with placebo-treated patients. In other studies, however, the abstinence rates are somewhat lower. Unfortunately, in several studies acamprosate shows no benefit compared with placebo. It is not evident that acamprosate reduces the amount of drinking once relapse occurs. We consider acamprosate a second- or third-line treatment of alcoholism.

Pharmacology and Mechanism of Action

Acamprosate is an analog of homotaurine, a GABAergic agonist, although its exact mechanism of action is unknown. It is proposed that acamprosate may stimulate GABAergic neurotransmission and antagonizes excitatory amino acids, such as glutamate. Acamprosate, however, does not directly affect $GABA_A$ receptors. Acamprosate is not a sedative, has little or no abuse potential, and does not induce physiologic dependence.

Adverse Effects and Toxicity

Acamprosate is generally well tolerated; however, some patients suffer adverse effects. Gastrointestinal side effects are most common, although generally mild and time limited, and can be minimized by slow dose titration or dose reduction. Contraindications include pregnancy, lactation, and significant kidney or liver disease.

Side effects are as follows:

CNS effects: Insomnia, headache, and confusion are uncommon side effects.
Gastrointestinal effects: Diarrhea, nausea, and flatulence are not uncommon and are dose dependent. Vomiting is an uncommon effect.
Genitourinary effects: Sexual dysfunction, including erectile dysfunction and decreased libido are uncommon side effects.
Dermatologic effects: Pruritus is an uncommon adverse effect.

Overdose

There are limited data regarding overdose, although the drug appears to be relatively benign in overdose. No cardiac toxicity is known, and following gastric lavage, the only significant adverse effect was time-limited diarrhea.

Teratogenicity

There are no data in humans, and acamprosate does not appear to be a teratogen in rodents.

Drug Interactions

The only known drug interaction is with the tetracyclines, which may be partially inactivated by the calcium component in acamprosate.

Laboratory Abnormalities

Acamprosate has no known clinically relevant effects on laboratory parameters.

Pharmacokinetics

Acamprosate plasma levels reach steady state after approximately 7 days of treatment. The drug is slowly absorbed in the gastrointestinal tract and has low bioavailability, with only approximately 10% absorption. Taking medication with food increases absorption modestly. The drug does not appear to be protein bound, and the drug is excreted unchanged through the kidney and through the feces. Acamprosate has a short elimination half-life, in some as short as 3 hours.

Dosage

To help patients maintain alcohol abstinence, the recommended oral daily dose is 1,333 mg per day for patients weighing less than 60 kg and 1,998 mg per day for patients weighing more than 60 kg. The daily dose should be given in three divided doses with meals, starting at 333 mg t.i.d. and gradually increasing as tolerated.

Acamprosate should be started after alcohol detoxification and should not be stopped if the patient relapses into drinking. Although the exact duration of treatment is not known, 6 months to 1 year appears reasonable when combined with psychosocial treatments.

Because acamprosate is excreted unchanged by the kidneys, it is contraindicated in patients with renal failure. The manufacturer suggests that acamprosate not be used in elderly patients.

Doses Available
Acamprosate pills include 333 mg of drug and 33 mg of calcium.

Disulfiram
One strategy in the treatment of alcoholism is the use of sensitizing agents that produce noxious physical symptoms when the patient consumes ethanol; the rationale for this strategy is that the threat of an aversive reaction will deter alcohol consumption. Disulfiram is one of several compounds that is used for sensitization to alcohol; however, it is the only one commonly used in the United States. Although controlled clinical trials do not favor the use of sensitizing agents as effective treatments for alcoholism, disulfiram continues to be prescribed in the United States.

Controlled trials do not indicate any advantage of disulfiram over placebo in achieving total abstinence, in delaying resumption of drinking, or in improving employment status or social stability. At dosages of 250 mg per day, however, the drug appears to increase the proportion of days in which no alcohol is consumed. Some clinicians believe that this modest benefit may decrease the medical complications associated with alcoholism over time, but there are no controlled studies to confirm this impression.

Although disulfiram has only limited value in the general population, some clinicians believe that the drug is useful for selected individuals who remain employed, are highly motivated for abstinence, and are socially stable. Because these patients have the best outcomes in any case, it is unclear that disulfiram actually contributes to therapeutic success.

Pharmacology and Mechanism of Action
Disulfiram is 80% to 90% absorbed after an oral dose. Although it has a short half-life (because it is rapidly metabolized by the liver), it is an irreversible inhibitor of aldehyde dehydrogenase, resulting in a longer biologic effect than one might predict. Aldehyde dehydrogenase is a hepatic enzyme involved in the intermediary metabolism of ethanol. In normal ethanol metabolism, acetaldehyde is produced but does not accumulate because it is rapidly oxidized by aldehyde dehydrogenase. However, when this enzyme has been inhibited by disulfiram, acetaldehyde levels accumulate to 5 to 10 times higher than usual. It is acetaldehyde that is responsible for most of the noxious symptoms.

Disulfiram inhibits other hepatic enzymes including the microsomal enzymes, thus interfering with the metabolism of a variety of drugs, including the following:

Phenytoin
Isoniazid
Warfarin
Rifampin
Barbiturates
Long-acting benzodiazepines (e.g., diazepam, chlordiazepoxide)

Disulfiram also inhibits dopamine β-hydroxylase, thus potentially decreasing the concentrations of norepinephrine and epinephrine in the sympathetic nervous system. This may be partly responsible for the severity of hypotension observed in the disulfiram—alcohol reaction. Inhibition of dopamine β-hydroxylase is also theorized to be the mechanism underlying the rare consequence of psychosis associated with disulfiram use.

The Disulfiram—Alcohol Reaction

Almost 5 to 10 minutes after consuming alcohol, the patient taking disulfiram develops a feeling of heat in the face, followed by facial and then whole-body flushing due to vasodilation. This is accompanied by throbbing in the head and neck and a severe headache. Sweating, dry mouth, nausea, vomiting, dizziness, and weakness usually occur. In more severe reactions, there may be chest pain, dyspnea, severe hypotension, and confusion. Death has been reported, usually in patients who have taken more than 500 mg of disulfiram but occasionally with lower doses. After the symptoms pass, the patient is usually exhausted and often sleeps, after which the patient usually recovers entirely. The symptoms last from 30 minutes to 2 hours. The length and severity depend both on the dose of disulfiram and on the amount of ethanol consumed. The threshold for the reaction is approximately 7 mL of 100% ethanol or its equivalent. After a dose of disulfiram, sensitization to ethanol lasts for 6 to 14 days, the time required for recovery of the aldehyde dehydrogenase enzymatic apparatus.

Diphenhydramine, 50 mg intramuscularly or intravenously, has been reported to be helpful for the symptoms induced by disulfiram. Severe reactions may require emergency supportive treatment, most often with intravenous fluids for hypotension and dehydration. Shock, requiring pressors, may occur, as may arrhythmias. Respiratory distress often improves with the administration of oxygen.

Therapeutic Use

Disulfiram should only be prescribed to alcoholics who seek total abstinence, agree to use the drug, and appear able to comply with its use. Its use is therefore not recommended in severely impulsive, psychotic, or suicidal patients. In addition, patients should have no medical contraindications to its use. These contraindications include the following:

Pregnancy
Moderate to severe hepatic dysfunction
Renal failure
Peripheral neuropathies
Cardiac disease

Patients must understand the dangers of drinking alcohol while taking the drug and should be warned to avoid ethanol in any form, including such disguised forms as sauces, cough syrups, and even topical preparations such as aftershave.

There is no evidence that disulfiram or any alcohol-sensitizing agent is effective long term (months to years). In individual patients, the agent may be useful as an adjunct to a comprehensive psychosocial treatment plan in which the maintenance of complete abstinence is sought. Disulfiram may also be useful in alcoholics with a history of long-term sobriety followed by a relapse or in sober alcoholics who are faced with situations that may lead to relapse (e.g., vacations or winter holiday season).

Patients should be thoroughly detoxified before starting the drug. The usual dosage is 250 mg per day, usually taken in the morning (a time when the patient's resolve to remain abstinent is often greatest). Patients who feel drowsy on taking the drug may prefer to take their dose at bedtime. An optimal dosage that is both safe and effective is not known. Doses above 250 mg are associated with more severe side effects and do not appear to be warranted. Doses as low as 100 mg have been used when side effects do not permit higher doses.

Once therapy is established, it is important to assess compliance at regular intervals. A complete blood count and liver function tests should be done every 3 to 6 months; however, most patients will take the drug for less than 6 months. Disulfiram may be teratogenic and should not be used by pregnant women.

Side Effects and Toxicity
The most common adverse effects are fatigue and drowsiness, which can be managed by taking the dose at bedtime or reducing the dosage. Some patients complain of body odor or halitosis, which also may improve with dosage reduction. Other reported side effects include tremor, headache, impotence, dizziness, and a foul or metallic taste in the mouth. Rare but severe side effects include hepatotoxicity and neuropathies. Psychiatric side effects appear to be rare, although psychosis and catatonic-like reactions have been reported.

An isolated report of a disulfiram overdose with apparently no other drugs involved described delirium with prominent hallucinations, tachycardia, and hypertension. The patient recovered in 7 days with supportive care plus haloperidol to control delirium.

Drug Interactions
Because hepatic microsomal enzymes are inhibited by disulfiram, levels of several drugs (i.e., vasodilators, α- or β-adrenergic antagonists, antidepressants, antipsychotic agents) may be increased with a risk of toxicity. Hepatic glucuronic acid conjugation is not affected; thus, the metabolism of such drugs as oxazepam and lorazepam is not affected. Certain drugs increase the severity of the disulfiram—alcohol reaction, and their use should be considered as a relative contraindication for disulfiram. The following drugs may worsen the disulfiram—alcohol reaction:

MAOIs
Vasodilators
α- or β-Adrenergic antagonists
Tricyclic antidepressants
Antipsychotic drugs

Ondansetron
Ondansetron is a serotonin antagonist, specific for the 5-HT_3 receptor subtype. Its principal uses have been for control of nausea related to cancer chemotherapy and for postoperative nausea and vomiting. That use has been extended and tested in the treatment of persons with alcohol, based on the findings that there are abnormalities in serotonergic function in alcoholics. Limited controlled data suggest that ondansetron may play a role in reducing drinking in early-onset alcoholics. In the clinical trials, however, patients were enrolled in weekly cognitive-behavioral therapy and a large drop in drinking behavior occurred at the start of treatment, suggesting that nonspecific factors related to motivation to stop drinking may play a role. Those limitations aside, patients with early-onset alcoholism show modest improvement in alcohol consumption while taking ondansetron, both in the amount of drinking and in the number of days abstinent. In the largest study, 70% of the ondansetron-treated patients and 50% of placebo-treated patients were abstinent for the 12-week study, suggesting nonspecific factors may have contributed to treatment success. It does not appear that late-onset alcoholics improve with ondansetron treatment, and the use of ondansetron in clinical settings in which there are multiple psychiatric and/or medical comorbidities has not been sufficiently studied.

Pharmacology and Mechanism of Action
Ondansetron is moderately well absorbed (50% to 70% bioavailability) and reaches peak concentration within 1 to 2 hours. The liver via hydroxylation and

glucuronide conjugation metabolizes it extensively. The mean elimination half-life is approximately 4 hours and increases significantly in advanced liver disease. Although ondansetron is generally well tolerated, occasionally patients may have liver function test elevations, and infrequent side effects include constipation, diarrhea, dry mouth, headache, malaise, and fatigue. To date, there have been no reports of serious drug interactions.

Ondansetron is a selective 5-HT$_3$ antagonist and is not known to affect any other receptors. Receptors for 5-HT$_3$ are found throughout the brain but are in highest concentrations in the chemoreceptor trigger zone of the area postrema and in the vagal nerve terminals peripherally. It is not known if its antiemetic benefits are mediated via central or peripheral effects. The mechanism for its potential benefits for alcoholism is unknown. Ondansetron has not been reported to be a drug of abuse.

Method of Use
Because of the high cost of ondansetron (>$15 for 4-mg tablet) and the lack of established dosing, regular clinical use of ondansetron cannot be supported at this time.

Dose Forms Available
Ondansetron is available at 4-, 8-, and 24-mg tablets. The trade name is Zofran. The dosage is not established in the treatment of alcoholism.

Topiramate
Topiramate is a sedating anticonvulsant with proven benefit for epilepsy and migraine that may reduce the likelihood of alcohol use in several ways. Not only does it appear to reduce withdrawal symptoms via its blockade of excitatory amino acid (glutamate and kainate) receptors but it also inhibits dopamine release indirectly through stimulating GABA release, thereby potentially decreasing alcohol's reward effects. Unlike some other abstinence treatments for alcohol, **topiramate may be useful initiating while patients are still in withdrawal.**

There has been limited controlled clinical study of topiramate, although the initial controlled studies are promising. In a study of 150 chronic, heavy-drinking alcoholics, patients were randomized to topiramate, up to 300 mg daily, or placebo and followed for 3 months. At the start of the study, patients drank approximately nine alcohol drinks per day. At the end of the trial, patients taking topiramate drank an average of three drinks per day and placebo-treated patients drank an average of 5.5 drinks per day. More importantly, topiramate-treated patients were much more likely to have abstinent days than placebo-treated patients. During the study period, topiramate-treated patients reported not drinking 44% of the days compared with placebo-treated patients who reported abstinence only 18% of the days. Topiramate-treated patients also reported less craving for alcohol and were much more likely to report greater physical health and life satisfaction. Another 14-week controlled study found similar results, with topiramate leading to a reduction in heavy drinking days compared with placebo. On the other hand, sustained abstinence over 3 months was achieved by less than 20% of patients, and topiramate-treated patients reported being abstinent only 40% of the trial days. Although many patients receiving topiramate report cognitive dulling, patients in most studies tolerate topiramate well. In most studies, topiramate was associated with modest weight loss.

Pharmacology and Mechanism of Action
The exact mechanism of action is unknown, although topiramate appears to potentiate GABA mediated chloride currents and antagonize excitatory amino acid receptors. It is unclear if either of these effects contributes to decreased alcohol drinking or seizure prevention.

Kinetics

Topiramate reaches peak concentration in 2 to 4 hours. Eating food does not significantly affect absorption. Only 10% to 20% is protein bound. Much of the drug is eliminated unchanged in the urine, although some is hydroxylated and then solubilized by the addition of glucuronide. The elimination half-life is between 18 and 24 hours.

Adverse Effects

CNS Effects. CNS adverse effects occur commonly with topiramate. Sedation, ataxia, somnolence, slurred speech, paresthesias, and nystagmus are common; however, slow dose escalation may limit these effects and patients may accommodate to the CNS effects over time. Many patients also report cognitive dulling, and in our experience, this adverse effect may be less likely to improve over time, although dose reduction may be helpful. Cognitive impairment from topiramate appears worse than with other anticonvulsants. Rarely, patients have been reported to develop psychotic symptoms while taking topiramate. Unpleasant taste or alteration of food taste is common.

Metabolic Effects. Weight loss is common with topiramate use. Most patients will lose some weight, some to a striking degree. The mechanism responsible for weight loss is unclear, although topiramate appears to reduce appetite and have a diuretic effect. Topiramate inhibits carbonic anhydrase, which leads to renal bicarbonate wasting that in some cases may cause hyperchloremic, nonanion gap, and metabolic acidosis. Patients with renal disease or diarrhea may be at greater risk for developing metabolic acidosis. Chronic, untreated metabolic acidosis may lead to the formation of kidney stones or osteoporosis.

Gastrointestinal Effects. Nausea is somewhat common at the onset of treatment, although it generally resolves. Abdominal pain and diarrhea are uncommon side effects. As noted previously, loss of appetite is common. Elevated transaminase levels occur uncommonly with topiramate use. Topiramate is associated with mild drops in serum cholesterol levels in some patients.

Cardiovascular Effects. Topiramate has uncommonly been associated with hypotension, bradycardia, palpitations, and bundle branch block.

Ocular Effects. Acute angle glaucoma is a rare side effect, although visual blurring and diplopia are common.

Drug Interactions

Because topiramate is a weak inhibitor of carbonic anhydrase, combining it with other carbonic anhydrase inhibitors such as acetazolamide or dichlorphenamide may further increase the risk of metabolic acidosis.

Topiramate does not inhibit hepatic microsomal enzymes and appears to be a weak inducer of microsomal enzymes. Used in combination with drugs that induce hepatic enzymes (e.g., phenytoin or carbamazepine), topiramate concentrations may fall. Topiramate may slightly reduce the effectiveness of oral contraceptive agents because of its weak induction of microsomal enzymes.

Overdose

Topiramate overdose may be associated with metabolic acidosis, coma, seizures, or even death. Treatment is supportive, and because the drug is not significantly protein bound, renal dialysis may be used to reduce plasma concentration.

Dose Forms Available
Topiramate is available as 25-, 50-, 100-, and 200-mg tablets. It is also available as 15- and 25-mg sprinkle capsules.

Dosage
The dosage of topiramate is not established for alcohol dependence. Clinical studies and practice suggest a dosage between 200 to 400 mg daily in divided doses or as a single dose in the evening.

Method of Use
For selected patients, start topiramate at a dose of 25 mg at bedtime and gradually titrate every 3 to 4 days, as tolerated, over several weeks to 200 to 300 mg per day. The gradual titration leads to less CNS toxicity. Obtain blood for electrolytes and check chloride and bicarbonate concentrations at baseline and after reaching target dose. Encourage the patient to attend Alcoholics Anonymous meetings or other psychosocial rehabilitation.

Baclofen
Baclofen is a $GABA_B$ agonist primarily used to treat spasticity. Several small studies found that it reduced alcohol craving and use, and a recent larger study ($N = 84$) found that among alcoholics with liver cirrhosis, baclofen was clearly superior to placebo for preventing relapse into heavy drinking and providing prolonged abstinence. In this 12-week study, patients were seen weekly for the first month and then every 2 weeks. Patients received counseling during each visit to help them with sobriety and were given either baclofen or placebo, titrated to 10 mg three times daily. Alcohol use was determined from patient self-reports as well as family reports and the findings from blood and urine tests. During the study period, 71% of baclofen-treated patients achieved abstinence, whereas only 29% of placebo-treated patients refrained from drinking. Baclofen-treated patients were less likely to have any days of heavy drinking (19%) compared with placebo-treated patients (46%). In our experience, baclofen is very well tolerated and appears clinically useful.

Pharmacology and Mechanism of Action
The mechanism of action of baclofen is unknown for alcoholism, although it appears to reduce spasticity by reducing neural transmission in the spinal cord via agonist effects at $GABA_B$ receptors. It is readily absorbed through the gastrointestinal tract and is eliminated through the urine unchanged. Its plasma half-life is approximately 4 hours.

Adverse Effects
The most common adverse effect is sedation, though at lower doses this is generally not a problem. Slow dose titration improves tolerance to sedation. Other sedating drugs or alcohol may compound sedation. Gastrointestinal irritation or vomiting along with cognitive impairment, weakness, and ataxia are relatively common dose-dependent side effects. The most serious uncommon side effect is hypotension, particularly when it is combined with an antihypertensive agent. Abrupt withdrawal from prolonged use of baclofen may lead to a discontinuation syndrome with hallucinations, anxiety, and mild confusion.

Method of Use
Baclofen is best started as a single bedtime dose of 5 mg for several days. It should be gradually increased, given two or three times per day because of its short half-life to a total dose of 30 mg per day, with most of the dose given at bedtime. Patients report that the bedtime dose helps with sleep. The dose for alcoholism is not

established. The highest daily dose recommended for spasticity is 80 mg. Discontinuation should be done over several weeks to avoid withdrawal symptoms.

Overdose
Respiratory depression, coma, and seizures have been reported with overdose.

Dose Forms Available
Baclofen is available as 10- and 20-mg tablets.

Dosage
The dosage of baclofen is not established for the treatment of alcohol dependence. Clinical studies and practice suggest a dosage between 15 and 30 mg daily in divided doses. Higher doses may be useful, though a maximum dose of 80 mg is suggested for spasticity.

Combination Treatments
Emerging evidence suggests that the combination of treatments may be more beneficial than individual treatments, theoretically because of the effects of different mechanisms. For example, naltrexone plus ondansetron shows early promise as an effective combination treatment for maintaining alcohol abstinence. Nicotine replacement treatment may enhance alcohol treatment. Other combinations may also prove beneficial, though a large study found that acamprosate does not improve outcomes when combined with naltrexone.

PSYCHOSTIMULANT DEPENDENCE
In predisposed individuals, psychostimulant use may lead to severe intoxication, abuse, and dependence. Amphetamines are abused orally and intravenously, and methylphenidate is abused orally. Pemoline does not appear to be commonly abused. Stimulants include amphetamine, methamphetamine, cocaine, nicotine, and methylphenidate; these drugs produce feelings of euphoria and enhanced self-confidence. Some may improve cognitive performance briefly in some individuals. When these drugs are used in the high dosage ranges, there are often signs of adrenergic hyperactivity (i.e., increased pulse and blood pressure, dry mouth, and pupillary dilatation). High doses of amphetamine may result in stereotyped behaviors, bruxism, formication, irritability, restlessness, emotional lability, hallucinations, and paranoia. With chronic abuse, a paranoid psychosis may develop, characterized by paranoid delusions; ideas of reference; and auditory, visual, or tactile hallucinations.

Withdrawal
Although the withdrawal syndrome from stimulants is not medically dangerous, dependent individuals usually experience neuropsychiatric symptoms, including fatigue, hypersomnia or insomnia, hyperphagia, irritability and mood symptoms ranging from dysphoria to severe depression in the short term and anhedonia, dysphoria, and intense drug craving in the long term. Currently, there is no proven pharmacologic treatment for dependence to cocaine and amphetamines and behavioral treatment is the standard of care. Patients should be observed for the emergence of a major depressive syndrome and suicidal behavior or alternatively for recurrent drug abuse. There are effective treatments for nicotine dependence.

Overdose
Overdose with psychostimulants results in a syndrome of marked sympathetic hyperactivity (i.e., hypertension, tachycardia, hyperthermia) often accompanied by toxic psychosis or delirium. Patients may be irritable, paranoid, or violent. Grand

mal seizures may occur. Death may result from hypertension, hyperthermia, cardiac arrhythmias, or uncontrollable seizures.

Treatment consists of supportive care and blockade of adrenergic receptors. If the patient is unconscious or seizing, the airway must be protected. High fevers should be treated with cooling blankets. Seizures can be controlled with an intravenous benzodiazepine, such as lorazepam (1 to 2 mg) or diazepam (5 to 10 mg), repeated as necessary.

Delirium or psychosis usually responds to an antipsychotic agent. If the patient is also hypertensive, risperidone or chlorpromazine has the advantage of blocking both α-adrenergic and dopamine receptors. Risperidone dosages of 1 to 2 mg b.i.d. are reasonable if this agent is chosen. Dosages of chlorpromazine 50 mg intramuscularly q.i.d. are usually adequate, although dosages up to 100 mg q.i.d. may be necessary. Otherwise, haloperidol might be a better choice; 5 mg b.i.d. will usually suffice. Additional sedation can be provided by benzodiazepines, such as lorazepam, 1 to 2 mg orally or 1 mg intramuscularly, or diazepam, 5 to 10 mg orally every 1 to 2 hours as needed. Delirium usually clears in 2 to 3 days, but paranoid psychoses due to long-term, high-dose abuse may take longer to clear. Severe hypertension or tachyarrhythmias can usually be treated with propranolol, 1 mg intravenously every 5 to 10 minutes as needed up to a total of 8 mg.

TREATMENT OF CHRONIC COCAINE USE

Although a number of agents, including antidepressants, baclofen, and dopamine agonists have been touted as potentially useful for the treatment of stimulant withdrawal or to maintain abstinence, there are no controlled studies supporting their efficacy over placebo. Several other agents, however, including disulfiram, modafinil, and topiramate, have shown preliminary promise in controlled studies for at least curtailing cocaine use in motivated patients. The patient is best treated in a rehabilitation program or through a support group such as Cocaine Anonymous. In addition, comorbid conditions such as alcohol dependence or mood disorders should be treated with established treatments.

Disulfiram

In addition to inhibiting aldehyde dehydrogenase, disulfiram also inhibits an enzyme in dopamine metabolism, dopamine-β hydroxylase, which leads to a relative increase in CNS dopamine. This property is conjectured to blunt cocaine craving or alter cocaine subjective experience and therefore reduce cocaine use. The pharmacology of disulfiram is covered in the section on alcohol dependence.

Although the initial studies examined cocaine use in alcohol-dependent patients, it appears that disulfiram may reduce cocaine use even in the absence of alcohol use. In the largest clinical trial ($N = 121$), cocaine-dependent patients, with or without concurrent alcoholism, were randomized to placebo or disulfiram, 250 mg, along with weekly interpersonal or cognitive behavioral therapy. Patients were studied for 12 weeks and gave urine samples weekly. About half of the patients completed the trial. Among those who completed the trail, there was a reduction in cocaine use, which was greater for disulfiram-treated patients than placebo-treated patients. At baseline, cocaine was used approximately three times per week, but at endpoint disulfiram-treated patients used 0.5 times per week and placebo-treated patients used twice per week. This study does not answer the question if disulfiram would play a role with less intensive treatment, but it appears a reasonable and inexpensive option for motivated patients.

Modafinil

Modafinil is a wake-promoting drug established for the treatment of narcolepsy whose mechanism of action is unknown, though *in vitro* studies show that it inhibits reuptake of dopamine and stimulates glutamate receptors. The pharmacology of modafinil is covered in Chapter 3. Modafinil is postulated to reduce cocaine withdrawal symptoms and craving during early abstinence. In the biggest clinical trial, 62 patients addicted to cocaine without other alcohol or drug dependence were randomized to placebo or modafinil, 400 mg once daily for 8 weeks. Subjects attended the clinic three times a week and gave urine samples each visit. They also participated in cognitive behavioral therapy twice per week. Approximately 66% completed the study and modafinil was well tolerated. For any given week, approximately 45% of modafinil-treated patients provided "clean" urines compared with 25% of placebo-treated patients. More prolonged sobriety was less common among these patients. Only 33% attained abstinence for 3 or more weeks, though this was better than the 13% abstinence rate achieved by the placebo-treated patients. As with the other pharmacologic agents used in drug addiction, this should only be a part of the treatment. High price of modafinil may limit its utility in clinical practice.

Topiramate
Topiramate is an anticonvulsant that enhances GABA activity while antagonizing glutamate pathways. It has already shown promise in treating alcoholism and some recent studies suggest it may provide benefit for cocaine addiction as well. In a 13-week pilot trial ($N = 40$), topiramate was compared with placebo in treating patients addicted to cocaine. Patients had to be 3 days sober before starting the treatment because of topiramate's potential for worsening acute cocaine withdrawal. Patients received twice-weekly psychotherapy to assist in attaining abstinence and were gradually titrated on topiramate or placebo, up to a dose of 200 mg per day, starting at 25 mg with a dose increase of 25 mg every week. The slow titration was intended to enhance compliance because of topiramate's well-known cognitive and neurological side effects. (Pharmacology of topiramate is covered in the section on alcohol dependence.) The primary outcome was abstinence as proved by twice-weekly urine drug tests for cocaine. Nearly 80% of subjects completed the study. In any given week, more topiramate-treated patients were abstinent from cocaine than placebo-treated patients, but even in the best week, more than half of the patients still used cocaine. Using the "continuous abstinence" definition of abstinence for 3 more weeks, 59% of topiramate-treated patients attained this milestone compared with 26% of placebo-treated patients. Hence, topiramate may offer some benefits in this very difficult to treat condition.

NICOTINE DEPENDENCE
Nicotine is probably the most lethal addiction and accounts for over 440,000 premature deaths related to heart disease and various cancers annually in the United States alone. Tobacco smoking accounts for most of nicotine dependence. Because of the rapid absorption of smoked nicotine through the pulmonary circulation and the reinforcing effects of multiple daily doses that lead to sustained effects on the brain, it is one of the most difficult addictions to overcome. It is routine for nicotine-dependent patients to require up to five trials of effective combined pharmacologic and behavioral treatment before they attain sustained abstinence. With pharmacologic treatment, abstinence rates following several months of treatment are 40% to 60% in many studies, double to triple the placebo rates. However, the relapse rate at 1 year following discontinuation of pharmacologic treatment is high. Most treatment studies have tested only brief treatment periods of 4 to 12 weeks; there is limited evidence that treatment up to 2 years is effective and safe. Further study of chronic treatment to prevent relapse to smoking is underway. Because of the profoundly detrimental long-term effects of tobacco smoking, however, all smokers should be encourage to accept treatment.

In contrast to popular lore, **successful smoking cessation may also improve the outcome for patients with other addictive disorders.** Indeed, a meta-analysis found that smoking cessation treatment led to a 25% improvement in long-term drug and alcohol abstinence. Success of the treatment is dependent on the patient's desire to quit smoking and is much more likely when the person is actively involved in a smoking cessation program.

Patients with comorbid psychiatric disorders, particularly depression, schizophrenia, and other substance use disorders, are more likely than those in the general population to smoke tobacco and in general their abstinence rates with treatment are lower. Patients with a history of depression are less likely to quit and may even suffer depressive recurrence during the period when they try to quit smoking. Smokers who are depressed often use nicotine as a means to modulate depressive symptoms, complicating even further any efforts to help them withdraw; antidepressants can often be helpful in these situations. In persons with substance abuse or schizophrenia, nicotine dependence is extremely common, prompting some to hypothesize that there may be an underlying genetic or biological propensity for the high rates and refractory nature of nicotine abuse in these populations.

First-line treatments for smoking cessation are varenicline, nicotine replacement therapy, and sustained-release bupropion. Second-line treatments include combination of two forms of nicotine replacement therapy, tricyclic antidepressants and clonidine. Nicotine replacement strategies for treatment serve to replace nicotine from inhaled sources with nicotine absorbed through the skin or mucous membranes, thus reducing the craving and withdrawal symptoms associated with smoking cessation. Varenicline is a partial agonist at a subtype of nicotinic receptors, the $\alpha_4\beta_2$ receptor. Bupropion, on the other hand, is not as effective in reducing craving as nicotine is, although it appears that bupropion may be more effective than nicotine for prolonged abstinence, and the combination of bupropion and nicotine replacement is more effective than either alone. Other pharmacologic treatments used in addiction treatment, such as naltrexone, show preliminary promise of increasing the likelihood of smoking cessation when combined with nicotine replacement treatment, suggesting that patients with multiple addictions may benefit from combined pharmacotherapy.

The preponderance of data for treating nicotine dependence has been gleaned from studies on tobacco smoking. It is not clear whether these agents work for chewing tobacco, although the current established agents appear to be reasonable options given the lack of specific data.

Pharmacology

Nicotine is a naturally occurring compound with many pharmacologic effects. It is best known as a cholinergic agonist, specific for receptors of the nicotinic subtype. Because these receptors are found widely in peripheral nerve ganglia and in the CNS, nicotine use leads to a wide range of central and peripheral effects. Through its action as a direct agonist at nicotinic cholinergic receptors, nicotine causes release of a wide range of neurotransmitters including serotonin, norepinephrine, dopamine, GABA, vasopressin, and glutamate. This effect on multiple receptor systems may help explain its varied effects, including reduction in anxiety and depression, improved cognition, and alertness.

Peripheral and Autonomic Nervous System Effects

Nicotine may stimulate the sympathetic nervous system or inhibit the parasympathetic nervous system and exert effects on the peripheral organs, especially the heart, through the autonomic and peripheral nervous system. Nicotine also causes release of catecholamines from the adrenal medulla, which leads to sympathomimetic effects at peripheral organs such as peripheral tremors when used at the higher doses.

CNS Effects

Nicotine is a CNS stimulant, increasing arousal and respiration at lower doses, effects commonly experienced by smokers. Similarly, nicotine also improves attention and concentration and improves short- and long-term memory on a range of cognitive tasks. Nicotine causes increased release of dopamine in the brain, which may contribute to its propensity for causing addiction in susceptible individuals. In addition, nicotine receptors are found on the dopamine-containing cells of the ventral tegmental area, a brain region that projects, in part, to the nucleus accumbens, a brain area associated with pleasure and reward, likely linked to addiction. Activation of these dopamine neurons is likely involved in the neurochemical mechanisms that reinforce nicotine abuse. Nicotine may also serve as an agonist in the chemoreceptor area and induce nausea and/or vomiting.

Cardiovascular Effects

Nicotine increases heart rate and blood pressure acutely, although this tends to normalize over time. The cardiovascular effects are due to stimulation of sympathetic ganglia and the adrenal medulla. Nicotine also activates chemoreceptors in the carotid and aortic bodies, which results in vasoconstriction, tachycardia, and elevated blood pressure.

Gastrointestinal Effects

Nicotine stimulates parasympathetic neurons in the gastrointestinal system, leading to increased tone and bowel activity. Nausea, vomiting, and diarrhea are common physiologic toxic effects of nicotine.

Nicotine Formulations

Nicotine is available in several preparations: a slowly acting formulation, the transdermal patch and faster acting forms, polacrilex gum, oral inhaler, and nasal spray. Although an individual preparation is the preferred starting treatment, some smokers may require two forms at once, usually the patch used daily combined with one of the faster acting formulations used as needed for craving. Indeed the nicotine patch combined with the inhaler, gum, or nasal spray leads to higher abstinence rates than the patch alone. In all forms, nicotine affects central and peripheral cholinergic (nicotinic) receptors. The inhaled or nasal sprays more closely mimic the immediate effects of smoking compared with the gum or patch. Nicotine replacement is only approved for use as replacement treatment to facilitate nicotine withdrawal and smoking cessation.

Nicotine Polacrilex

In the gum or lozenge form, nicotine is bound in an ion-exchange resin known as nicotine polacrilex. It is rapidly absorbed through the mucous membranes of the mouth and reaches peak concentration within 15 to 30 minutes. Absorption is decreased by swallowing the gum or lozenge and by drinking acidic beverages such as colas or coffee while chewing the gum. Nicotine is metabolized by the liver via oxidation and there are no active metabolites. The mean elimination half-life is approximately 1 hour.

In the gum form, nicotine has minimal cardiovascular effects; however, in higher concentrations, nicotine may cause tachycardia or hypertension. The most consistent physiologic effects from nicotine gum are nausea and indigestion; infrequently, patients vomit from nicotine gum chewing. Irritations of the mouth and gum sores are common, as are complaints of flatulence. Hiccups may occur during early use of nicotine gum, although this is usually transient. Adverse effects of the lozenge are similar to the gum form, but this preparation is obviously easier for those with troubles chewing.

Signs of overt toxicity include cold sweats, nausea, vomiting, diarrhea, abdominal pain, headache, dizziness, tremor, mental confusion, and lethargy.

Doses Available. The formulations available are 2 and 4 mg of nicotine in gum and 2 and 4 mg of nicotine in lozenges.

Method of Use. Once the person decides to stop smoking, gum or lozenge use may begin. Heavy smokers (>20 cigarettes per day, or first cigarette within 30 minutes of waking) should start with the 4-mg gum or lozenge. Less heavy smokers can start with 2-mg gum or lozenge. The person should then use an additional gum or lozenge every 1 to 2 hours and use approximately 10 per day. The gum should be chewed briefly, to soften the gum, and be placed between the cheek and gum and kept there for 15 minutes, and swallowing should be limited. The lozenge should be allowed to slowly dissolve in the mouth more than 15 to 20 minutes and swallowing should be minimized. This high dosing should continue for at least 6 weeks.

Following the first 6 weeks, the daily dose of nicotine can be reduced gradually by lengthening the dose interval of either the gum or lozenge. The patient can modify the nicotine replacement from every 2 hours to every 4 hours, as tolerated. Over the next 4 weeks, this interval should be maintained at every 4 hours with the eventual goal of extending the interval to every 8 hours for several more weeks before stopping completely. Some patients do better using the gum for longer periods, perhaps up to 6 months.

The person attempting to quit smoking should also participate in psychosocial treatments such as participation in a smoking cessation group and/or working with trained therapists to change certain behaviors associated with smoking. For example, spending time with other smokers will increase the chances of relapse and taking walks during times of stress or eating hard candies may be a useful alternative to smoking.

Nicotine Nasal Spray

In this preparation, nicotine is absorbed through the mouth or nasal mucous membranes. Each nasal spray contains approximately 0.5 mg of nicotine, and each cartridge has 4 mg of nicotine. The spray is intended for absorption through the nasal mucosa not the lungs. Absorption is relatively fast, reaching peak concentration in 4 to 15 minutes. This preparation allows for absorption closest to cigarette smoking. Nicotine steady-state plasma concentrations, however, fall below that found in smokers.

Common adverse effects include mouth and throat irritation and dyspepsia. Severe toxicity is uncommon with the inhalers. Caution must be used in patients with asthma or obstructive lung disease or in patients with serious cardiac disease (vasospastic disease; i.e., Prinzmetal's angina, arrhythmia, angina, recent myocardial infarction). Care must also be taken in patients with hyperthyroidism or pheochromocytoma because nicotine causes release of catecholamines. Nicotine may delay healing in peptic ulcer disease and should be used judiciously in patients suspected of having peptic ulcers.

Doses Available. The preparation is available in a 10-mg cartridge that contains 4 mg of nicotine; each spray contains 0.5 mg of nicotine.

Method of Use—Nasal Inhaler. Once a "stop day" is decided, the nasal inhaler can start. The initial dose is two sprays (one in each nostril) every hour or two for the first 8 weeks. The user sprays the nasal mucosa and should not inhale the vapor. The person should use the spray at least 10 times per day during the first few weeks and then reduce as tolerated during this period. Over the next 6 weeks, the dose can be gradually reduced to every 4 to 6 hours. The maximum daily dosing should be 40 doses per day. The maximum recommended treatment length is 6 months.

Nicotine Oral Inhaler

As with the nasal spray, the oral inhaler is designed to allow nicotine absorption through the mucosa rather than through the lungs. In this case, the inhaler is puffed to allow buccal absorption. Common side effects include throat irritation and coughing. Less common side effects include nausea, vomiting, and heart palpitations. The inhaler consists of a plastic mouthpiece that accommodates a nicotine cartridge. Each cartridge contains approximately 4 mg of nicotine, and the average inhaled puff contains 13 mg of nicotine; hence, approximately 75 to 80 puffs are required to deliver 1 mg of nicotine.

Method of Use—Oral Inhaler. The oral inhaler requires time for gradual puffing. It takes approximately 20 minutes to allow for complete use of a cartridge that delivers 4 mg of nicotine. Peak concentration is reached in approximately 30 minutes. These cartridges should be used every 2 to 4 hours during the first few weeks. At least six cartridges should be used daily during the first 3 weeks, although some patients may need as many as 16 per day. After 8 weeks, the dose can be gradually tapered as tolerated and use may be stopped after 12 weeks; however, some patients may need a longer treatment period.

Nicotine Transdermal Patch

Nicotine is absorbed slowly through the transdermal patch, which limits acceptance in some smokers because of its lack of efficacy for initial craving. There is an initial time lag of 1 to 2 hours before nicotine is absorbed and peak concentration is not reached for 6 to 12 hours. Rash or local irritation uncommonly follows from the patch adhesive; otherwise, the patch is very well tolerated. When patients complain of nausea or palpitations, the clinician should consider toxicity and might formulate another strategy for smoking cessation.

Method of Use. On the day smoking stops, a patch can be placed. Patients smoking more than 10 cigarettes per day start with the 21-mg patch dose. The patch generally should not be worn while the patient is smoking, though some patients do smoke a few cigarettes when they start with the patch. The skin should be cleaned and dry and then the patch can be placed anywhere on the body, although ideally in a place with limited hair and low likelihood for being disrupted, such as the upper arm or abdomen. After the backing is removed, the patch should be held on the skin for 10 to 15 seconds to ensure that it sticks. The patch should then be worn for 16 to 24 hours; many patients initially need 24 hours to optimize outcomes.

A new patch should be placed at the same time each day, 24 hours after the previous patch was applied. The 21-mg strength should be used for the first 6 weeks of treatment and then the dose can be gradually reduced, first to 14 mg for several weeks and then to 7 mg for several weeks until the patch is discontinued.

Patients who smoke less than 10 cigarettes per day can be started on the 14-mg transdermal patch. They can be treated with this strength for 6 weeks and then tapered to the 7-mg patch for another 4 to 6 weeks before stopping.

Doses Available. The patches are available in 7, 14, and 21 mg of nicotine.

Varenicline

Varenicline (Chantix) is a recent pharmacologic treatment specifically developed and marketed for smoking cession. It is a selective nicotinic acetylcholine receptor partial agonist. It has been studied in a number of 12-week placebo-controlled trials, with bupropion as a comparison drug in two trials, and has been studied in a 12-month safety trial. Study subjects were generally moderate smokers (one pack per day) and had smoked for approximately 20 years. More serious smokers, or smokers with depressive or psychotic disorders have not been studied. Use of varenicline for tobacco chewing has not been studied. During the short-term trials, varenicline produced abstinence rates confirmed by carbon monoxide exhalation methods in approximately 60% of subjects, compared with a 20% placebo response rate and 40% abstinence rate on bupropion. Studies find varenicline to be superior to bupropion in the short term, but only marginally better at long-term follow-up. Despite the success rates in studies of 12-week treatment, at a 1-year follow-up, abstinence rates are considerably lower, usually around 20% to 25% compared with placebo response rates of 10% to 15%. The findings suggest that short-term use may not be adequate, and greater abstinence may follow longer use. Twenty-four weeks of treatment has been demonstrated to be superior to 12 weeks of treatment for abstinence when rates are compared at 1 year. For those able to quit smoking during the first 12 weeks of treatment, an additional 12 weeks of treatment is recommended for prevention of relapse.

There have been postmarketing concerns about the onset of depression or suicide attempts during varenicline or shortly after discontinuation. Clinical trial data do not suggest this as a legitimate concern, though there is a well known, if complex, association between smoking and depression. Suicidal feelings or depression may follow smoking cessation, and some patients seeking smoking cessation treatment may not report their depressive feelings. Therefore, past patient history of depression and past experience with smoking cessation must be included in the decision of treatment with varenicline or any other nicotine replacement therapy. Even though clinical trials have not addressed depressed patients trying to quit, it behooves the prescriber to address mood disorders in patients seeking smoking cessation treatment.

Pharmacology

Varenicline is a partial agonist at $\alpha_4\beta_2$ nicotinic acetylcholine receptors. These CNS receptors are reinforcing for nicotine use. Nicotine has high affinity for $\alpha_4\beta_2$ receptors in the ventral tegmentum, a region rich in dopamine neuron cell bodies, which are presumed important in the reinforcing and reward properties of nicotine and a number of addictive drugs. Varenicline competitively inhibits the effects of nicotine at the $\alpha_4\beta_2$ receptor and thereby reduces the effects of smoking in patients who smoke while taking the pill. In addition to stimulating these nicotine receptors, varenicline also stimulates other nicotine receptors ($\alpha_3\beta_4$ and α_7), though it is unclear if these are relevant to its salutary effects on smoking cessation. The drug does not have other known direct effects on non-nicotinic receptors other than modest blockade of 5-HT_3 receptors.

Pharmacokinetics

Varenicline has a half-life of approximately 1 day and reaches peak concentration after 3 hours. It is readily absorbed in the small intestine and excreted largely unchanged through the kidney. Dosage reductions are not needed for hepatic disease. Patients with significant renal dysfunction should be treated with 0.5 to 1 mg daily doses. Smoking does not affect its metabolism and it does not inhibit nor induce hepatic cytochrome enzyme responsible for drug metabolism. There are no known serious drug interactions. In particular, it does not affect metabolism of bupropion and nicotine.

Adverse Effects

The most common dose-dependent adverse effect is nausea, experienced by 30% to 40% of patients in clinical trials. Other gastrointestinal problems, including abdominal pain, diarrhea or nausea, and vomiting, are much less common. More highly addicted smokers are less prone to gastrointestinal side effects. Slow titration limits these side effects. In most cases, nausea subsides over 1 to 2 weeks, but it may persist and lead to drug discontinuation. Insomnia, abnormal dreams, anxiety, and headaches are the other common side effects, but these may be related to nicotine withdrawal. Chest pain and palpitations are uncommon. Hypersensitivity rash is rare.

Pregnancy
Varenicline is rated a category C risk when used during pregnancy. In high doses it produces reduced fetal weights in rabbits and rats. There are no data in humans regarding teratogenicity. In animals, varenicline passes through the placenta and into milk. The safety for the fetus in humans during pregnancy or during breast-feeding is unknown.

Method of Use
Varenicline should be started 1 to 2 weeks before smoking cessation. To limit gastrointestinal side effects, it should be taken on a full meal with a full glass of liquid. Dosing should be gradual and as tolerated, starting with 0.5 mg daily and increasing every 3 to 5 days by 0.5 mg to reach a total dose of 1 mg twice daily. Patients should be told to expect nausea to occur and then to resolve. In general, wait for nausea to resolve before increasing the dose. Some patients may not be able to tolerate 2 mg per day, and may have to stop at 1 mg per day. Highly addicted smokers (>30 cigarettes per day) may tolerate more rapid titration and may need higher than the 2 mg daily dose. Patients may need brief hypnotic treatment of insomnia that sometimes follows smoking cessation and varenicline treatment. Patients should be engaged in a smoking cessation program to help change behaviors and cope with the difficulties of not having smoking as a solution for stressful situations.

Doses Available
Varenicline is available as 0.5 and 1 mg tablets.

Bupropion
For smoking cessation, bupropion treatment approximately doubles quit rates compared to placebo. Although bupropion's mechanism of action to facilitate smoking cessation is unknown, it is theorized to assist in smoking cessation through blocking the reuptake of norepinephrine and dopamine. Because nicotine also increases brain catecholamines, these similar effects of bupropion may mimic nicotine's pharmacologic effects and thereby attenuate nicotine withdrawal.

Bupropion is a well-tolerated pharmacologic treatment of smoking cessation. In several large clinical trials, bupropion was equal to, or more effective than, nicotine replacement treatment of smoking cessation. In combination with the nicotine patch, bupropion was better than the patch alone. In one large study following 8 weeks of smoking cessation treatment, at the 1-year follow-up the abstinence rates were higher in bupropion-treated patients compared with patients treated with the nicotine patch (30% vs 16%), and the combination of nicotine and bupropion led to slightly higher abstinence rates (36%). Bupropion may not be as effective as varenicline, though it may improve smoking cessation rates when combined with varenicline, even if this combination has not yet been studied.

Although bupropion is effective for smoking abstinence in short-term trials, after a 1-year follow-up period, abstinence rates are still relatively low. The drop-off in abstinence rates suggests that treatment should continue longer than is currently recommended; however, there are no controlled trials to support long-term use. For patients with recurrent depression and smoking problems, however, bupropion appears a prudent choice for chronic treatment. Bupropion is also as helpful for smoking cessation in patients with a history of depression as it is for patients without a history of depression.

Pharmacology
The pharmacology of bupropion is covered in detail in Chapter 3. In smoking cessation clinical trials, bupropion is very well tolerated and may be better tolerated than in depressed patients. The most common side effects in these trials were dry mouth and insomnia. Sexual side effects are uncommon.

Method of Use
Unlike nicotine replacement therapy, the smoker should begin bupropion several weeks before stopping smoking. Bupropion SR (Zyban) is well studied, although the older and now generic formulation, bupropion immediate-release formulation, is also effective. Using bupropion SR, the patient can be started on 150 mg per day for 1 week and then increased to 150 mg b.i.d. The final dose is best given by midafternoon to reduce drug-induced insomnia. The extended-release bupropion formulation (Wellbutrin XL) may also be used, though it is unstudied for smoking cessation and it is more expensive than bupropion SR. Bupropion XL should also be started at 150 mg per day for several days and then increased to 300 mg per day in the morning. Some patients may require up to 450 mg per day. After the patient has been on bupropion without adverse effects for 2 or 3 weeks, the patient can quit smoking. As with the other treatments, the patient should be engaged in a smoking cessation program to help change behaviors and cope with the difficulties of not having smoking as a solution for stressful situations.

Bibliography

Drug Dependence
Cami J, Farre M. Drug addiction. *N Engl J Med* 2003;349:975.
Dackis CA, O'Brien CP. Cocaine dependence: a disease of the brain's reward centers. *J Subst Abuse Treat* 2001;21:111.
Koob GF, Nestler EJ. The neurobiology of drug addiction. *J Neuropsychiatry Clin Neurosci* 1997;9:482.

Ethanol Withdrawal Treatment
Anton RF. Pharmacologic approaches to the management of alcoholism. *J Clin Psychiatry* 2001;62(suppl 20):11.
Ntais C, Pakos E, Kyzas P, et al. Benzodiazepines for alcohol withdrawal. *Cochrane Database Syst Rev* 2005;(3):CD005063
Salloum IM, Cornelius JR, Daley DC, et al. The utility of diazepam loading in the treatment of alcohol withdrawal among psychiatric inpatients. *Psychopharmacol Bull* 1995;31:305.

Opioid Replacement Treatment
Anglin MD, Conner BT, Annon J, et al. Levo-alpha-acetylmethadol (LAAM) versus methadone maintenance: 1-year treatment retention, outcomes and status. *Addiction* 2007;102:1432–1442.
Eissenberg T, Bigelow GE, Strain EC, et al. Dose-related efficacy of levomethadyl acetate for treatment of opioid dependence: a randomized clinical trial. *JAMA* 1997;277:1945.
Fiellin DA, Pantalon MV, Chawarski MC, et al. Counseling plus buprenorphine-naloxone maintenance therapy for opioid dependence. *N Engl J Med* 2006;355(4):365–374.
Fudala PJ, Bridge TP, Herbert S, et al. Office-based treatment of opiate addiction with a sublingual-tablet formulation of buprenorphine and naloxone. *N Engl J Med* 2003;349:949.
Gowing LR, Farrell M, Ali RL, et al. Alpha2-adrenergic agonists in opioid withdrawal. *Addiction* 2002;97:49.
Johnson RE, Cutup MA, Strain EC, et al. A comparison of levomethadyl acetate, buprenorphine, and methadone for opioid dependence. *N Engl J Med* 2000;343:1290.

Ling W, Wesson DR, Charuvastra C, et al. A controlled trial comparing buprenorphine and methadone maintenance in opioid dependence. *Arch Gen Psychiatry* 1996;53:401.

Smith MY, Bailey JE, Woody GE, et al. Abuse of buprenorphine in the United States: 2003–2005. *J Addict Dis* 2007;26:107–111.

Alcohol Dependence Treatment

Addolorato G, Leggio L, Ferrulli A, et al. Effectiveness and safety of baclofen for maintenance of alcohol abstinence in alcohol-dependent patients with liver cirrhosis: randomised, double-blind controlled study. *Lancet* 2007;370(9603):1915–1922.

Anton RF, O'Malley SS, Ciraulo DA, et al. Combined pharmacotherapies and behavioral interventions for alcohol dependence: the COMBINE study: a randomized controlled trial. *JAMA* 2006;295(17):2003-2017.

Fuller RK, Branchey L, Brightwell DR, et al. Disulfiram treatment of alcoholism. A Veterans Administration cooperative study. *JAMA* 1986;256:1449.

Garbutt JC, Kranzler HR, O'Malley SS, et al. Efficacy and tolerability of long-acting injectable naltrexone for alcohol dependence: a randomized controlled trial. *JAMA* 2005;293(13):1617–1625.

Johnson BA, Ait-Daoud N, Bowden CL, et al. Oral topiramate for treatment of alcohol dependence: a randomised controlled trial. *Lancet* 2003;361:1677.

Johnson BA, Ait-Daoud N, Prihoda TJ. Combining ondansetron and naltrexone effectively treats biologically predisposed alcoholics: from hypotheses to preliminary clinical evidence. *Alcohol Clin Exp Res* 2000;24:737.

Johnson BA, Roache JD, Javors MA, et al. Ondansetron for reduction of drinking among biologically predisposed alcoholic patients: a randomized controlled trial. *JAMA* 2000;284:963.

Johnson BA, Rosenthal N, Capece JA, et al. Topiramate for treating alcohol dependence: a randomized controlled trial. *JAMA* 2007;298(14):1641–1651.

Krystal JH, Cramer JA, Krol WF, et al. Naltrexone in the treatment of alcohol dependence. *N Engl J Med* 2001;345:1734.

Morley KC, Teesson M, Reid SC, et al. Naltrexone versus acamprosate in the treatment of alcohol dependence: a multi-centre, randomized, double-blind, placebo-controlled trial. *Addiction* 2006;101(10):1451–1462.

O'Malley SS, Garbutt JC, Gastfriend DR, et al. Efficacy of extended-release naltrexone in alcohol-dependent patients who are abstinent before treatment. *J Clin Psychopharmacol* 2007;27(5):507–512.

Rubio G, Jimenez-Arriero MA, Ponce G, et al. Naltrexone versus acamprosate: one year follow-up of alcohol dependence treatment. *Alcohol Alcohol* 2001;36:419.

Sass H, Soyka M, Mann K, et al. Relapse prevention by acamprosate: results from a placebo-controlled study on alcohol dependence. *Arch Gen Psychiatry* 1996;53:673.

Suh JJ, Pettinati HM, Kampman KM, et al. The status of disulfiram: a half of a century later. *J Clin Psychopharmacol* 2006;26(3):290–302.

Nicotine Dependence Treatment

Bolliger CT, Zellweger J, Danielsson T, et al. Smoking reduction with oral nicotine inhalers: double blind, randomized clinical trial of efficacy and safety. *BMJ* 2000;321:329.

Gonzales D, Rennard SI, Nides M, et al. Varenicline, an alpha4beta2 nicotinic acetylcholine receptor partial agonist, vs sustained-release bupropion and placebo for smoking cessation: a randomized controlled trial. *JAMA* 2006;296(1):47–55.

Hayford KE, Patten CA, Rummans TA, et al. Efficacy of bupropion for smoking cessation in smokers with a former history of major depression or alcoholism. *Br J Psychiatry* 1999;174:173.

Jorenby DE, Leischow SJ, Nides MA, et al. A controlled trial of sustained-release bupropion, a nicotine patch, or both for smoking cessation. *N Engl J Med* 1999;340:685.

O'Malley SS, Cooney JL, Krishnan-Sarin S, et al. A controlled trial of naltrexone augmentation of nicotine replacement therapy for smoking cessation. *Arch Intern Med* 2006;166:667–674.

Oncken C, Gonzales D, Nides M, et al. Efficacy and safety of the novel selective nicotinic acetylcholine receptor partial agonist, varenicline, for smoking cessation. *Arch Intern Med* 2006;166(15):1571–1577.

Prochaska JJ, Delucchi K, Hall SM. A meta-analysis of smoking cessation interventions with individuals in substance abuse treatment or recovery. *J Consult Clin Psychol* 2004;72: 1144–1156.

Cocaine Dependence Treatment

Carroll KM, Fenton LR, Ball SA, et al. Efficacy of disulfiram and cognitive behavior therapy in cocaine-dependent outpatients: a randomized placebo-controlled trial. *Arch Gen Psychiatry* 2004;61(3):264–272.

Johnson BA, Roache JD, Ait-Daoud N, et al. A preliminary randomized, double-blind, placebo-controlled study of the safety and efficacy of ondansetron in the treatment of cocaine dependence. *Drug Alcohol Depend* 2006;84(3):256–263.

Kampman KM, Pettinati H, Lynch KG, et al. A pilot trial of topiramate for the treatment of cocaine dependence. *Drug Alcohol Depend* 2004;75:233–240.

Kenna GA, Nielsen DM, Mello P, et al. Pharmacotherapy of dual substance abuse and dependence. *CNS Drugs* 2007;21:213–237.

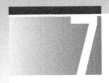

Drugs for the Treatment of Sleep Disorders

To understand sleep disorders, one needs to be familiar with sleep stages. Sleep can be broadly divided into two major states: rapid eye movement (REM) sleep and non–rapid eye movement (NREM) sleep. NREM sleep accounts for 75% to 80% of the total sleep period, whereas REM sleep comprises the rest of the sleep. NREM sleep is subdivided into four stages. Stage 1 is the transitional state between the wake state and sleep. Stage 2 is typically viewed as the true onset of sleep. Stages 3 and 4 are considered the "deep sleep"; based on the electroencephalogram, they are also called "slow wave sleep." **Deep sleep decreases with age,** leading many elderly individuals to complain about the quality of their sleep.

Sleep disorders can be primary, secondary to psychiatric disorders, or related to pharmacologic treatment or to psychoactive substance use. Sleep disorders also become more common in persons older than 65 years, when the ability to sleep typically diminishes, especially NREM stages 3 and 4. Therefore, in evaluating sleep disorders, it is essential to complete the following:

1. A sleep history: prospective data, such as those obtained with a sleep-wake diary, can sometimes be more informative than a sleep history alone.
2. A psychiatric and medical assessment.
3. An assessment of psychoactive substance use (e.g., alcohol, caffeine, stimulants, and cocaine, especially in proximity to attempts to sleep).
4. An assessment of concomitant medications use, including antidepressants and those obtained over the counter.
5. An important diagnostic tool is polysomnography, which comprises the overnight recording of electroencephalography, eye movements, and electromyography. Polysomnography allows the determination of the characteristics and duration of the various stages of sleep and the duration of REM and NREM sleep. Additional measures include oral/nasal airflow, respiratory effort, chest and abdominal wall movement, and oxyhemoglobin saturation.
6. Another diagnostic test, commonly used to study excessive sleepiness, is the Multiple Sleep Latency Test (MSLT), in which the individual is asked to lie down in a dark room and not resist falling sleep. Sleep latency (the amount of time required to fall asleep) is assessed five times during the day to provide an index of sleepiness.

BREATHING-RELATED SLEEP DISORDER

Breathing-related sleep disorder is characterized by sleep disruption, leading to excessive daytime sleepiness, and is caused by abnormalities of ventilation during sleep, such as sleep apnea or central alveolar hypoventilation. Partial respiratory cessations are defined as hypopneas, and complete respiratory cessations are defined as apneas. Apneas and hypopneas can be classified as central, obstructive, or mixed. The number of apnea episodes per hour of sleep is the apnea index, and the number of hypopnea episodes per hour of sleep is called the hypopnea index. The total number of apnea and hypopnea episodes per hour of sleep is called the respiratory disturbance index.

Three forms of breathing-related sleep disorder have been described:

1. Obstructive sleep apnea syndrome, characterized by repeated apneas or hypopneas during sleep caused by airway obstruction. It usually occurs in overweight and obese individuals and is accompanied by normal central drive for respiration and respiratory movements. Loud snores or brief gasps alternating with episodes of silence lasting 20 to 30 seconds are common. The termination of the apneas may be associated with loud snores, gasps, or moans.

2. Central sleep apnea syndrome, characterized by apneas and hypopneas during sleep without airway obstruction. In contrast to obstructive sleep apnea syndrome, central sleep apneas are not associated with continued chest wall and abdominal breathing movements and often occur in individuals with cardiac or neurological conditions. Insomnia due to repeated awakenings is often the chief concern, and individuals may or may not report breathing difficulties. Snoring may be present, but it is usually not a prominent symptom.

3. Central alveolar hypoventilation syndrome, characterized by an impairment in ventilatory control during wake, resulting in abnormally low arterial oxygen levels that tend to worsen during sleep. It typically occurs in very obese individuals. Insomnia and excessive sleepiness are the chief concerns.

Epidemiology

In middle-aged populations, sleep-disordered breathing is present typically in 2% of women and 4% of men, whereas in older adults, the prevalence rates often increase up to 25%. Approximately one third of subjects with hypertension have sleep-disordered breathing; sleep-disordered breathing events are associated with transient elevations in blood pressure and perhaps systemic hypertension and cardiac arrhythmias. In addition, this sleep-disordered breathing has been linked to increased mortality in some studies, particularly from cardiovascular conditions. This is not surprising, given the association of sleep-disordered breathing and obesity and higher body mass index.

Alcohol, as well as sedative-hypnotics, narcotics, and barbiturates, may exacerbate respiratory problems at night and reduce the patient's ability to wake up and breathe. Therefore, these pharmacologic agents should not be used at all or should be used with extreme caution in these patients.

Diagnosis of Obstructive and Central Sleep Apnea Syndromes

1. Symptoms of snoring and daytime sleepiness. Snoring tends to be milder in central sleep apnea, whereas it is prominent in the obstructive form. Excessive sleepiness is the chief concern of patients with both forms of sleep apnea syndrome and is due to the frequent awakenings at night. The sleepiness is most apparent during relaxing situations, such as watching television and reading. The MSLT (mentioned previously) and/or the Epworth Sleepiness Scale, a self-rating scale assessing the degree of sleepiness, are often used to evaluate daytime sleepiness. The mean sleep latency on the MSLT is often less than 10 minutes.

2. On polysomnography, an apnea index greater than 4 or a respiratory disturbance index greater than 9 and a reduction in oxyhemoglobin saturation are supportive of the diagnosis. In central sleep apnea, there may be episodes of Cheyne-Stokes respiration, characterized by a pattern of periodic breathing, with an apnea followed by hyperventilation for 10 to 60 seconds, followed by a gradual decrease in ventilation culminating in another apnea episode.

3. Imaging studies or endoscopic procedures may reveal airway obstruction, in the case of obstructive sleep apnea syndrome.

Diagnosis of Central Alveolar Hypoventilation Syndrome

On polysomnography, periods of decreased respiration lasting up to several minutes, with sustained arterial oxygen desaturation and increased carbon dioxide levels.

Sleep apnea is frequently associated with cognitive functioning problems (e.g., difficulties with memory, concentration, and attention), and some (but not all) studies have suggested a relationship between these symptoms and the degree of oxygen desaturation. Cardiac arrhythmias, such as sinus arrhythmias and premature ventricular contractions, often occur during sleep in these patients.

Treatment

Positive Airway Pressure

Nasal continuous positive airway pressure (CPAP) and bilevel positive airway pressure are probably the most commonly used nonsurgical approaches for obstructive sleep apnea. Both systems use a mask that is connected with a machine that generates positive air pressure. CPAP uses continuous pressure throughout inspiration and expiration, and bilevel positive airway pressure uses higher pressures during inspiration than expiration. Autoadjusting PAP is a variation of CPAP that incorporates various algorithms to automatically adjust air pressure based on persistence of apneas/hypopneas, snoring, and airflow limitation. It has not been found clinically superior to standard CPAP in the treatment of obstructive sleep apnea.

Surgical Interventions

Surgical interventions such as the uvulopharyngopalatoplasty and the laser-assisted uvulopalatoplasty are typically considered appropriate for those patients with anatomic abnormalities and obstructive sleep apnea.

Oral Appliances

Several dental devices are used to open the airway by holding the tongue and mandible forward. These devices are typically used with patients who have difficulties using CPAP or as a substitute for CPAP.

Weight Loss and Other Behavioral Measures

Because excess fatty tissue in the neck area may be a contributing factor, weight loss has been considered a possible treatment approach, although controlled data are lacking. In mild cases of obstructive sleep apnea, eliminating evening alcohol and sedatives, and sleeping in a lateral or prone position may help symptoms.

Pharmacologic Treatment

Pharmacologic treatment has clearly a very limited role in this condition. There have been only anecdotal reports of the use of tricyclic antidepressants (TCAs) or selective serotonin reuptake inhibitors (SSRIs), such as protriptyline and fluoxetine (see Chapter 3 for a discussion of the pharmacology of TCAs and SSRIs), improving oxyhemoglobin saturation, and drugs such as theophylline, medroxyprogesterone, and acetazolamide have also been used with only very limited results. The overall evidence of efficacy for these drug treatments is lacking.

Pharmacologic Treatment of Excessive Sleepiness

In addition to treatment interventions aimed at eliminating the cause of the excessive sleepiness, it is not uncommon for clinicians to treat the excessive sleepiness pharmacologically with caffeine, psychostimulants (e.g., methylphenidate 20 to 80 mg per day), or modafinil (Provigil) (100 to 400 mg per day, usually once per day). For a discussion on the pharmacology of psychostimulants and modafinil, see Chapter 9.

PERIODIC LIMB MOVEMENTS IN SLEEP

Periodic limb movements in sleep (PLMS) consist of repeated leg movements and kicks during sleep, typically every 20 to 40 seconds, causing brief arousals from sleep.

Diagnosis

1. Symptoms of insomnia and/or daytime sleepiness.
2. Subjective reporting of leg kicks, either by the patient or by the bed partner.
3. Objective polysomnography recordings of frequent leg kicks, usually lasting 0.5 to 5 seconds. The number of leg jerks per hour of sleep is called the periodic leg movement index. An index greater than 4, with each jerk associated with arousal, is typically required for the diagnosis.

Epidemiology

The prevalence of PLMS in adults is estimated at 5% to 6%, with significant increases in prevalence (up to 30%) in older age. Iron deficiency, renal failure, peripheral neuropathy, rheumatoid arthritis, and fibromyalgia have all been associated with PLMS.

Restless legs syndrome (RLS) is a common but often underdiagnosed neurologic disorder characterized by an imperative desire to move the extremities associated with paresthesias (unpleasant sensations in legs that feel "achy," crawly," "tingly," and/or "painful"), motor restlessness, worsening of symptoms at rest in the evening or at night, and, as a consequence, sleep disturbances. In addition, most patients with RLS have periodic limb movements during both sleep and relaxed wakefulness. The etiology of RLS remains unknown.

Treatment

Pharmacotherapy of PLMS

The typical approach to the pharmacologic management is the use of dopaminergic agents [e.g., levodopa/carbidopa, cabergoline, pergolide, selegiline, pramipexole (Mirapex), and ropinirole (Requip)]. Because the newer dopamine D_2 and D_3 receptor agonists are usually better tolerated than the older agents, pramipexole or ropinirole (0.25 to 2 mg q. 8 p.m.) are typically used. Most common side effects of these two dopaminergic drugs may include dizziness, drowsiness, dry mouth, insomnia, lack of appetite, memory difficulties, nausea, and fatigue. Pramipexole is available as 0.125-, 0.25-, 0.5-, 1-, and 2-mg tablets, and ropinirole is available as 0.25-, 0.5-, 1-, 2-, 3-, 4-, and 5-mg tablets. Melatonin [3 mg at bedtime (q.h.s.)], the benzodiazepine, clonazepam (0.5 to 2 mg q.h.s.) (see later in this chapter), and the anticonvulsant valproic acid (125 to 600 mg q.h.s.) have also been used with some success in the treatment of PLMS. For a discussion on the pharmacology of valproic acid, see Chapter 4.

Pharmacotherapy of RLS

As in the case of PLMS, the first-line approach to the pharmacologic management is the use of dopaminergic agents; pramipexole or ropinirole (0.25 to 1 mg q. 8 p.m.) is typically used. In the event of partial response, opiates (e.g., acetaminophen with codeine 300 mg/30 mg q.h.s.) or gabapentin (Neurontin) (300 to 1,200 mg q.h.s.) is used as an augmentor. For a discussion of the pharmacology of gabapentin, see Chapter 4. In the event of persistent sleep disruption, the adjunctive use of hypnotics is common [e.g., trazodone (Desyrel) 25 to 150 mg q.h.s., zolpidem (Ambien) 5 to 10 mg q.h.s., eszopiclone (Lunesta) 2 to 3 mg q.h.s., temazepam 7.5 to 30 mg q.h.s., clonazepam 0.25 to 1 mg q.h.s., topiramate (Topamax) 100 to 300 mg q.h.s., and gabapentin 300 to 1,200 mg q.h.s.]. A discussion on the pharmacology of these hypnotics follows later in this chapter. High-dose intravenous iron is a promising, but yet rather experimental approach.

INSOMNIA

Insomnia is defined as difficulty falling asleep, staying asleep, and/or nonrestorative sleep with associated impairment or significant distress for at least 1 month. When insomnia does not occur exclusively during the course of another sleep disorder or psychiatric disorder, or as a consequence of psychoactive substance use or general medical condition, the *Diagnostic and Statistical Manual of Mental Disorders*, 4th edition (*DSM-IV*), uses the term primary insomnia. The inability to initiate sleep is typically called "sleep onset insomnia," whereas the inability to maintain sleep is termed "sleep maintenance insomnia." Another form of insomnia is characterized by early morning awakenings and is often termed "late insomnia." Patients who suffer from insomnia either may have only one form of insomnia or, more commonly, may experience any combination of these subtypes. Insomnia is frequently secondary to psychiatric disorders ("insomnia related to another mental disorder," according to the *DSM-IV*), medical disorders ("sleep disorder due to a medical condition, insomnia type," according to the *DSM-IV*), or the use of medications or psychoactive substances ("substance-induced sleep disorder, insomnia type," according to the *DSM-IV*). In particular, insomnia accompanied by daytime fatigue is one of the most common manifestations of depression, being experienced by 40% to 60% of outpatients with major depressive disorder. Insomnia related to depression often encompasses both sleep initiation and maintenance difficulties and sleep architecture abnormalities. Sleep electroencephalographic recordings of patients with major depressive disorder who have sleep initiation and maintenance problems most commonly show prolonged sleep latency (sleep onset insomnia), intermittent wakefulness, sleep fragmentation, and, in some cases, early morning awakenings. **Significant sleep architecture abnormalities are also detected by sleep electroencephalography,** including an increase in light, stage 1 sleep, a decrease in deep, slow-wave NREM sleep in stages 3 and 4, decreased REM sleep latency, prolonged first REM sleep cycle, and an increase in total REM sleep. Overall, electroencephalographic sleep abnormalities appear to occur less frequently in depressed adolescents and children than in depressed adults.

Epidemiology

It has been estimated that approximately one third of the U.S. population has suffered from insomnia in the previous year and nearly 10% of adults suffer from chronic insomnia, defined as insomnia lasting longer than 1 month. Approximately 40% of those with insomnia have one or more psychiatric disorders, with anxiety, depressive, and substance use disorders being the most common ones. However, it appears that only a relatively small percentage of individuals who suffer from insomnia actually seek treatment for it. The prevalence of chronic insomnia markedly increases in older populations, with up to 40% of those older than 60 years reporting symptoms of insomnia. Insomnia is typically more common among women than men, and this may reflect the higher rates among women of psychiatric disorders associated with insomnia, such as anxiety and depression.

There are both substantial economic and clinical implications of untreated insomnia. It has been estimated that insomnia costs tens of billions of dollars in the United States annually. In fact, untreated insomnia is associated with decreased productivity; reduced concentration; a higher risk of accidents; and an increased risk for the emergence of psychiatric disorders, such as major depressive disorder and generalized anxiety disorder. Thus, it has been suggested that early and **aggressive treatment of insomnia** may be an effective means of decreasing the morbidity associated with insomnia and improving quality of life for individuals predisposed to sleep difficulties.

Diagnosis

1. Difficulty falling asleep, staying asleep, and/or nonrestorative sleep, with associated impairment or significant distress for at least 1 month.
2. Associated symptoms of depression and anxiety are common, together with diminished energy and concentration.

When evaluating patients with insomnia, it is essential to complete the following:

1. A sleep history (e.g., obtaining specific details regarding the onset, duration, and time course of the insomnia and possible precipitants of the insomnia, such as environmental stress and shift work) and an assessment of sleep habits (e.g., the patient's bedtime routine, how long the patient stays in bed awake before falling asleep, and what the patient does in the middle of the night if he or she wakes up after having been asleep).
2. A psychiatric and medical assessment.
3. A psychoactive substance use (e.g., alcohol, caffeine, stimulants, cocaine) assessment.
4. An assessment of concomitant medications use, including those over the counter.
5. An evaluation of daytime functioning.
6. When available, sleep logs or diaries are useful diagnostic tools, although subjective.

As mentioned earlier, chronic insomnia may be comorbid with a number of medical and psychiatric conditions, necessitating a proper differential diagnosis to facilitate treatment planning. These include the following:

1. Pulmonary disorders (e.g., chronic obstructive pulmonary disease and asthma) and cardiac disorders (e.g., angina).
2. Gastrointestinal conditions (e.g., gastroesophageal reflux disease).
3. Medical disorders that are associated with pain during the night (e.g., arthritis) or frequent urination at night.
4. Neurological disorders (e.g., Parkinson's disease and dementia).
5. Psychiatric conditions (e.g., major depressive disorder, bipolar disorder, generalized anxiety disorder, panic disorder, posttraumatic stress disorder, and psychotic disorders).
6. Other sleep disorders (e.g., obstructive sleep apnea and upper airway restrictive syndrome, RLS, and periodic limb movement disorder).
7. Psychoactive drug withdrawal states (e.g., nicotine withdrawal, cocaine withdrawal, opioid withdrawal, and sedative/anxiolytic withdrawal).

Insomnia may also occur in the context of medication and psychoactive substance use, including the following:

1. Antidepressants (e.g., SSRIs, serotonin-norepinephrine reuptake inhibitors (SNRIs), bupropion)
2. Central nervous system (CNS) stimulants (e.g., methylphenidate, dextroamphetamine)
3. Corticosteroids
4. Bronchodilators
5. β-Blockers
6. Decongestants
7. Histamine H_2 blockers (e.g., cimetidine)
8. Antiparkinsonian drugs (e.g., carbidopa-levodopa, selegiline)
9. Alcohol (initial sleepiness followed by insomnia)
10. Nicotine
11. Caffeine

Finally, insomnia may be associated with major life events and lifestyle changes, high levels of chronic stress, and poor sleep hygiene practices.

Behavioral Interventions

Behavioral interventions for the treatment of insomnia are indicated when the insomnia is not secondary to another sleep disorder or to comorbid medical or psychiatric disorders and there is evidence of inadequate sleep hygiene. Inadequate sleep hygiene refers to maladaptive behaviors or attitudes that interfere with sleep onset or maintenance, such as taking daytime naps, drinking caffeine during the day, and drinking alcohol before going to bed. Caffeine increases sleep latency and sleep fragmentation and decreases total sleep time. Alcohol use is discouraged because, although it promotes sleep onset, alcohol leads to sleep fragmentation, decreased REM sleep, and early morning awakenings, thereby predisposing one to wake up frequently during the night.

Sleep Hygiene

In contrast, good sleep hygiene refers to behaviors and environmental factors that facilitate sleep onset and maintenance. Sleep hygiene may be promoted by eliminating naps, caffeine consumption, and alcohol use. Other strategies include not exercising within 5 to 6 hours of bedtime, eliminating noise or temperature extremes (i.e., being very warm or very cold while in bed), encouraging the use of window blinds (to eliminate light), and turning the clock around to avoid "clock watching," a behavior associated with performance anxiety about sleep, which in turn might make it difficult to fall or stay asleep.

Stimulus Control and Sleep Restriction

Following multiple failed attempts at sleeping, many people become classically conditioned to pair their bed and bedrooms with not sleeping. To break this association, patients are encouraged to engage in stimulus control, a behavioral paradigm in which patients are instructed to use their bed and bedroom only for sleep and for sex—they are not to watch television or to do work in bed, and, at night, they are to go to bed only when they are sleepy and after a set bedtime. If they have trouble falling asleep after 20 minutes, they are to exit the bed and to return again only when sleepy. Patients are encouraged to arise in the morning at the same time, regardless of the amount of sleep obtained during the previous night. Stimulus control is often used in conjunction with sleep restriction, which entails cutting average time in bed to increase sleep drive. Research supports the use of these strategies as individual behavioral interventions for insomnia.

Cognitive Restructuring, Paradoxical Intention, and Relaxation Therapy

Cognitive restructuring aims at changing and correcting maladaptive and distorted cognitions about sleep with more logical, reality-based thoughts. For example, people with insomnia often overemphasize the importance of sleep and make overly negative and catastrophic predictions about a poor night's sleep. Cognitive therapy seeks to set more realistic expectations about sleep and to decatastrophize the consequences of sleeping fewer hours on a given night.

Paradoxical intention is another cognitive-behavioral strategy that seeks to decrease performance anxiety related to sleep. This approach is based on the following rationale: Patients with insomnia often lie awake, worrying about sleeping, thereby contributing to physiologic arousal, which in turn might make it more difficult to fall or stay asleep. To counteract this performance anxiety, patients are instructed to stay awake. By forcing themselves to stay awake, anxiety about sleep is decreased, and sleep, as a result, comes more easily.

Relaxation therapy such as progressive muscle relaxation and imagery training (e.g., imagining oneself lying on a beach listening to the sound of the waves crashing on the shore) may also be used to target and decrease the physiologic hyperarousal that is often characteristic of individuals with insomnia and may be useful adjuncts to sleep hygiene, stimulus control, sleep restriction, and cognitive therapy.

Pharmacologic Interventions

Pharmacotherapy may be indicated for the treatment of primary insomnia when behavioral interventions alone are insufficient or when a patient prefers medication to behavior therapy. Medications may also be indicated for insomnia secondary to psychiatric or medical conditions when the treatment of the underlying condition proves ineffective or when patients become sufficiently distressed or impaired by their untreated insomnia that to not treat it would lead to increased distress or dysfunction.

The currently available hypnotics are typically approved by the Food and Drug Administration (FDA) for short-term use only, and a common concern among clinicians about prescribing hypnotics is that patients will increase the dose of the hypnotic medication over time. Although tolerance can occur with almost all hypnotics, there is evidence that a **substantial proportion of patients will continue to benefit from continued treatment without dosage escalation.**

The benzodiazepines are often used as hypnotics, particularly given the relatively low cost of their generic formulations. Not all benzodiazepines are FDA approved for the treatment of insomnia, but off-label use is common, given the pharmacologic similarities among the compounds in this class.

Tolerance is considered to be less likely to occur in the newer, nonbenzodiazepine hypnotics zolpidem, eszopiclone, and zaleplon (Sonata), a finding consistent with recent research indicating that patients receiving intermittent dosing with zolpidem were not more likely than those administered placebo to increase the number of pills taken over time. Other studies that have examined the efficacy of intermittent dosing with zolpidem have also found sustained efficacy and a lack of rebound insomnia among patients treated for either 2 or 3 months.

Ramelteon (Rozerem) is a selective MT1/MT2 melatonin receptor agonist approved by the U.S. FDA for treatment of insomnia; its use is primarily limited to the treatment of early insomnia. The antidepressant trazodone is commonly prescribed off-label for the treatment of insomnia; however, it is not approved as a hypnotic by the FDA and limited data exist to support its efficacy as a hypnotic. The antihistamine, diphenhydramine (Benadryl), although commonly used as an over the counter sleep aid, is not a reliable treatment of insomnia because it often loses its sedative effect over time. It also exposes people to significant anticholinergic side effects.

Benzodiazepines

A large number of benzodiazepines (Table 7.1) are currently available. Prior to the introduction of the benzodiazepines in the 1960s, a variety of other compounds were used to treat insomnia. These included bromides early in the century; ethanol and structural analogs such as paraldehyde and chloral hydrate in the 1940s; followed by the barbiturates and propanediol drugs, including meprobamate, in the 1950s.

Benzodiazepines, like the older sedative-hypnotics, are CNS depressants, with sedative-hypnotic effects (i.e., induction of drowsiness or sleep) at higher doses. Compared with barbiturates and similarly acting drugs, benzodiazepines have a higher ratio of the median dose producing lethality to median effective dose (LD_{50}:ED_{50}). Indeed, the barbiturates and similarly acting drugs are dangerous in overdose, potentially causing coma, respiratory depression, and death, whereas the benzodiazepines are rarely associated with death from overdose in the absence of other drugs. Since the introduction of benzodiazepines, the number of

Handbook of Psychiatric Drug Therapy

TABLE 7.1 Available Benzodiazepine Preparations for Insomnia

Preparations	Regular Oral Dose Forms (mg)	FDA-Approved	Available Parenteral Forms	Active Metabolite(s)
Clonazepam (Klonopin) (off-label)	0.5, 1.0, 2.0 (tablet) 0.125, 0.25, 0.5, 1.0, 2.0 (wafer)	No		Yes
Estazolam (ProSom)	1, 2 (tablet)	Yes		No
Flurazepam (Dalmane)	15, 30 (capsule)	Yes		Yes
Lorazepam (Ativan)	0.5, 1.0, 2.0 (tablet)	No	20 mg/10 mL; 40 mg/10 mL (vial) 2 mg/mL, 4 mg/mL (syringe)	No
Midazolam (Versed) (Dormicum—Europe)	7.5, 15 (tablets)	No	1 mg/mL/5 mg/mL (vial)	Yes
Oxazepam (Serax)	10, 15, 30 (capsule)	No		Yes
Quazepam (Doral)	7.5, 15.0 (tablet)	Yes		Yes
Temazepam (Restoril)	7.5, 15.0, 30 (capsule)	Yes		No
Triazolam (Halcion)	0.125, 0.25 (tablet)	Yes		No
Chlordiazepoxide	5, 10 and 25	No		Yes

[a]Available with clidinium bromide (Librax, Clipoxide) and amitriptyline (Limbitrol).

hypnotic-related suicides and accidental deaths has decreased markedly. Given the advantages of benzodiazepines, the use of most of the older compounds (e.g., secobarbital, pentobarbital, meprobamate, glutethimide, or ethchlorvynol) for the treatment of insomnia is irrational. The effectiveness and relative safety of the benzodiazepines have led to their extensive use in the treatment of insomnia. Benzodiazepines should be avoided in patients with a history of alcohol or drug abuse unless there is a compelling indication, no good alternative, and close follow-up.

Chemistry
The benzodiazepines are a group of closely related compounds. The name benzodiazepine is derived from the fact that the structures are composed of a benzene ring fused to a seven-member diazepine ring.

Pharmacology

Pharmacokinetics. Most benzodiazepines are well absorbed when given orally on an empty stomach; many achieve peak plasma levels within 1 to 3 hours, although there is a wide range among the benzodiazepine drugs (Table 7.2). Antacids seriously interfere with benzodiazepine absorption; thus, benzodiazepines should be taken well ahead of any antacid dose.

The rate of onset of action after an orally administered benzodiazepine (Table 7.2) is an important variable in choosing a drug for the treatment of insomnia. For

TABLE 7.2	Pharmacologic Characteristics of Available Benzodiazepines for Insomnia			
Preparations	**Oral Dose Equivalency (mg)**	**Onset After Oral Dose**	**Distribution Half-life**	**Elimination Half-life (h)**[a]
Clonazepam (Klonopin)	0.25	Intermediate	Intermediate	18–40
Estazolam (ProSom)	2.0	Intermediate	Intermediate	10–24
Flurazepam (Dalmane)	30.0	Rapid–intermediate	Rapid	50–160
Lorazepam (Ativan)	1.0	Intermediate	Intermediate	10–20
Midazolam (Versed; Dormicum— Europe)	—	Intermediate	Rapid	2–3
Oxazepam (Serax)	15.0	Intermediate–slow	Intermediate	8–12
Quazepam (Doral)	15.0	Rapid–intermediate	Intermediate	50–160
Temazepam (Restoril)	30.0	Intermediate	Rapid	8–20
Triazolam (Halcion)	0.25	Intermediate	Rapid	2–5

[a]The elimination half-life represents the total for all active metabolites; elderly patients tend to have the longer half-lives in the range reported. Flurazepam and quazepam share *N*-desalkylflurazepam as a long-acting active metabolite. With chronic dosing, these active metabolites represent most of the pharmacodynamic effect of these drugs.

example, rapid onset is important for the individual who has trouble falling asleep. On the other hand, a more slowly acting drug might be prescribed when insomnia occurs later in the night. Drugs with a rapid onset achieve higher peak levels than equivalent doses of drugs with slow onset, whose peaks are spread over time. The available benzodiazepines differ markedly in the rate of onset of their therapeutic effect (Table 7.2), offering a wide choice of drugs to fit the patient's needs.

For benzodiazepines, simple half-life data are potentially misleading regarding duration of clinical effect. Clinical efficacy depends on the presence of at least a minimum effective concentration in the blood, which is reflected by levels in well-perfused tissues such as those in the brain. After a single dose, the levels may decrease to ineffective concentrations, either (a) by being distributed into peripheral tissues, such as fat (α-phase) or (b) by metabolic inactivation or elimination from the body altogether (β-phase).

The volume of distribution represents the size of the pool of tissues into which the drug may be drawn; this is determined by the drug's lipid solubility and tissue-binding properties. With repeated drug dosing, its volume of distribution becomes saturated, and the elimination half-life becomes the more important parameter in describing its behavior. Benzodiazepines differ markedly in their half-lives of distribution and elimination, producing varying clinical effects.

These pharmacokinetic considerations have clear clinical relevance in the use of benzodiazepines for the treatment of insomnia. Short half-life benzodiazepines work well for early insomnia, whereas benzodiazepines with longer half-life are better suited for middle or late insomnia. These points can be demonstrated in the clinical use of two commonly used drugs, triazolam and temazepam. Triazolam has a relatively short half-life (2 to 5 hours) and is typically used for the treatment of early insomnia, while temazepam, with a half-life of 8 to 20 hours, is typically used for the treatment of middle and late insomnia.

Another important clinical issue related to duration of effect applies to the use of the high-potency, short-acting benzodiazepines, triazolam, midazolam, and, to a lesser extent, lorazepam. Such drugs pose a potential clinical problem because their high potency may make them more liable to cause dependence and their rapid termination of effect unmasks any dependence that develops. Patients may therefore experience rebound symptoms. For example, patients treated with triazolam for insomnia may develop rebound symptoms, as manifested by early morning awakening or anxiety. Such problems can be addressed by switching to longer-acting drugs when indicated (e.g., replacing triazolam with temazepam or flurazepam for the treatment of insomnia).

Metabolism

Except for lorazepam, oxazepam, and temazepam, the commonly used benzodiazepines are metabolized by hepatic microsomal enzymes to form demethylated, hydroxylated, and other oxidized products that are pharmacologically active. Most of the benzodiazepines are substrates of the cytochrome P450 3A4; therefore, they tend to accumulate when coadministered with inhibitors of such pathways. The active metabolites of benzodiazepines are, in turn, conjugated with glucuronic acid; the resulting glucuronides are inactive and, because they are more water soluble than the parent compounds, they are readily excreted in the urine.

Some of the active metabolites of benzodiazepines, such as desalkylflurazepam, have extremely long half-lives and with repeated dosing may come to represent most of the pharmacologically active compound in serum. In contrast, under normal circumstances (e.g., excluding cirrhosis) the active metabolic products of triazolam and midazolam are of little clinical importance. Lorazepam, oxazepam, and temazepam are metabolized only by conjugation with glucuronic acid with no intermediate steps, and they have no active metabolites. Unlike the pathways involved in the initial metabolism of other benzodiazepines, **glucuronidation is less affected by aging and liver disease**; thus, if benzodiazepines are to be used in elderly patients or those with cirrhosis, lorazepam and oxazepam are the drugs of choice. In cirrhosis, the elimination of benzodiazepines metabolized by oxidation and demethylation may be reduced by as much as fivefold; thus, routine doses could lead to toxicity. In cirrhosis, even triazolam and midazolam may accumulate to dangerous levels.

Mechanism of Action

Acting through its γ-aminobutyric acid A ($GABA_A$) receptor, the amino acid neurotransmitter GABA is the major inhibitory neurotransmitter in the brain. $GABA_A$ receptors are ligand-gated channels, meaning that the neurotransmitter-binding site and an effector ion channel are part of the same macromolecular complex. Because $GABA_A$ receptor channels selectively admit the anion chloride into neurons, activation of $GABA_A$ receptors hyperpolarizes neurons and thus is inhibitory on neuronal firing. Benzodiazepines produce their effects by binding to a specific site on the $GABA_A$ receptor.

The pharmacology of $GABA_A$ receptors is complex; $GABA_A$ receptors are the primary site of action not only of benzodiazepines but also of barbiturates and of some of the intoxicating effects of ethanol. $GABA_A$ receptors are composed of multiple subunits. $GABA_A$/benzodiazepine receptors have a pentameric structure made up of a coassembly of subunits. There are six known α, four β, three γ, two ρ, and one δ subunits. $GABA_A$ receptors in the brain are most commonly composed of different subtypes of α, β, and γ subunits, with different subunit composition in different brain regions. Series of transgenic mice have been constructed in which each α subunit was genetically disrupted by a point mutation. This selective inactivation strategy revealed that $GABA_A$ receptors containing the α-1 subunit mediate sedation, anterograde amnesia, and part of the seizure protection, whereas $GABA_A$ receptors containing α-2 subunits are thought to mediate the anxiolytic effects of benzodiazepines. This finding has led to attempts to develop drugs that selectively interact with different $GABA_A$ receptor subtypes.

Benzodiazepines, barbiturates, and alcohol allosterically regulate the $GABA_A$ receptor (changing its conformation) so that it has a greater affinity for its neurotransmitter GABA. At higher doses, barbiturates and ethanol, but not benzodiazepines, also can open the chloride channel within the receptor independent of GABA. The fact that benzodiazepines, barbiturates, and ethanol all have related actions on a common receptor explains their pharmacologic synergy (and therefore the dangers of combined overdose) and their cross-tolerance. Their cross-tolerance is exploited in detoxification of alcoholics with benzodiazepines.

Dependence

Clinically, the major pharmacologic problem with benzodiazepines is their tendency to cause dependence, that is, a risk of significant discontinuation symptoms, especially with long-term use. Long-term benzodiazepine use typically occurs in the context of treatment of chronic insomnia. Discontinuation symptoms may pose a serious clinical problem in some patients, causing worsening of (rebound) insomnia, distress, or inability to discontinue treatment.

Choosing a Benzodiazepine

All benzodiazepines have similar mechanisms of action and side effects. Of all of the drugs used in psychiatry, benzodiazepines are the class in which pharmacokinetic considerations play the greatest role in selecting a drug for a particular situation. The dose forms, rate of onset of action, duration of action, and tendency to accumulate in the body vary considerably and can influence both side effects and the overall success of the treatment.

Side Effects

The most common side effects of benzodiazepines are sedation, drowsiness, memory difficulties, fatigue, and muscle weakness. Uncommon side effects include dysarthria, confusion, abnormal coordination, ataxia, depression or worsening of mood, dry mouth, constipation, nausea, slurred speech, dizziness, and tremor. Side effects due to rapid decrease or abrupt withdrawal from benzodiazepines may include agitation, heightened sensory perception, paresthesias, muscle cramps, muscle twitching, diarrhea, reduced concentration, worsening of mood, anxiety, nervousness, restlessness, sleeping difficulties, insomnia, tremors, and, in rare cases, seizures and hallucinations.

Overdoses

Overdoses from benzodiazepines are typically safe, although there have been occasional reports of lethal overdoses. Drowsiness, dysarthria, diplopia, ataxia, lethargy, and dizziness are the most common symptoms of benzodiazepine overdosing. Coma and severe respiratory depression are uncommon complications of these overdoses.

Therapeutic Use

Benzodiazepines typically reduce sleep latency and intermittent wakefulness during sleep. Their effect on sleep stages is variable, in that most benzodiazepines suppress stages 3 and 4 NREM sleep, increase stage 2 sleep, and mildly suppress REM sleep.

For short-term insomnia, benzodiazepines are effective symptomatic treatments but should follow the use of nonpharmacologic interventions. If prescribing a benzodiazepine for short-term insomnia, a small amount should be given, usually no more than a 2- or 4-week supply. For long-term insomnia for which no primary medical or psychiatric cause can be found or for which no effective treatment of the underlying condition has been effective, long-term use of benzodiazepines also may be helpful, but the ratio of benefit (long-term efficacy) to risk (dependence, impairment of psychomotor performance, memory difficulties, subtle changes in mood) must be considered.

The greatest benefit of benzodiazepines used as hypnotics appears to be **reduced sleep fragmentation during the night**. Benzodiazepines have many effects of unknown clinical significance: They suppress REM sleep; prolong REM latency; increase stage 2 sleep; and decrease stages 1, 3, and 4 sleep. Flurazepam, temazepam, triazolam, quazepam, and estazolam are specifically marketed for insomnia, although, as noted, the benzodiazepine hypnotics have no special features to distinguish them from other benzodiazepines that are often used in off-label fashion such as lorazepam (Table 7.3). Outside the United States, a variety of other benzodiazepines are marketed as hypnotics, including brotizolam, loprazolam, lormetazepam, and nitrazepam. In healthy adults, the standard hypnotic dose of flurazepam and temazepam is 30 mg, although 15 mg is effective for some individuals. Quazepam is given at 15 mg; 7.5 mg may be adequate for some individuals and is the manufacturer's recommended dose for elderly patients. Because of the risk of accumulation, flurazepam and quazepam should not be used in elderly patients if more than a few days' use is contemplated, in which case temazepam, 15 mg, would be a better choice. Triazolam is given at dosages of 0.125 to 0.25 mg nightly (0.125 mg in elderly patients).

The two major considerations in choosing a benzodiazepine hypnotic are **rapidity of onset and half-life**. For patients who report difficulty in falling asleep, the rapidity of onset of the drug is particularly important. After oral administration, flurazepam acts rapidly, achieving peak plasma concentrations in 0.5 to 1.0 hour. Triazolam (1.3 hours to peak) and quazepam (1.5 hours to peak) have intermediate

TABLE 7.3	Available Benzodiazepine Preparations: Common Doses for the Treatment of Insomnia
Preparation	**Regular Bedtime Doses (mg q.h.s.)**
Marketed as Hypnotics	
Estazolam (ProSom)	1–2
Flurazepam (Dalmane)	7.5–30
Quazepam (Doral)	7.5–30
Temazepam (Restoril)	7.5–30
Triazolam (Halcion)	0.125–0.25
Marketed as Antianxiety Drugs	
Clonazepam (Klonopin)	0.5–2.0
Lorazepam (Ativan)	1.0–3.0
Oxazepam (Serax)	10–30

rates of absorption. Temazepam has a slower rate of onset, with peak levels achieved only after 3 hours, making it less helpful for sleep-latency insomnia unless taken 1 hour prior to bedtime. To improve absorption, all benzodiazepines should be administered at bedtime on an empty stomach.

The other important consideration in choosing a hypnotic is half-life. Flurazepam has a long-acting metabolite, N-desalkylflurazepam, which reaches its peak plasma concentration approximately 10 hours after an oral dose. After 2 weeks of nightly administration, this metabolite (which has a half-life of 50 to 160 hours; 200 hours or more in elderly patients) accumulates to levels seven to eight times its peak level on the first night. Although only 3.5% of N-desalkylflurazepam is free (not protein bound), after 2 weeks this represents a great deal of pharmacodynamic activity; indeed, with repeated dosing, this metabolite may represent most of the active compound in plasma. Quazepam is metabolized to oxoquazepam and then to N-desalkylflurazepam, which, as in the case of flurazepam, represents most of the drug's pharmacodynamic activity with chronic dosing. With repetitive administration, this drug is not likely to differ significantly from flurazepam in its effects.

Two advantages of long-acting drugs are that they may decrease early morning awakening and treat daytime anxiety. However, the trade-off may be residual daytime drowsiness; possible cognitive impairment; and possible interactions with other CNS depressants, such as ethanol, that might be consumed during the day (although most patients develop tolerance to daytime effects and experience no hangover and little impairment). In elderly patients, the level of accumulation may be greater and thus more likely to produce intoxication or delirium; therefore, in elderly patients, repetitive dosing with long-acting compounds, such as flurazepam and quazepam, is not recommended.

Short-acting benzodiazepines do not accumulate but may be more associated with rebound insomnia after treatment discontinuation. Rebound insomnia may occur when short-acting benzodiazepines (e.g., triazolam or lorazepam) are used on several consecutive nights. The shortest period necessary to produce rebound is unclear, but it may be only several days. Rebound is common when triazolam is used at dosages of 0.5 mg nightly; it is less of a problem at a dosage of 0.25 mg nightly but is still reported by many patients. On the first or second night after discontinuation of short-acting benzodiazepines, patients may complain of increased sleep latency and increased total wake time. Especially if misinterpreted as reemergence of underlying chronic insomnia, rebound may reinforce chronic benzodiazepine use and risk of dependence. In addition to rebound after discontinuation, triazolam, which has a very short half-life, may occasionally cause rebound symptoms within the same night, manifested by early morning awakening and morning anxiety symptoms. Rebound side effects from triazolam may occur even if it was ineffective for the original complaint of insomnia. Rebound insomnia appears to be uncommon with temazepam and with very long-acting drugs such as flurazepam. If rebound insomnia occurs with flurazepam, it might not be expected until 4 to 10 nights after discontinuation.

Zolpidem, Zaleplon, and Eszopiclone

Both zolpidem (Ambien), a nonbenzodiazepine hypnotic of the imidazopyridine class, and zaleplon (Sonata), a pyrazolopyrimidines, exhibit preferential affinity for benzodiazepine α-1 receptors in binding assays. They are therefore pharmacologically cross-reactive with the benzodiazepines to a degree and are effective for short-term treatment of insomnia but, relative to the benzodiazepines, lack significant anxiolytic, muscle relaxant, or anticonvulsant effects. They are rapidly and completely absorbed from the gastrointestinal tract, reaching peak serum levels in 1 to 2 hours. Absorption is delayed by food, so for optimal hypnotic effect, they should be ingested on an empty stomach. Both are metabolized by the liver, with short elimination half-lives of 2 to 3 hours for zolpidem and 1 to 2 hours for zaleplon. Because of their short half-lives, there is very little carryover of daytime sedation. Rebound would have been expected with zolpidem and zaleplon, but their more selective mechanism of action may be responsible for less than expected observation of rebound insomnia. The half-life is prolonged in elderly patients and in patients with liver disease. Zolpidem is available as a 10-mg tablet for usual adult dosing, but the 5-mg strength should be selected for elderly patients and is often adequate for other adults with insomnia. Because of its relatively short half-life, zolpidem is also available in a controlled-release formulation (Ambien CR) at 6.25 and 12.5 mg doses. The FDA has recently approved an oral spray formulation of zolpidem at 5 and 10 mg for the short-term treatment of insomnia characterized by difficulties with sleep initiation. Zolpidem has little effect on stages of sleep perhaps because of its binding profile for a subset of benzodiazepine receptors. The lower doses are recommended for elderly patients or possibly for initiation of treatment, especially in the patient naive to hypnotics. Zaleplon is available in 5- and 10-mg capsules. The recommended doses are 5 to 10 mg q.h.s. for zolpidem, 6.25 to 12.5 mg q.h.s. for zolpidem CR, and 5 to 20 mg q.h.s. for zaleplon. Given its rapid clearance, zaleplon in doses up to 20 mg has been observed to be safe and effective without residual daytime impairment. Although there are few clear, consistent differences between these two drugs, evidence suggests that zaleplon gives shorter duration of sleep than zolpidem, reflecting the pharmacologic profiles of the drugs. Some studies suggest that rapid tolerance does not occur with these drugs, interaction with alcohol may be less than the benzodiazepines, and amnestic and residual effects at therapeutic doses are minimal, although zolpidem at higher doses may produce some next-day anterograde amnesia. The safety profile of these agents with respect to risk for dependence and withdrawal appears to be greatly improved over the benzodiazepines, but vigilance is still indicated, especially if patients are taking high dosages. These agents may be safely coprescribed with the SSRIs or other nonsedating antidepressants for short-term management of insomnia. Possible side effects of these drugs, in addition to drowsiness, are nausea, vomiting, diarrhea, headache, and dizziness. Their safety in overdose appears to be high, and liability for abuse appears to be low.

Eszopiclone (Lunesta) is a single enantiomer formulation of zopiclone, a hypnotic agent currently available in Europe. Eszopiclone interacts with various a number of $GABA_A$ receptor subtypes, and has shown a balanced selectivity for the α-1, α-2, α-3, and α-5 subtypes. Research has shown that, compared to placebo, eszopiclone is associated with improvements in sleep onset, maintenance, and quality and with effects that have been sustained for a year. A study has indicated that the sleep-improving effects of nightly eszopiclone at doses of 3 mg are **sustained for 6 months** and are also associated with improvements in next-day functioning. In addition, eszopiclone's longer duration of action may make it an attractive option for patients whose insomnia is characterized by difficulties with sleep maintenance. Another study evaluated the efficacy and safety of eszopiclone in a 6-month open label extension of the previous study. Patients in the original double-blind placebo study continued to receive nightly eszopiclone if they had originally received eszopiclone or were switched to eszopiclone if they had originally received placebo. Results indicated that patients switched from placebo to eszopiclone reported significant improvements in sleep and daytime functioning. These improvements were comparable to those noted by patients who had originally received eszopiclone and were sustained for the remainder of the 6-month extension study. Patients who remained on eszopiclone for the entire 12 months (6-month double-blind, placebo-controlled portion and 6-month open extension) maintained the improvements in sleep that they had demonstrated earlier. In addition, among patients completing the study, there was not significant evidence of tolerance with nightly eszopiclone over the course of the study. In a second, 6-month study, eszopiclone was abruptly discontinued and demonstrated a relative lack of rebound insomnia and withdrawal effects. Eszopiclone is available in 1-, 2-, and 3-mg tablets. For elderly patients, the recommended doses are 1 and 2 mg q.h.s., and for adults younger than 65 years, the doses are 2 and 3 mg q.h.s. Its most common side effects are drowsiness, dizziness, unpleasant taste, and memory difficulties.

Ramelteon

Ramelteon (Rozerem) is a melatonin receptor agonist with both high affinity for melatonin MT1 and MT2 receptors, which are thought to be involved in the maintenance of the circadian rhythm underlying the normal sleep-wake cycle. The major metabolite of ramelteon, M-II, is active and has approximately one tenth and one fifth the binding affinity of the parent molecule for the human MT1 and MT2 receptors, respectively, and is 17- to 25-fold less potent than ramelteon in *in vitro* functional assays. Although the potency of M-II is lower than that of the parent drug, M-II circulates at higher concentrations than the parent producing 20- to 100-fold greater mean systemic exposure compared with ramelteon. M-II has weak affinity for the serotonin $5-HT_{2B}$ receptor but no appreciable affinity for other receptors or enzymes. Similar to ramelteon, M-II does not interfere with the activity of a number of endogenous enzymes. All other known metabolites of ramelteon are inactive. Metabolism of ramelteon consists primarily of oxidation to hydroxyl and carbonyl derivatives, with secondary metabolism producing glucuronide conjugates. CYP1A2 is the major isozyme involved in the hepatic metabolism of ramelteon; the CYP2C subfamily and CYP3A4 isozymes are also involved to a minor degree. The rank order of the principal metabolites by prevalence in human serum is M-II, M-IV, M-I, and M-III. These metabolites are formed rapidly and exhibit a monophasic decline and rapid elimination. Repeated once daily dosing with ramelteon does not result in significant accumulation due to the short elimination half-life of ramelteon (on average, approximately 1 to 2.6 hours). The half-life of M-II is 2 to 5 hours and independent of dose. Ramelteon is not classified as a controlled substance. In patients with chronic insomnia, objectively assessed latency to persistent sleep at week 1 was improved with oral ramelteon 8 mg administered 30 minutes before bedtime, compared with placebo, and this effect was maintained throughout the duration of 5-week and 6-month clinical studies. Subjectively assessed sleep latency improved in some, but not all, studies. Improvements in objectively assessed total sleep time and sleep efficiency were only reported during the first week of treatment. It is available in 8 mg tablets; the recommended dosing is 8 mg q.h.s. and should not be taken with or immediately after a high-fat meal. Ramelteon is generally well tolerated, with very low rates (3% to 4%) of spontaneously reported side effects, such as somnolence, fatigue, dizziness, and nausea. It does not impair next-day cognitive or motor performance and is not associated with withdrawal symptoms, rebound insomnia, or abuse potential. Thus, ramelteon provides a well-tolerated option for the treatment of patients with insomnia characterized **primarily by difficulty in sleep onset.**

Antihistamines

For patients with a history of adverse reactions to benzodiazepines or a history of alcohol or sedative-hypnotic abuse, sedating antihistamines are sometimes used, but they are less effective in reducing sleep latency than benzodiazepines and are associated with residual daytime sedation and anticholinergic effects. Antihistamine drugs greatly vary in the degree of penetration into the CNS. Diphenhydramine is most commonly used, often at a dose of 50 mg (range 25 to

100 mg). Its half-life is 3.4 to 9.3 hours. Hydroxyzine (Atarax) (dosing: 50 to 200 mg q.h.s.) with a half-life of 7 to 20 hours, and doxylamine (Unisom) (dosing: 25 to 100 mg q.h.s.) with a half-life of 4 to 12 hours are also sometimes used as hypnotics. All sedating antihistamines are strongly anticholinergic, and caution should be used in prescribing them in combination with other anticholinergic compounds. It is important to monitor elderly patients for emergence of anticholinergic toxicity.

Trazodone

Trazodone (Desyrel) is a serotonin 5-HT$_2$ receptor antagonist antidepressant with mild inhibition of the serotonin transporter. This drug, whose pharmacology is discussed in Chapter 3, is often used in an off-label modality in the treatment of insomnia at dosages lower than those necessary to treat depression. It has been shown to be better than placebo in treatment of insomnia induced by other antidepressants. The disadvantages are that trazodone is also an antagonist of α_1-adrenergic receptors and is thereby associated with **orthostatic hypotension** and, less commonly, with priapism in men and that it has a long half-life and may cause daytime sedation. The doses of trazodone used for the treatment of insomnia typically range between 50 and 300 mg q.h.s.

Mirtazapine

Mirtazapine (Remeron) is an α_2-receptor antagonist and a serotonin 5-HT$_2$ and 5-HT$_3$ antagonist antidepressant, which is commonly used in the treatment of insomnia induced by other antidepressants or associated with depression and, more rarely, as off-label monotherapy for primary insomnia. The disadvantages are that mirtazapine is also an antagonist of histamine H$_1$ receptors and is thereby associated with increased appetite and weight gain and has a long half-life and may cause daytime sedation (see Chapter 3 for a discussion of its pharmacology). The doses of mirtazapine used for the treatment of insomnia typically range between 15 and 45 mg q.h.s.

Tricyclic Antidepressants

The sedating tertiary-amine TCAs amitriptyline (Elavil), trimipramine (Surmontil), and doxepin (Adapin and Sinequan) have often been used off-label in the treatment of insomnia at dosages lower than those necessary to treat depression. Compared with the benzodiazepines, they have not been well studied for primary insomnia with respect to efficacy and the development of tachyphylaxis, but they appear to be safe among patients with insomnia and sleep apnea. The disadvantages are that they are strongly anticholinergic, have a long half-life and may cause daytime sedation, are dangerous in overdose, and have cardiac side effects (see Chapter 3 for a discussion of their pharmacology). The doses of TCAs used for the treatment of insomnia typically range between 25 and 100 mg q.h.s. The tertiary-amine TCAs trimipramine, amitriptyline, and doxepin and the secondary-amine TCA nortriptyline (Pamelor) are, among TCAs, those probably used the most in the treatment of insomnia. The FDA is currently reviewing the application with the indication of insomnia for a newer formulation of doxepin, at oral doses of 1, 3, and 6 mg.

Anticonvulsants

Anticonvulsants are commonly used off-label in the treatment of insomnia induced by antidepressants or associated with mood disorders and, more rarely, as monotherapy for primary insomnia. The disadvantages are that many of the sedating anticonvulsants have fairly long half-lives. Daytime sedation and sleepiness are therefore common side effects. Gabapentin (at doses between 300 and 2,100 mg q.h.s.), topiramate (at doses between 100 and 400 mg q.h.s.), and tiagabine (Gabitril) (at doses between 4 and 24 mg q.h.s.) may be used to treat insomnia. For a review of the pharmacologic properties of these anticonvulsants, see Chapter 4.

Atypical Antipsychotics
Atypical antipsychotics are uncommonly used off-label in the treatment of insomnia. Their use for this indication should be limited primarily because of their side effects. Quetiapine (at doses between 25 and 200 mg q.h.s.), olanzapine (at doses between 2.5 and 10 mg q.h.s.), and risperidone (at doses between 0.5 and 4 mg q.h.s.) may be used to treat insomnia in patients refractory to treatment. For a review of the pharmacologic properties of these agents, see Chapter 2.

Barbiturates
Barbiturates, such as secobarbital, pentobarbital, and amobarbital, and related drugs, glutethimide and ethchlorvynol, essentially have no place in the treatment of insomnia because of their high risk of causing tolerance and dependence and their danger in overdose. Of the barbiturate-like drugs, chloral hydrate appears to be the least problematic, with relatively low abuse potential. Thus, it is still used as an alternative to benzodiazepines by some physicians.

Conclusions
Epidemiologic studies indicate that insomnia is a relatively common condition associated with significant morbidity and comorbidity. However, with proper differential diagnosis and treatment, its severity may be attenuated and quality of life improved considerably. Clinicians have treatment options available to them that include both cognitive-behavioral strategies and pharmacotherapy with hypnotics.

PRIMARY HYPERSOMNIA
Primary hypersomnia is characterized by excessive sleepiness for at least 1 month, not better accounted for by an inadequate amount of sleep, insomnia, or another sleep disorder. The duration of the major sleep episode may range from 8 to 12 hours and is often followed by difficulty awakening in the morning. The excessive sleepiness is evidenced by either prolonged sleep episodes or daytime sleep episodes that occur almost daily. More specifically, during normal waking hours, excessive sleepiness manifests itself as intentional naps or inadvertent episodes of sleep. The hypersomnia must cause significant distress or psychosocial impairment and the disturbance may not occur exclusively during the course of another mental disorder, such as major depressive disorder, or as the result of drug use or a general medical condition. As a consequence of the daytime sleepiness, patients may report inattentiveness, poor memory, and automatic behaviors, such as driving without awareness.

Diagnosis
1. Symptoms of hypersomnia and/or daytime sleepiness.
2. Objective polysomnography recordings of prolonged sleep duration, short sleep latency, and normal distribution of REM and NREM sleep. The MSLT has sleep latency values of 5 to 10 minutes.

Prevalence
In the National Institute of Mental Health Epidemiologic Catchment Area study, 3.2% of the respondents noted hypersomnia at the first interview. Of those, 46.5% had a psychiatric disorder, compared with 16.4% of those with no sleep complaints. Typically, only 5% to 10% of those presenting to sleep disorders clinics with hypersomnia as a chief concern are diagnosed with primary hypersomnia.

Treatment

Behavioral Interventions

Regularizing sleep-wake schedules, ensuring adequate sleep duration, and taking short daytime naps are the typical elements of the behavioral treatment of primary hypersomnia.

Pharmacologic Treatments

Regimens typically include wake-promoting drugs such as methylphenidate (dosing: 10 to 80 mg per day), dextroamphetamine (dosing: 10 to 60 mg per day), and modafinil [dosing: 100 to 400 mg everyday (q.d.)]. For a discussion on the pharmacologic properties of these drugs, see Chapter 9.

NARCOLEPSY

Narcolepsy is characterized by irresistible attacks of refreshing sleep during the day, resulting in brief naps. The excessive sleepiness typically decreases after a sleep attack, only to return a few hours later. The sleep attacks must occur daily for at least 3 months. In addition to the sleep attacks, patients may experience cataplexy (brief episodes of sudden, bilateral loss of muscle tone, most often associated with intense emotion) and/or recurrent intrusions of REM sleep into the transition between sleep and wakefulness, as manifested by either hypnopompic-hypnagogic hallucinations or sleep paralysis (profound weakness occurring at the onset of sleep or on awakening) at the beginning or end of sleep episodes. These sleep attacks may not occur exclusively as the result of drug use or a general medical condition. As a consequence of the daytime sleepiness, patients may report inattentiveness, poor memory, and automatic behaviors, such as driving without awareness.

Diagnosis

1. Sleep attacks.
2. Cataplexy and/or hypnopompic-hypnagogic hallucinations or sleep paralysis (although not required).
3. Objective polysomnography recordings of short sleep latency (less than 10 minutes), sleep-onset REM periods, increased REM sleep and density.
4. MSLT: average sleep latency less than 5 minutes.
5. Human leukocyte antigen (HLA) typing of narcolepsy patients often shows HLA-DRQw6 and DQw1.
6. It is important to rule out conditions associated with sleep attacks, such as breathing-related sleep disorder, general medical conditions (e.g., hypothalamic tumors, hypothalamic sarcoidosis), substance-induced sleepiness, and use of dopaminergic agents.

Prevalence

The prevalence of narcolepsy has been estimated to hover around 0.05% of the general population. First-degree relatives have a 40-fold increase in the risk of having narcolepsy.

Treatment

Behavioral Interventions

Scheduling short daytime naps (e.g., two to four 15-minute naps) represents the typical element of the behavioral treatment of primary hypersomnia, although typically only adjunctive in nature.

Pharmacologic Treatments

Regimens typically include wake-promoting drugs such as methylphenidate (dosing: 10 to 80 mg per day), dextroamphetamine (dosing: 10 to 60 mg per day), and modafinil (dosing: 100 to 400 mg q.d.). For a discussion on the pharmacologic properties of these drugs, see Chapter 9.

Although most patients with narcolepsy do not require treatment of cataplexy, those with significant symptoms of cataplexy may require pharmacologic treatment, typically in the form of a drug suppressing REM sleep, such as SSRIs (e.g., fluoxetine), SNRIs (e.g., venlafaxine), and TCAs (e.g., protriptyline, imipramine, and clomipramine). All these antidepressants are typically used at 50% to 75% lower doses than those used for the treatment of depression (see Chapter 3 for a discussion on the pharmacology of these drugs). γ-Hydroxybutyrate (sodium oxybate) (Xyrem) may decrease symptoms of sleepiness, hallucinations, and cataplexy in patients with narcolepsy. The most commonly observed adverse events associated with the use of sodium oxybate are headache, nausea, dizziness, nasopharyngitis, somnolence, vomiting, and urinary incontinence. Symptoms of a sodium oxybate overdose may include sleepiness, dizziness, confusion, sweating, vomiting, difficulty breathing, seizures, and unconsciousness. Because of the potential for abuse of this medication and the serious side effects that may occur, sodium oxybate should be prescribed with great caution. The recommended starting dose is 4.5 g per night divided into two equal doses of 2.25 g. The starting dosage can then be increased to a maximum of 9 g per night in increments of 1.5 g per night (0.75 g per dose). One to two weeks are recommended between dosage increases to evaluate clinical response and minimize adverse effects. The effective dose range of sodium oxybate is 6 to 9 g per night. Each dose of sodium oxybate must be diluted with two ounces (60 mL, ¼ cup, or 4 tablespoons) of water in the child-resistant dosing cups provided prior to ingestion. The first dose is to be taken at bedtime and the second taken 2.5 to 4 hours later; both doses should be taken while seated in bed. After ingesting each dose, patients should then lie down and remain in bed. Patients should be informed that sodium oxybate is associated with urinary and, less frequently, fecal incontinence, and that they **should not take alcohol or other sedative-hypnotics with sodium oxybate.** Because food significantly reduces the bioavailability of sodium oxybate, the patient should allow at least 2 hours after eating before taking the first dose of sodium oxybate and should try to minimize variability in the timing of dosing in relation to meals.

CIRCADIAN RHYTHM SLEEP DISORDER

Circadian rhythm sleep disorder is characterized by a persistent or recurrent pattern of sleep disruption leading to excessive sleepiness or insomnia, due to a mismatch between the sleep-wake cycle schedule of the individual's environment and one's circadian sleep-wake pattern. Individuals may complain of insomnia at certain times of the day and of excessive sleepiness at other times, with subsequent distress and psychosocial impairment. There are four subtypes: the delayed sleep phase type (e.g., "night owls"), the jet lag type, the shift work type, and the unspecified type.

Diagnosis

1. Symptoms of insomnia and/or excessive sleepiness.
2. Objective polysomnography recordings of prolonged sleep latency in the delayed sleep phase type and normal to short sleep latency in the shift work type.

Prevalence

The prevalence of this disorder has not been well established.

Treatment

Behavioral Interventions

Regularizing sleep-wake schedules and strict adherence to an early and regular rising time have been used for the treatment of the delayed sleep phase syndrome.

With the jet lag and shift work types, preventive (e.g., gradually changing one's schedule before traveling across time zones), environmental (e.g., elimination of noises and stimuli during the day), and rescheduling measures are common.

Light Therapy
Appropriately timed bright white light may shift endogenous circadian rhythms to more closely match the required environmental rhythms. For example, bright light in the morning may advance circadian rhythms.

Pharmacologic Treatments
Short-acting benzodiazepines as well as melatonin may help symptoms of jet lag. Short-acting benzodiazepines have also been used to help with the shift work type (e.g., by administering them only on the first 2 days of a particular night shift) and may also be used to reinforce a particular time of sleep onset in patients with delayed sleep phase syndrome. Modafinil (dosing: 100 to 400 mg q.d.) has recently been approved for the treatment of shift work sleep disorder.

PARASOMNIAS
Parasomnias are sleep disorders characterized by abnormal behavioral or physiologic events occurring in association with sleep, specific sleep stages, or sleep-wake transitions. Nightmare disorder, for example, is characterized by repeated awakenings from the major sleep period or naps with detailed recall of extended and frightening dreams. The sleep terror disorder is characterized by recurrent episodes of abrupt awakening from sleep, accompanied by intense fear and signs of autonomic arousal, amnesia for the episode, and beginning with a panicky scream. Finally, sleepwalking disorder is characterized by recurrent episodes of rising from bed during sleep and walking about, typically with amnesia on awakening.

Treatment of Nightmare Disorder
Most behavioral approaches have used relaxation and systematic desensitization (exposure-based intervention aimed at facilitating emotional processing of the underlying anxiety). Anecdotal observations suggest the usefulness of benzodiazepines or REM-suppressing antidepressants such as SSRIs or SNRIs, although treatment with these two classes of antidepressant drugs has also been associated with the emergence of nightmares.

Treatment of Sleep Terror and/or Sleepwalking
Hypnosis has shown some benefit in the treatment of these two conditions. Most behavioral approaches for sleepwalking have used awakening the individual just before the typical time of sleepwalking episodes. Anecdotal observations suggest the usefulness of benzodiazepines and TCAs.

Bibliography

Ellenbogen JM, Hu PT, Payne JD, et al. Human relational memory requires time and sleep. *Proc Natl Acad Sci U S A* 2007;104(18):7723–7728.

Lee-Chiong TL Jr. Sleep and sleep disorders: an overview. *Med Clin North Am* 2004;88:xi.

Qureshi A, Lee-Chiong T Jr. Medications and their effects on sleep. *Med Clin North Am* 2004;88:751.

Insomnia

Dundar Y, Dodd S, Strobl J, et al. Comparative efficacy of newer hypnotic drugs for the short-term management of insomnia: a systematic review and meta-analysis. *Hum Psychopharmacol* 2004;19:305.

Kierlin L. Sleeping without a pill: nonpharmacologic treatments for insomnia. *J Psychiatr Pract* 2008;14(6):403–407.

Neubauer DN. The evolution and development of insomnia pharmacotherapies. *J Clin Sleep Med* 2007; 3(5 suppl): S11–S16.

Ringdahl EN, Pereira SL, Delzell JE Jr. Treatment of primary insomnia. *J Am Board Fam Pract* 2004;17:212.

Roth T, Drake C. Evolution of insomnia: current status and future direction. *Sleep Med* 2004;5(suppl 1):S23.

Restless Legs Syndrome

Hening WA, Allen RP, Earley CJ, et al.; Restless Legs Syndrome Task Force of the Standards of Practice Committee of the American Academy of Sleep Medicine. An update on the dopaminergic treatment of restless legs syndrome and periodic limb movement disorder. *Sleep* 2004;27:560.

Satija P, Ondo WG. Restless legs syndrome: pathophysiology, diagnosis and treatment. *CNS Drugs* 2008;22(6):497–518.

Breathing-Related Sleep Disorder

Ballard RD. Management of patients with obstructive sleep apnea. *J Fam Pract* 2008;57(8 suppl):S24–S30.

Doghramji PP. Recognition of obstructive sleep apnea and associated excessive sleepiness in primary care. *J Fam Pract* 2008;57(8 suppl):S17–S23.

Merritt SL, Berger BE. Obstructive sleep apnea-hypopnea syndrome. *Am J Nurs* 2004;104:49.

Quinnell TG, Smith IE. Obstructive sleep apnea in the elderly: recognition and management considerations. *Drugs Aging* 2004;21:307.

Verse T, Pirsig W, Stuck BA, et al. Recent developments in the treatment of obstructive sleep apnea. *Am J Respir Med* 2003;2:157.

Narcolepsy

Billiard M. Narcolepsy: current treatment options and future approaches. *Neuropsychiatr Dis Treat* 2008;4(3):557–566.

Naumann A, Daum I. Narcolepsy: pathophysiology and neuropsychological changes. *Behav Neurol* 2003;14:89.

Wise MS. Narcolepsy and other disorders of excessive sleepiness. *Med Clin North Am* 2004;88:597.

8 Drugs for the Treatment of Dementia

OVERVIEW OF DEMENTIA AND DRUGS FOR ITS TREATMENT

The most common forms of dementia are Alzheimer's disease, vascular dementia, and Alzheimer's and vascular dementia. Alzheimer's disease typically starts with memory loss and gradually progresses to include multiple cognitive impairments and neuropsychiatric symptoms. Psychological manifestations such as social withdrawal, depression, anxiety, and paranoia are common. Vascular dementia manifests with memory loss and a wide range of cognitive and behavioral abnormalities depending on the affected brain regions. In addition, a variety of other neurodegenerative diseases produce dementia, such as frontotemporal dementia and Parkinson's disease with dementia. There has been remarkable progress in understanding the pathophysiology of Alzheimer's disease and other neurodegenerative diseases during the last decade, but treatments based on such growing understanding, ultimately influencing the course of the disease, are still some years in the future. Thus, existing treatments remain palliative.

Briefly, insights derived from rare early-onset familial cases of Alzheimer's disease due to single mutations appear to be applicable to the far more common sporadic and late-onset forms (although these forms also clearly have genetic modifiers such as the apolipoprotein E locus). The emerging story suggests that oligomeric forms of a peptide fragment called Aβ are highly toxic to neurons. Ultimately, aggregates of Aβ form the amyloid plaques that mark the late stages of the disease. Treatment development is currently focused on blocking the enzymes that liberate Aβ or enhancing its degradation. Such drugs are nearing the stage of clinical trials, but there is not yet evidence of safety and efficacy in humans. Another strategy has been to vaccinate individuals against Aβ; an early trial was suggestive of efficacy but produced serious autoimmune toxicities. New approaches to vaccine strategies are being pursued.

Neuroinflammation and its effects on neurodegeneration have also been explored for possible therapeutics in Alzheimer's dementia. Tissue necrosis factor–α has been examined because it is known to increase expression of interleukin-1, which subsequently leads to the production of proteins used to form amyloid plaques and neurofibrillary tangles. Therefore, tissue necrosis factor-blockers used in treating arthritis are being investigated for their possible benefit in Alzheimer's dementia. Indeed, a recent case report found that etanercept, a tissue necrosis factor blocker effective for treating rheumatoid arthritis, proved to markedly improve cognitive test scores when given perispinally over several weeks. Further controlled studies are required, but this may be the start of new treatments focused on the immune system.

The workup for dementia and the differential diagnosis are beyond the scope of this chapter, but workup includes a detailed history, physical examination, and neuropsychiatric testing. Imaging studies may be appropriate based on the findings. At present, imaging to detect early Alzheimer's disease is still experimental; studies using magnetic resonance imaging measurements of hippocampus or positron emission tomography studies of hippocampal metabolism and other approaches using probes for brain amyloid appear promising, but they are not yet ready for clinical use. Table 8.1 outlines some medical, psychiatric, and drug-induced conditions that are in the differential diagnosis of a person presenting with dementia.

TABLE 8.1 Differential Diagnosis of Dementia

I. Diseases associated with dementia
   Alzheimer's disease
   Vascular dementia
   Dementia with Lewy bodies
   Pick's disease
   Huntington's disease
   Creutzfeldt-Jakob disease
   Parkinson's disease
   Traumatic brain injury
   Multiple sclerosis
   HIV-related dementia
   Chronic alcoholism

II. Reversible conditions appearing like dementia
   A. Medical illnesses
      Adrenal diseases (Addison's disease, Cushing's syndrome)
      Thyroid diseases (hyper- and hypothyroidism)
      Hepatic failure
      Renal diseases (renal failure, volume depletion, hyponatremia)
      Pulmonary diseases (hypercarbia of COPD)
      Normal pressure hydrocephalus
      Primary or metastatic brain tumors
      Hyperparathyroidism
      Hypoglycemia
   B. Psychiatric illnesses
      Depression
      Psychotic disorders
      Drug withdrawal (benzodiazepines, phenobarbital)
   C. Drug-induced causes
      Drugs used in medical illnesses
         Antihypertensives
         Corticosteroids
         Digitalis
      Opioids
         Nonsteroidal antiinflammatory drugs (NSAIDs)
         Phenytoin
         Anticholinergics
      Drugs used in psychiatric illnesses
         Antipsychotics
         Anticholinergics
         Sedative-hypnotics
   D. Infectious diseases
      Syphilis
      Meningitis
   E. Deficiency conditions
      Vitamin B_{12} deficiency
      Folate deficiency

COPD, chronic obstructive pulmonary disease.

ACETYLCHOLINESTERASE INHIBITORS

The findings that cholinergic neurons were affected early in the course of Alzheimer's disease and that acetylcholine plays a critical role in cognitive processes, including memory, resulted in clinical trials of drugs that block acetylcholinesterase, the synaptic enzyme that breaks down acetylcholine. Although the preponderance of agents available for the treatment of Alzheimer's disease are cholinesterase inhibitors, their clinical effect is modest. Nonetheless, lacking alternatives at present, they are in wide use. Cholinesterase inhibitors that are sufficiently lipophilic to cross the blood–brain barrier can effectively increase the availability of central acetylcholine. Although several well-designed clinical trials have indicated that these cholinesterase inhibitors may be useful in slowing the progression of symptoms, **these drugs are at best palliative,** provide only modest benefit, and have no known effects on the underlying disease process. Although the cholinesterase inhibitors have been considered a candidate for delaying the onset of dementia, prospective study of patients with mild cognitive impairment find that cholinesterase inhibitors do not delay the onset of dementia. Although cholinesterase inhibitors may not change the course of dementia, they may slow the onset of neuropsychiatric signs and symptoms (e.g., paranoia or agitation) associated with dementia. Unfortunately, patients who stop cholinesterase inhibitors quickly return to the cognitive level of the placebo group. It remains unclear how long the treatment should continue with the cholinesterase inhibitors.

Four cholinesterase inhibitors, tacrine, donepezil, galantamine, and rivastigmine, are currently available for the treatment of cognitive impairment of dementia of the Alzheimer's type. Because of significant liver toxicity, the first approved agent, tacrine, should not be used. Despite the mild variations in their mechanism of action, the drugs are similar in efficacy. Only tolerability separates them; donepezil is best tolerated.

Donepezil

Donepezil is a reversible inhibitor of acetylcholinesterase and has become a drug of choice for mild to moderate Alzheimer's disease because it is well tolerated and easy to administer. The drug has been shown to modestly improve cognitive performance and enhance activities of daily living in patients with Alzheimer's disease, compared with placebo. In more behaviorally disturbed patients, donepezil may improve mood and psychotic symptoms, though a recent study ($N = 272$) found that donepezil was ineffective for treating agitation in Alzheimer's dementia.

The drug is well tolerated at both 5- and 10-mg dose per day. Possible adverse effects include nausea, diarrhea, insomnia, muscle cramps, fatigue, and anorexia, but these are typically mild and time limited. More worrisome cholinergic side effects include bradycardia, worsening of chronic obstructive pulmonary disease, and exacerbation of urinary obstruction. Donepezil or other cholinesterase inhibitors should be **avoided in patients with bradycardia**. Both 5- and 10-mg doses were efficacious, but treatment is begun with 5 mg for several months. Frail patients can be started at 2.5 mg per day. Although 10 mg is not proven to be more efficacious than 5 mg, an increase to 10 mg can be considered. Donepezil is usually given in the evening. Donepezil is a substrate for metabolism by cytochrome P450 2D6 and 3A4; medications that inhibit these enzymes (e.g., paroxetine or fluoxetine for 2D6 or erythromycin or cimetidine for 3A4) may lead to higher concentrations of donepezil and cholinergic toxicity. Although follow-up studies suggest sustained benefit for almost 2 years, there is no clear evidence that the drug alters the course of the disease, and, with progression of the illness, the efficacy of the drug could diminish. Because the drug lacks hepatotoxicity, has a long elimination half-life that permits single daily dosing, is well absorbed without significant influence of food, and is relatively selective for brain (versus gastrointestinal) acetylcholinesterase, donepezil is a first-line treatment alternative for Alzheimer's disease.

Donepezil also appears to have benefit for patients with other dementias including those with mixed vascular and Alzheimer's dementia, Lewy body dementia, and possibly dementia associated with Down's syndrome. Although donepezil has been primarily studied in mild to moderate dementia, a limited number of studies find that it may have a role for **behavioral disturbances** and cognition in more advanced cases of dementia. Donepezil is the only cholinesterase inhibitor approved by the Food and Drug Administration for the treatment of severe Alzheimer's disease. In these cases, as with milder cases, the benefits of donepezil remain modest.

Galantamine

Galantamine, like donepezil, inhibits the intrasynaptic enzyme that deactivates acetylcholine. Galantamine has a short half-life, approximately 7 hours, and requires at least twice daily dosing. It is partially protein bound, is metabolized through the cytochrome P450 2D6 pathway, and, like donepezil, its concentration may be increased by drugs such as paroxetine that inhibit the 2D6 enzyme. Elimination kinetics is linear throughout the recommended dosage range, whereas in hepatically impaired patients clearance is decreased slightly. In patients with renal disease, clearance may be decreased by as much as two thirds. Galantamine is **not as well tolerated as donepezil** and requires gradual dose titration, starting at 4 mg twice daily with meals; increased after several weeks, as tolerated, to 8 mg twice daily; and finally up to 8 mg thrice daily. Patients unable to reach 16 mg per day should be tried on another medication. Nausea and vomiting are more common than with donepezil, although this may be ameliorated with very slow titration. The drug is otherwise reasonably well tolerated.

In addition to inhibiting acetylcholinesterase, galantamine is believed to modulate the **nicotinic acetylcholine receptor**. Because brain nicotinic receptors have a role in memory and attention, this property may be important, although the direct benefits of these nicotinic effects have not been proved in patients with Alzheimer's disease.

Like donepezil, galantamine is postulated to slow the progression of Alzheimer's dementia and has been shown to be effective in trials over a 1-year period. Generally, the cognitive improvement is modest, offering the most benefit for patients with mild to moderate dementia. For severe, mixed, and Alzheimer's-type dementias, galantamine is less likely to offer relief and, in light of its more complex side-effect profile, should be used cautiously.

Rivastigmine

Rivastigmine reversibly inhibits two enzymes, acetylcholinesterase and butyrylcholinesterase, that regulate brain acetylcholine. This property may be of clinical significance because butyrylcholinesterase activity becomes relatively greater during the later stages of Alzheimer's dementia as acetylcholinesterase activity declines. Rivastigmine, thus, may be of greater value in more advanced stages of dementia, although this is yet to be confirmed by clinical trials.

Rivastigmine has a **short half-life**, approximately 1.5 hours, which requires at least twice daily dosing. It is not highly protein bound and unlike many drugs, is not metabolized through the hepatic P450 system, but rather is inactivated via hydrolysis at the site of its target enzyme, acetylcholinesterase. This metabolic pathway greatly limits its drug interactions. For unknown reasons, however, clearance is decreased by half or more in patients with significantly impaired renal or hepatic function. Elimination kinetics is linear in the lower dosage range (0 to 6 mg per day) and nonlinear in the higher dosage range (6 to 12 mg per day).

Unfortunately, rivastigmine has **considerable gastrointestinal side effects** and many patients have difficulty with nausea, vomiting, or diarrhea. In comparison studies, it is not as well tolerated as donepezil, though very gradual titration helps reduce toxicity. Because of the gastrointestinal side effects, it should be started very slowly, beginning at 1.5 mg once or twice daily. The dose should be increased gradually after several weeks by 1.5 mg per dose, up to 6 mg twice daily. Some patients, who are unable to tolerate the target dose of 12 mg per day, should reach at least 6 mg per day.

As with other cholinesterase inhibitors, controlled trials with rivastigmine has proven to be of only modest benefit for cognitive and behavioral symptoms associated with Alzheimer's dementia, although other controlled trials indicate that rivastigmine may benefit patients with Lewy body dementia as well as patients with mixed vascular and Alzheimer's dementia.

Tacrine

Because of the high incidence of **hepatic toxicity** and the protracted period necessary to initiate and maintain treatment to avoid serious hepatic injury, we recommend that tacrine be avoided unless other alternatives have been exhausted.

Tacrine is an acridinamine derivative for the treatment of cognitive deficits due to Alzheimer's disease. It is a noncompetitive, reversible inhibitor of acetylcholinesterase.

Tacrine is a highly lipid soluble, unlike many acetylcholinesterase inhibitors; thus, it produces high levels in the brain. Oral absorption produces highly variable plasma levels, which peak at approximately 2 hours after administration. The drug is extensively metabolized in the liver; its half-life is prolonged in elderly patients and in individuals with liver disease. In healthy volunteers, the elimination half-life is 2 hours; in elderly patients, it is approximately 3.5 hours.

Double-blind, placebo-controlled trials of tacrine have demonstrated its benefit in a minority of mildly to moderately impaired patients with probable Alzheimer's disease.

Tacrine is begun at 10 mg four times daily for 6 weeks, with hepatic transaminase levels monitored every other week. If the patient is able to tolerate the drug and the transaminase levels have not gone over three times normal, the dose may be increased to 20 mg four times daily for an additional 6 weeks. The same process ensues with increases every 6 weeks to 30 mg, then to 40 mg four times daily. This is the Food and Drug Administration–approved protocol for treatment with tacrine based on the clinical trial data that were reviewed.

Approximately 50% of patients taking tacrine develop elevations in hepatic aminotransferase activity. In short-term studies of tacrine, these elevations have usually returned to normal within 6 weeks of drug discontinuation. Approximately 25% of patients studied have had marked abnormalities (at least three times the upper limit of normal). Several patients on dosages of 100 to 200 mg per day have had biopsy-proven hepatitis, which resolved clinically on drug discontinuation. Other side effects include nausea, vomiting, diarrhea, headache, and ataxia.

Tacrine may interact with drugs metabolized by the hepatic P450 pathway; it has been shown to increase levels of theophylline.

OTHER DRUGS FOR TREATMENT OF DEMENTIA

As the baby-boom generation transitions into senior status over the next 30 years, the need for more effective agents for the treatment of Alzheimer's disease has prompted investigators, clinicians, and pharmaceutical firms to pursue a variety of strategies to combat this illness. The most active areas have addressed a variety of the possible etiologies cited previously, including: (a) normalizing glutaminergic transmission using antagonists for the N-methyl-D-aspartate (NMDA) receptor;

TABLE 8.2	Drugs Indicated for Alzheimer's Dementia		
Drug	**Doses Available**	**Starting Dose (mg)**	**Final Dose Range (mg)**
Donepezil (Aricept)	5-, 10-mg tablets	5	5–10
Galantamine (Reminyl)	4-, 8-, 12-mg tablets, 4 mg/mL oral solution	4	12–24
Rivastigmine (Exelon)	1.5-, 3.0-, 4.5-, 6.0-mg capsules	1.5	6–12
Memantine (Namenda)	5-, 10-mg tablets	5	10–20

(b) reducing oxidative processes using *Ginkgo biloba*, a popular antioxidant used in nontraditional and alternative medicine practice; (c) reducing inflammatory processes using nonsteroidal antiinflammatory drugs (NSAIDs), including novel and commonly used compounds; and (d) treating mood or psychotic symptoms associated with dementia.

Memantine (Namenda)

Recently, memantine, an antagonist of NMDA glutamate receptors, has been added to the dementia treatment armamentarium (Table 8.2). Glutamate-mediated over-activation of NMDA receptors may contribute to cell death in Alzheimer's dementia. Memantine is an **NMDA noncompetitive antagonist** with low to moderate affinity for the central receptor. It is hypothesized that memantine blocks pathologic but not physiologic activation of NMDA receptors. There is, however, no evidence that memantine alters the pathologic progression of Alzheimer's disease. Like the cholinesterase inhibitors, it provides modest clinical benefit for dementia and does not reverse the course of the disease. In two 6-month studies, memantine showed modest improvement compared with placebo for moderate to severe dementia across several domains. Patients in both drug and placebo groups showed progression of symptoms, though patients treated with memantine showed less deterioration. In clinical practice, memantine may improve behavioral disturbances of dementia. Effects on cognition are typically modest. Memantine may also provide modest improvement when combined with donepezil. In milder cases of dementia, however, memantine has not established benefit over placebo. Sufficient data exist to justify the combined use of memantine and cholinergic agents for patients with moderate to severe Alzheimer's disease, particularly for those refractory to more standardized monotherapies. Because this drug, like the cholinesterase inhibitors, is relatively expensive and its expected benefits are modest, its cost may not be justifiable for some patients.

Pharmacology

As noted above, memantine is an uncompetitive NMDA antagonist is the central nervous system. It does not affect acetylcholinesterase, and it does not appear to have any direct effects on glycine, γ-aminobutyric acid, histamine, or dopamine receptors. It is readily absorbed in the gastrointestinal tract and is eliminated unchanged in the urine, in part by tubular excretion, or by the addition of a glucuronide. Accumulation of memantine occurs in patients with moderate to severe renal failure, and dose reduction is required for patients with a creatinine clearance below 50 mL per minute. Hydrochlorothiazide does not affect its clearance. Drugs that make the urine more alkaline, such as carbonic anhydrase, reduce clearance; dose reduction is required if memantine is used in combination with carbonic anhydrase or other similarly acting drugs.

It is not highly protein bound, and therefore not prone to displace drugs such as warfarin when used in combination. Its elimination half-life is approximately 60 hours, allowing for once daily dosing. It does not inhibit cytochrome enzymes and is not known to cause significant drug–drug interactions. Because the drug is partially eliminated via glucuronide addition in the liver, dose reduction should be made for patients with moderated to severe liver disease.

Adverse Effects
Memantine is generally very well tolerated. Some patients may experience sedation or confusion with rapid dose escalation. In clinical trials, very few patients discontinue because of side effects; the rate of adverse effects is low, no different than placebo. Memantine does not affect blood pressure, pulse, or electrocardiogram parameters.

Method of Use
The usual starting dose is 5 mg once daily for a week, with weekly increases of 5 mg until the target dose of 20 mg per day is reached, generally after 3 or 4 weeks. The drug is available as in pill or oral solution form.

Dosages Available
Memantine is available in 5- and 10-mg tablets and in a titration starter pack. It is also available in a 2 mg/mL oral solution.

Treatment of Neuropsychiatric Symptoms Associated with Dementia
Alzheimer's dementia clinically requires management in two broad areas—cognitive symptoms and behavioral and neuropsychiatry symptoms. Although various symptoms such as irritability, depression, apathy, anxiety, delusions, disinhibition, elation, agitation and aggression, aberrant motor behavior, and hallucinations are often listed as problematic in the management of these patients, apathy, agitation and aggression, delusions, irritability, and depression are the most common symptoms leading to disturbed behavior needing pharmacologic intervention. As common as these behavioral problems arise, the controlled studies to match them are quite few, and the practitioner is often left to best guess which treatments might be reasonable. Much remains to be studied regarding using psychotropics for the neuropsychiatric complications of dementia. Because this patient group is frequently frail from dementia and an accumulation of other diseases, extreme caution must be taken before adding still unproven drug treatments for the behavioral and psychopathologic manifestations of dementia. The added conundrum for selecting treatment is that many of the studies find little benefit for drugs to treat these frequent behavioral problems.

Antipsychotics
The psychotic symptoms of dementia that do not respond to cholinesterase inhibitors incline the clinician to use medications if other treatments (e.g., treatment of pain or delirium; environmental adjustments and cues) are ineffective. For these situations, second-generation antipsychotics have been favored because of their limited propensity for extrapyramidal symptoms. Several small placebo-controlled studies support their use for the psychosis and agitation associated with dementia. On the other hand, recent larger studies suggest that caution should be exercised before using these drugs. A meta-analysis of treatment trials of elderly patients with dementia found slightly higher death rates (3.5% vs 2.3%) for second-generation antipsychotics compared with placebo. This mortality risk is amplified by the slightly increased risk of cerebrovascular accidents that was found with several of the second-generation antipsychotics. Both findings are now noted as the

Food and Drug Administration "black box warnings" and have created concern for using such medications clinically. As a result of these findings, clinicians should weigh the risks and benefits of using antipsychotics for each patient with dementia, and obtain informed consent from patient or their health care proxy or guardian (when the patient lacks capacity to give such consent).

In addition, the lack of benefit of second-generation antipsychotics for behavioral disturbance in a large ($N = 421$) randomized trial (Clinical Antipsychotic Trial of Intervention Effectiveness Study for Alzheimer's Disease) designed to study the effectiveness of treating agitation, aggression, or psychosis in dementia, makes us realize that we must **proceed thoughtfully when using antipsychotics** for behavioral problems in dementia. The older first-generation antipsychotics, unfortunately, carry the same mortality risk as the newer second-generation antipsychotics in patients with dementia. In this population, the older drugs are often more problematic for neurological side effects and therefore less desirable. The antipsychotic drugs, in general, should therefore be reserved for cases in which nonpharmacologic treatments fail, knowing that antipsychotic drug treatments at times may not be effective. Drug treatment should be time limited if observable benefits are not obvious. The lowest possible dose should be used to limit toxicity, and these drugs should not be used first line for sleep or anxiety.

Any of the antipsychotics may be used for the appropriate indication. Doses must be lower than those for treating psychotic disorders (Table 8.3). Olanzapine, quetiapine, and risperidone are commonly used because of their familiarity in treating psychotic disorders, though any are reasonable for the treatment of psychotic symptoms in dementia. Thus, risperidone 0.25 to 2.0 mg may be effective in elderly patients requiring control of behavioral and psychotic symptoms arising from Alzheimer's disease, vascular dementia, or mixed dementia pictures; the higher dosage range, 1.0 to 2.0 mg daily, will be needed for those patients whose conditions are more difficult to manage or those who have not responded satisfactorily at lower doses. Alternatively, olanzapine dosage ranging from 2.5 to 10 mg per day, or quetiapine dosage ranging from 12.5 to 200 mg per day may be administered to patients with dementia struggling with agitation, aggression, hallucinations, or delusions. This patient population is often sensitive to the sedating and orthostatic properties of the second-generation antipsychotics, so titration should be done slowly and the doses should be given before bedtime to limit side effects. Older first-generation antipsychotics with greater anticholinergic properties should be used only when trials with second-generation antipsychotics have failed.

Antidepressants

Antidepressants can improve anxiety and depression as well as agitation or hostility in dementia. For depression, the SSRI antidepressants, because of their relatively benign side-effect profile, have become the drug treatment of choice. These

TABLE 8.3	Antipsychotic Doses Used in Dementia	
Drug	**Starting Dose (mg)**	**Final Dose Range (mg)**
Haloperidol	0.25	0.5–2
Risperidone	0.25	0.5–2
Quetiapine	12.5	12.5–200
Olanzapine	2.5	2.5–10
Aripiprazole	2.5	2.5–10
Ziprasidone	20	20–60

compounds, however, have not been rigorously studied in large placebo-controlled trials for dementia; small studies found that venlafaxine and fluoxetine were not better than placebo. Interestingly, citalopram appears to improve depression as well as psychotic symptoms in dementia, though further study will be needed to confirm this benefit. Of the SSRIs, those with fewer drug interactions (e.g., citalopram, escitalopram, and sertraline) are usually the best choices, though they are not side effect free. In elderly patients with dementia, nausea or cognitive impairment may be quite problematic. If used, dosing should begin at the lowest doses (e.g., citalopram 10 mg) with gradual titration.

Mirtazapine may also prove helpful in depressed patients with dementia, and its properties of increasing appetite and improving sleep often prove useful. It has not been studied in a controlled fashion in patients with dementia, but its lack of significant side effects makes it a reasonable antidepressant choice. Sedation and falls associated with sedation may be problematic; starting doses should be low, generally 7.5 mg, and titration should be gradual over several weeks, upward to 30 mg per day. Mirtazapine at low doses may also be helpful for insomnia in patients with dementia. Bupropion has not been studied in patients with dementia, though we have found its alerting qualities useful in some patients. Trazodone is frequently used as a sleep aid in patients with dementia, and while this practice is reasonable, its propensity for causing orthostasis must be taken seriously to prevent falls during the night. The lowest possible doses (e.g., 12.5 to 25 mg) should be used if trazodone is prescribed. The tricyclic antidepressants should generally be avoided because of their anticholinergic effects.

Anticonvulsants

Carbamazepine and valproate as well as other anticonvulsants have been used to treat agitation associated with dementia. There is very limited data to support the use of any of these agents, and there are good reasons to avoid most of them. They all cause neurological toxicity and increase the risk of confusion and falls. Carbamazepine has a high risk for drug–drug interactions and the possibility for causing bone marrow suppression or the syndrome of inappropriate antidiuretic hormone secretion. Valproate, though better tolerated than carbamazepine, has proved no better than placebo for agitation in dementia in several placebo-controlled studies when used at typical doses. The lack of benefit for valproate is surprising considering its widespread use for this purpose, though the negative results caution against using a drug with clear risk for toxicity and no clear evidence for benefit. If used, valproate should be started at very low doses, generally 125 mg per day and gradually increased as tolerated to a target dose of 750 mg per day or a plasma concentration of 50 mg/nL, with behavioral response being the primary determinant of dose. Other anticonvulsants, each with a range of toxicities, including gabapentin, topiramate, lamotrigine, oxcarbazepine, and levetiracetam, are best avoided until studies proving benefit are accomplished. In cases of vascular dementia or traumatic brain injury causing behavioral disturbances by partial seizures, the use of anticonvulsants may be helpful.

Benzodiazepines

Benzodiazepines should generally be avoided for patients with dementia. Although they may be effective for the treatment of anxiety, side effects in this population include worsening memory and increased risk for falls. (The benzodiazepines are covered in Chapters 5 and 7.) In selected situations, preferably in an inpatient setting where patients can be carefully observed, the benzodiazepines may help reduce anxiety or agitation not amenable to other treatments. Using multiple drugs (e.g., antipsychotic, antidepressant, and benzodiazepines) to control agitation is best avoided because of the increased risk of toxicity with combination treatment.

The benzodiazepines should be used for short periods and then discontinued. Occasionally, long-term anxiety disorders predating the onset of dementia may warrant continued benzodiazepine use, though dose reduction should still be considered given the risk for side effects of impairing cognition. If used, lorazepam or temazepam are the reasonable choices because they require only glucuronide addition before excretion and have relatively short half-lives. Doses are best kept low and given for short periods. Typical starting doses are 0.5 mg for lorazepam and 7.5 mg for temazepam. Long half-life drugs such as diazepam and clonazepam are best avoided in this population.

OTHER COMPOUNDS USED FOR DEMENTIA

Ginkgo biloba

Several well-designed, randomized, blinded, placebo-controlled clinical trials using *Ginkgo biloba* in patients with cognitive and behavioral symptoms of Alzheimer's and other uncomplicated dementias show that patients may have slower clinical deterioration than the placebo-control group over a 1-year period; the ginkgo must be a purified form of 120 mg per day of the EGb 761 *Ginkgo biloba* extract. Another similar trial using two doses, 160 and 240 mg per day, found no effect as compared with placebo at either dose over a 24-week period. Compared with placebo, *Ginkgo biloba* appears to be safe for use regarding side effects. Although larger trials are ongoing, the limited data to date suggest that the benefits of ginkgo are modest. Further studies are needed to clarify what role ginkgo may provide. Chronic use of properly purified ginkgo preparations might serve a protective function for worsening disease over a period of several years, though research is limited. Regarding drug–drug interactions, there have been case reports implicating *Ginkgo biloba*'s interacting with warfarin (potentially through inhibition of cytochrome 2C9), causing increased risk for bleeding. Recently, however, several controlled studies find that *in vivo* ginkgo does not affect the metabolism of warfarin. Given the limited proven benefits of ginkgo for dementia, we cannot recommend its clinical use at this time.

NSAIDs

At present, although the evidence for the use of NSAIDs in the treatment of the behavioral and cognitive symptoms of the various dementias is reasonably compelling, their use should be reserved as a preventive strategy in management of Alzheimer's disease rather than for control of the behavioral, cognitive, or affective symptoms that often complicate the management. The NSAIDs have not been studied prospectively for the treatment of dementia.

Bibliography

Birks J, Grimley Evans J. Ginkgo biloba for cognitive impairment and dementia. *Cochrane Database Syst Rev* 2007;CD003120.

Cummings JL, McRae T, Zhang R, et al. Effects of donepezil on neuropsychiatric symptoms in patients with dementia and severe behavioral disorders. *Am J Geriatr Psychiatry* 2006;14(7):605–612.

Doraiswamy PM, Bieber F, Kaiser L, et al. The Alzheimer's disease assessment scale: patterns and predictors of baseline cognitive performance in multicenter Alzheimer's disease trials. *Neurology* 1997;48:1511.

Greenblatt DJ, von Moltke LL, Luo Y, et al. Ginkgo biloba does not alter clearance of flurbiprofen, a cytochrome P450-2C9 substrate. *J Clin Pharmacol* 2006;46:214–221.

Howard RJ, Juszczak E, Ballard CG, et al. Donepezil for the treatment of agitation in Alzheimer's disease. *N Engl J Med* 2007;357(14):1382–1392.

Jellinger KA, Bancher C. Neuropathology of Alzheimer's disease: a critical update. *J Neural Transm Suppl* 1998;54:77–95.

Katz IR, Jeste DV, Mintzer JE, et al. Comparison of risperidone and placebo for psychosis and behavioral disturbances associated with dementia. *J Clin Psychiatry* 1999:60:107.

Kavirajan H, Schneider LS. Efficacy and adverse effects of cholinesterase inhibitors and memantine in vascular dementia: a meta-analysis of randomised controlled trials. *Lancet Neurol* 2007;6:782–792.

LeBars PL, Katz MM, Berman N, et al. A placebo-controlled, double-blind, randomized trial of an extract of ginkgo. *JAMA* 1997;278:1327.

Lyketsos CG, Steinberg M, Tschanz JT, et al. Mental and behavioral disturbances in dementia: findings from the Cache County Study on Memory in Aging. *Am J Psychiatry* 2000;157:708.

Pollack BG, Mulsant BH, Sweet RA, et al. Comparison of citalopram, perphenazine, and placebo for the acute treatment of psychosis and behavioral disturbances in hospitalized, demented patients. *Am J Psychiatry* 2002;159:460.

Raschetti R, Albanese E, Vanacore N, et al. Cholinesterase inhibitors in mild cognitive impairment: a systematic review of randomised trials. *PLoS Med* 2007;4(11):e338.

Reisberg B, Doody R, Stoffler A, et al. Memantine in moderate-to-severe Alzheimer's disease. *N Engl J Med* 2003;348:1333.

Scharf S, Mander A, Ugoni A, et al. A double-blind, placebo-controlled trial of diclofenac/misoprostol in Alzheimer's disease. *Neurology* 1999;53:197.

Schneider LS, Dagerman KS, Insel P, et al. Risk of death with atypical antipsychotic drug treatment for dementia: meta-analysis of randomized placebo-controlled trials. *JAMA* 2005;294:1934–1943.

Schneider LS, Tariot PN, Dagerman KS, et al. Effectiveness of atypical antipsychotic drugs in patients with Alzheimer's disease. *N Engl J Med* 2006;355(15):1525–1538.

Street JS, Clark WS, Gannon KS, et al. Olanzapine treatment of psychotic and behavioral symptoms in patients with Alzheimer's disease in nursing care facilities. *Arch Gen Psychiatry* 2000;57:968.

Tariot PN, Farlow MR, Grossberg G, et al. Memantine/donepezil dual-therapy is superior to placebo/donepezil therapy for treatment of moderate to severe Alzheimer's disease [abstract]. *J Am Geriatr Soc* 2003;51(suppl 4):S225.

Tariot PN, Raman R, Jakimovich L, et al. Divalproex sodium in nursing home residents with possible or probable Alzheimer disease complicated by agitation: a randomized, controlled trial. *Am J Geriatr Psychiatry* 2005;13:942–949.

Tobinick EL, Gross H. Rapid cognitive improvement in Alzheimer's disease following perispinal etanercept administration. *J Neuroinflammation* 2008;5:2.

9 Drugs for the Treatment of Attention Deficit Disorder

Attention-deficit/hyperactivity disorder (ADHD) is a developmental neurobehavioral disorder characterized by excessive inattentiveness, impulsivity, and hyperactivity. By definition, ADHD begins during childhood, with symptoms typically recognized before 7 years of age. The *Diagnostic and Statistical Manual of Mental Disorders*, 4th edition (*DSM-IV*), criteria for inattention are met when an individual displays often six or more of the following symptoms: inattention to details/making careless mistakes, difficulty sustaining attention in tasks or play activities, seems not to listen to what is being said, does not follow through and fails to finish tasks, difficulty organizing tasks and activities, avoids or strongly dislikes tasks requiring sustained attention, loses things necessary for tasks and activities, easily distracted, and forgetful. Similarly, the impulsivity and hyperactivity criteria are met when an individual displays often six or more of the following: blurts out answer before question is finished, difficulty awaiting turn or waiting in lines, interrupts or intrudes on others, fidgets, unable to stay seated, inappropriate running or climbing, difficulty in engaging in leisure activities quietly, "on the go"/driven by a motor, and talks excessively. When the criteria are met for inattention but not impulsivity and hyperactivity, the diagnosis of ADHD predominantly inattentive type is made. On the other hand, when the criteria are met for impulsivity and hyperactivity but not inattention, the diagnosis of ADHD predominantly hyperactive/impulsive type is made. When the criteria are met for both, the diagnosis of ADHD combined type is made. ADHD is a disorder that significantly impacts school performance, occupational functioning, and family and social functioning. Untreated, children with ADHD often have poor outcomes, including poor academic outcomes, increased risk of substance use disorders (SUDs) and other psychiatric disorders, and even a greater risk of arrest.

EPIDEMIOLOGY

A current estimate of the prevalence of ADHD in school-aged children and adolescents is approximately 5% to 9%. The increased awareness and recognition of the predominantly inattentive type of ADHD is thought to be a major contributing factor to the recent increase in the rates of diagnosis and treatment of ADHD in children. In addition, differences in criteria between the *Diagnostic and Statistical Manual of Mental Disorders*, 3rd edition, revised (*DSM-III-R*), and the *DSM-IV* classifications, namely, that the *DSM-III-R* required 8 of 14 symptoms, whereas the *DSM-IV* requires only 6 symptoms in either category, may have also contributed to the increased prevalence. As a result of the increased recognition of ADHD, there has also been an increase in the number of children treated for this condition. In fact, a recent study has shown a 2.9-fold increase in the rate of children with ADHD prescribed medications. In community epidemiologic samples, the male-to-female ratio in younger populations is closer to 2:1, although in clinical samples boys tend to greatly outnumber girls. In adults, the prevalence is thought to be somewhat lower and hovers around 4%, with a gender ratio of approximately 1:1.

ETIOLOGY

ADHD is thought to have multiple possible etiologic factors, including genetic, environmental, and neurologic ones. There is a highly significant association between maternal smoking during pregnancy and ADHD in the offspring (but it is unclear whether the smoking might be causal or a marker of maternal risk). Interestingly, adults with ADHD are more likely to smoke than the general population and their quit rate is significantly lower. Cerebral ischemia at birth may be a risk factor for ADHD, but it does not explain the vast majority of cases. It has also been postulated that abnormalities in dopaminergic, noradrenergic, and/or cholinergic neurotransmission may underlie ADHD, but the evidence is scant, and the nature of the putative abnormalities is unclear. All of these neurotransmitters are involved in higher cognitive function, with dopamine (DA) clearly playing important roles in executive function mediated by the prefrontal cortex. A more specific dopaminergic hypothesis states that cognitive impairments associated with ADHD result from a hypodopaminergic state in the prefrontal cortex, whereas hyperactivity and impulsivity result from a hyperdopaminergic state in the striatum, possibly secondary to the prefrontal hypodopaminergic state.

IMAGING STUDIES

Although neuroimaging techniques cannot be used to make a diagnosis of ADHD, they have revealed abnormalities in frontal lobe function and in cortical-subcortical circuits. A study has suggested abnormal morphology in the frontal cortices of patients with ADHD, with reduced regional brain size localized mainly to inferior portions of dorsal prefrontal cortices bilaterally and in anterior temporal cortices bilaterally. In another study, ADHD subjects demonstrated smaller total brain size, superior prefrontal, and right superior prefrontal volumes, as well as significantly smaller areas for cerebellar lobules I-V and VIII-X, total corpus callosum area, and splenium.

Dopamine transporter (DAT) densities seem to be particularly elevated in the brain of ADHD patients, particularly in the striatum, and tend to decrease after treatment with **methylphenidate** (MPH). A study examined DA D(2/3) receptor binding with positron emission tomography using [11C] raclopride as a tracer and found that high DA receptor availability was predicted by a history of low neonatal cerebral blood flow, supporting the hypothesis of cerebral ischemia at birth as a risk factor for ADHD.

Functional neuroimaging studies have evidenced deficits in striatal and prefrontal activation, as well as changes in activation in parietal areas, confirming the postulated importance of frontostriatal networks in ADHD, as deficits in this network have now been associated with a wide range of cognitive tasks. A recent study used diffusion tensor imaging to show that reduced frontostriatal activation during a go/no-go task was related to reduced white matter integrity in both children with ADHD and their affected parents.

GENETIC AND FAMILY STUDIES

Family studies have clearly shown an increase in the risk for ADHD in first-degree relatives of probands with ADHD compared with relatives of controls, and twin studies have demonstrated higher concordance among monozygotic twins rather than dizygotic twins. The heritability of ADHD tends to range between 0.6 and 0.9, depending on the study. ADHD families can include individuals with differing phenotypes, including both more inattentive and impulsive subtypes. Among the various genes investigated, the human thyroid receptor-β gene has been linked to an increased risk for ADHD. A fairly recent meta-analysis concluded that, to date, only seven candidate genes have risk alleles where the pooled odds ratio is significantly >1.0 and that are therefore overtransmitted in ADHD. These genes include five catecholamine genes [DA 4 (*DRD4*) and DA 5 (*DRD5*) receptors, dopamine transporter (*DAT1*), dopamine-β-hydroxylase (*DBH*), and synaptosomal-associated protein of 25 kDa (*SNAP-25*) genes] and two in the serotonin system [serotonin transporter (*5-HTT*) and serotonin 1B-receptor (*HTR1B*) genes]. Results from studies using a mouse model of ADHD using a combination of genetic and pharmacologic approaches demonstrated that DR4R signaling is essential for the expression of juvenile hyperactivity and impaired behavioral inhibition. A study suggests that variation in the glutamate receptor, ionotropic, *N*-methyl D-aspartate 2A (*GRIN2A*) gene may confer an increased risk for ADHD and that this, at least in part, might be responsible for the previously reported linkage results suggesting the presence of a susceptibility locus on chromosome 16p13.

COMORBIDITY

Comorbidity tends to be the rule more than the exception in ADHD, with approximately two thirds of patients with ADHD having comorbid psychiatric conditions. Conduct disorder and oppositional defiant disorder are often present in children with ADHD, as well as major depressive disorder, multiple anxiety disorders, and, to a lesser degree, bipolar disorder. The risk for developing substance use disorder (SUD) is higher in ADHD probands than controls, although pharmacologically treated ADHD probands have rates of SUD closer to controls. In fact, stimulant therapy does not increase but rather reduces the risk for cigarette smoking and SUDs in adolescents with ADHD. Furthermore, there is no evidence that stimulant treatment increases or decreases the risk for subsequent SUDs in children and adolescents with ADHD when they reach young adulthood. A significant proportion of children with ADHD have learning disabilities in the areas of spelling, mathematics, or reading (20% to 30%). Tourette's syndrome is also not uncommon in patients with ADHD and, certainly, ADHD is common in patients with Tourette's syndrome.

COURSE

Although ADHD may remit in childhood or adolescence, approximately 40% to 80% of patients diagnosed with ADHD will continue to exhibit symptoms during young adulthood. ADHD may persist as a disorder or as residual symptoms. Residual symptoms of ADHD in adulthood are an increasingly recognized condition, offering challenges both diagnostically and therapeutically. **The diagnosis requires an established diagnosis of ADHD in childhood,** with residual inattention and impulsiveness in adulthood. The difficulty in diagnosing and studying this condition reflects, in part, the difficulty of making a retrospective diagnosis of childhood ADHD based on the memories of the patient, the patient's parents, and teachers. Although adults with ADHD are generally reliable reporters of their past symptoms, they may tend to underreport compared with reports from their parents. Another difficulty with this diagnosis is that adults with residual symptoms of ADHD frequently suffer from one or more comorbid psychiatric disorders, most frequently mood disorders and SUDs, that may have significant symptom overlap with ADHD.

By themselves, the typical adult residual symptoms of ADHD are nonspecific, including restlessness, difficulty in concentrating, excitability, impulsiveness, and irritability. These symptoms are often associated with poor job or academic performance, anxiety, temper outbursts, antisocial behavior, and substance abuse. When untreated, ADHD is often accompanied by significant academic, familial, and social dysfunction at all ages, and may put those who suffer at risk for SUD. Although those treating children may be focused on conflicts with peers, poor academic performance, and oppositional behavior at school and at home, those treating adults tend to be focused on job and school difficulties.

DIAGNOSIS

ADHD is typically diagnosed clinically, on the basis of reported symptomatology and associated impairments. Collateral informants are very important to the diagnosis, in both children and adolescents. Diagnostic criteria described earlier require that symptoms be pervasive and have persisted for at least 6 months to a degree that is maladaptive and inconsistent with the developmental level, **manifested before age 7 years,** and cause significant academic and/or social impairment. Several scales are used to support the clinical diagnosis of ADHD: the ADD-H Comprehensive Teacher Rating Scale, the Barkley Home Situations Questionnaire and School Situations Questionnaire, the parent-completed Child Behavior Checklist, the Teacher Report Form of the Child Behavioral Checklist, the Conners' Parent and Teacher Rating Scales, and the ADHD Rating Scale. Although these scales can be useful clinically in supporting the diagnosis, they are not used in the real world as frequently as one would expect.

When the diagnosis of ADHD is made in an adult or an adolescent, the clinician needs to assess current symptoms and must also obtain a childhood history of ADHD. Self-report rating scales, such as the Brown Attention Deficit Disorder Scale, can be used to help assess whether ADHD was present during childhood, as well as the Conners' Adults ADHD Rating Scale. School records and report cards can also be used to support the diagnosis, as well as collateral informants. The clinician-rated ADHD rating scale and the Adult ADHD Self-Report Scale Symptom Checklist are often used in clinical trials to track the effects of treatment.

A number of conditions can mimic or complicate ADHD, including head injury, substance abuse, learning disabilities, Asperger's syndrome, autism, mood disorders, hearing or visual impairment, and mental retardation. It is important to be aware of these differential diagnoses when assessing patients for ADHD.

MANAGEMENT
The first step in the management of patients with ADHD involves psychoeducation. When the subject diagnosed as having ADHD is a child, most of the educational effort typically focuses on the parents, although the child may benefit greatly from an age-appropriate explanation of what ADHD is and how it can be helped. When the subject diagnosed as having ADHD is an adolescent or an adult, clinicians typically discuss with the patient some of the basic aspects of ADHD, including symptoms, nature, course of the illness, and available treatments. It is also helpful to provide both patients and their families with written materials such as brochures or review articles, so that they have the opportunity of supplementing the information derived from their interaction with the clinician. There are several Web sites that can be used for this purpose (e.g., www.chadd.org and www.add.org). Treatment usually involves education, psychosocial interventions, and pharmacologic treatments.

Psychosocial Approaches
Most of the psychosocial treatment studies in ADHD have focused primarily on behavioral and cognitive-behavioral therapies. Behavioral therapies are typically considered the initial treatment of choice for preschoolers with ADHD, and they can be effectively delivered by parents and teachers. However, they require high motivation on the part of those involved in their administration, and they require training in the use of contingency management, such as point/token economy reward systems. A large, randomized study has shown that carefully delivered medication management alone was superior to behavioral treatment and that there was only a modest benefit of adding intensive behavioral treatment to medications alone. Despite these findings, many clinicians favor the combination approach, and there is some evidence that such combined approach may allow for the administration of lower doses of stimulants. As far as ADHD in adults is concerned, a recent review of the literature concludes that the available data support the use of structured, skills-based psychosocial interventions as a viable treatment for adults with residual symptoms of ADHD. Common elements across the various treatment packages include psychoeducation, training in concrete skills (e.g., organization and planning

strategies), and emphasis on outside practice and maintenance of these strategies in daily life.

Pharmacologic Treatments

Psychostimulants and atomoxetine (Strattera) are typically considered the first-line pharmacologic agents for the treatment of ADHD. Bupropion, tricyclic antidepressants (TCAs), and modafinil (Provigil) are considered off-label, second-line agents, and a number of other classes of psychotropic drugs may have potential use in this condition.

PSYCHOSTIMULANTS

A wide variety of compounds (e.g., caffeine and strychnine) can produce central nervous system stimulation. However, the stimulant drugs that have found use in ADHD are sympathomimetic amines, of which the prototype is amphetamine. Amphetamine was first used as a bronchodilator, respiratory stimulant, and analeptic during the 1930s. Psychostimulants were then used in the treatment of depression until they were supplanted by TCAs and monoamine oxidase inhibitors (MAOIs) in the 1960s.

The clinical utility of stimulants had been limited by the perception of their risk to cause tolerance and psychological dependence and by their abuse potential. In 1970, the U.S. Food and Drug Administration (FDA) reclassified these drugs as schedule II, the most restrictive classification for drugs that are medically useful. They are currently approved only for the treatment of ADHD and narcolepsy. Their efficacy in ADHD has been demonstrated in all age groups, and the extensive experience with stimulant use in children, adolescents, and adults with ADHD has reassured the field about the safety of these agents when prescribed in a thoughtful way for those without a prior history of active substance misuse or abuse. In addition, the availability of extended-delivery preparations has reduced the risk of misuse of stimulants, although diversion remains a concern. Indeed, as mentioned earlier, meta-analytic data of children with ADHD followed from childhood, through adolescence and into adulthood show that **longitudinal treatment with stimulants may reduce the risk of substance abuse,** with greater protection conferred through adolescence than adulthood. Stimulants are currently the most frequently prescribed psychotropic agents in pediatric psychopharmacology, and they are increasingly prescribed to adults with ADHD as well. They also have several off-label uses in psychiatric practice (Table 9.1). Stimulants are the first-line choice for pharmacologic therapy of ADHD. Those psychostimulants that are most widely used in clinical practice are MPH, mixed amphetamine salts, and dextroamphetamine (DEX).

 Indications for Stimulants

Indications
  Narcolepsy
  ADHD

Off-label uses
  Treatment of apathy and withdrawal (in the medically ill and elderly patients)
  Potentiation of narcotic analgesics
  Antidepressant augmentation for nonresponders and partial responders
  Treatment of SSRI-induced fatigue, apathy, and sexual dysfunction

ADHD, attention deficit disorder with hyperactivity; SSRI, selective serotonin reuptake inhibitor.

Chemistry

Amphetamine is a racemic compound, with DEX being the D-isomer, which is three to four times more potent than the L-isomer as a central nervous system stimulant. MPH is a piperidine derivative that is structurally similar to amphetamine, while dexmethylphenidate hydrochloride is the D-threo enantiomer of racemic MPH hydrochloride. Adderall is an amphetamine mixture containing equal parts of DEX sulfate, D,L-amphetamine sulfate, D,L-amphetamine aspartate, and DEX saccharate. Lisdexamfetamine is a prodrug of DEX. After oral administration, lisdexamfetamine is rapidly absorbed from the gastrointestinal tract and converted to DEX, which is responsible for the drug's activity.

Pharmacology

Absorption and Metabolism

Amphetamine and DEX are well absorbed after oral administration. Immediate-release amphetamines (i.e., DEX and mixed amphetamine salts tablets) have a short half-life (3 to 6 hours); thus, they are usually administered two to three times daily. DEX and mixed amphetamine salts are available in extended-delivery preparations, which are usually administered once and sometimes twice daily. They cross the blood–brain barrier easily and develop high concentrations in the brain. Amphetamine and DEX are partly metabolized in the liver and primarily (80%) excreted unchanged in the urine. Their excretion is hastened by acidification of the urine.

As it was originally formulated in 1954, MPH was produced as an equal mixture of D,L-threo-MPH and D,L-erythro-MPH. Soon afterwards, it was found that the erythro form of MPH produced the cardiovascular side effects of the original formulation, and thus MPH is now manufactured as an equal mixture of D,L-threo-MPH. Studies have indicated that the primarily active form of MPH is the D-threo isomer. Therefore, the makers of brand name **MPH (Ritalin)** now produce the isomer of D,L-threo-MPH called Focalin (D-threo-MPH or dexmethylphenidate). Clinicians should note that, in terms of potency, 10 mg of D,L-threo-MPH (Ritalin) is biologically equivalent to 5 mg of D-threo-MPH (Focalin). Oral administration of immediate-release D,L-threo-MPH (available in generic MPH, Ritalin, Metadate ER, Methylin) results in a variable peak plasma concentration within 1 to 2 hours, with a half-life of 2 to 3 hours. Behavioral effects of immediate-release MPH peak 1 to 2 hours after administration and tend to subside within 3 to 5 hours. Although generic MPH has a similar pharmacokinetic profile to Ritalin, it may be more rapidly absorbed and may peak sooner. Oral administration of immediate-release D-threo-MPH (dexmethylphenidate, available as Focalin) results in peak plasma concentrations at about 1 to 1.5 hours postdose, with a **half-life of approximately 2.2 hours.** Behavioral effects of dexmethylphenidate peak 1 to 2 hours after administration and tend to subside within 3 to 5 hours.

Plasma levels of the sustained-release (SR) preparation of MPH (Ritalin SR) peak in 1 to 4 hours with a half-life of 2 to 6 hours. Clinicians observe significant variability in the absorption of the SR preparation and tend to use it less now that several alternative extended-delivery systems are available. Peak behavioral effects of this preparation occur 2 hours after ingestion and last up to 8 hours. Because of the wax-matrix preparation, absorption is clinically observed to be variable. Recently, several novel methods of delivering MPH and amphetamine have become available, with the goal of extending the clinical effectiveness of the stimulants. Although these medications all deliver stimulants, their pharmacokinetic profiles differ. Oros-MPH (Concerta), the first of these novel delivery systems, has been available since August 2000. Concerta uses the osmotic-controlled release oral delivery system technology to deliver a 50:50 racemic mixture of D,L-threo-MPH. An 18-mg caplet of Concerta delivers the equivalent of 15 mg of MPH (5 mg of MPH three times a day) providing 12-hour coverage. Initially, the 18-mg caplet provides 4 mg of MPH and delivers the additional MPH in an ascending profile over a total of 12 hours. Concerta is recommended to be dosed between 18 and 72 mg daily. If Concerta is cut or crushed, its delivery system is compromised. Metadate CD, available as 10-, 20- and 30-mg capsules, which may be sprinkled, contains two types of beads containing D,L-threo-MPH. The 20-mg Metadate CD capsule delivers 30% or 6 mg of D,L-threo-MPH initially and 70% or 14 mg in an ascending profile designed to simulate dosing MPH in the morning and again 4 hours later to provide 8 hours of coverage. Ritalin LA, available in capsules of 20, 30, and 40 mg that may be sprinkled, delivers 50% of its D,L-threo-MPH initially and another bolus approximately 3 to 4 hours later, thus providing approximately 8 hours of coverage. Recently, an MPH patch (Daytrana) was approved by the FDA. All these MPH preparations easily pass to the brain. Their concentrations in the brain appear to be higher than those in the blood. MPH is metabolized by plasma-based esterases.

Adderall, as mentioned earlier, is the brand name for a single-entity amphetamine product combining salts of DEX and amphetamine. It is available in two preparations—immediate-release and extended-release. It has a short **half-life (8 to 12 hours)** and is usually administered one or two times daily.

The T_{max} of DEX is approximately 3.5 hours following single-dose oral administration of 30, 50, or 70 mg lisdexamfetamine (Vyvanse) after an 8-hour overnight fast, whereas the T_{max} of lisdexamfetamine is approximately 1 hour. After oral administration, lisdexamfetamine is rapidly absorbed from the gastrointestinal tract. Lisdexamfetamine is converted to DEX and L-lysine, which is believed to occur by first-pass intestinal and/or hepatic metabolism. The plasma elimination half-life of lisdexamfetamine typically averaged less than 1 hour in studies of lisdexamfetamine dimesylate in volunteers.

Although data from the late 1960s suggest potential for drug interactions, the MAOIs remain the only contraindicated medication and usually the stimulants do not cause clinically significant medication interactions. It should be noted that when stimulants are administered with other sympathomimetics, patients may experience significant side effects. Tolerance to the sympathomimetic effects and to the drug-induced euphoria of amphetamine and MPH develops rapidly. Thus, chronic abusers often take very large doses that would be extremely toxic if taken by a nontolerant individual.

Mechanism of Action

Amphetamine and the similarly acting MPH are often termed indirectly acting amines. This is because they are thought to act primarily by causing release of amines. In particular, **amphetamine increases extracellular norepinephrine, DA, and serotonin.** Amphetamine enters different types of monoamine neurons via the DAT, norepinephrine transporter, and serotonin transporter, respectively. Acting on the vesicular transporter shared by all monoamine neurons [vesicular monoamine transporter (VMAT)], amphetamine causes monoamine neurotransmitters to exit their storage vesicles and to be released into the synapse via the uptake transporter. In other words, amphetamine-like drugs cause the DAT, norepinephrine transporter, and serotonin transporter to act in reverse. (In contrast, cocaine blocks these transporters, allowing already released monoamines to build up in the synapse.) Amphetamine-like drugs also have **modest and reversible inhibitory effects on monoamine oxidase A**. The main effect of amphetamines is thought to be through the dopaminerguic system: amphetamines inhibit DA transport by the DAT, stimulate DAT to move DA in the reverse direction, increase the rate of DA synthesis, inhibit monoamine oxidase, and redistribute DA from vesicles into the cytosol. MPH chiefly affects the prefrontal cortex and striatum by modulating catecholaminergic tone. MPH treatment produces an increase in DA signaling through multiple actions, including blockade of the DA reuptake transporter, disinhibition of DA D2 autoreceptors, and activation of DA D1 receptors on the postsynaptic neuron. The actions of MPH may also be mediated by stimulation of the noradrenergic α2 receptor and DA D1 receptor in the cortex. Therefore, the effects on DA are thought to be most important to the mechanism of action of both MPH and amphetamine in ADHD, since, when used at the high doses that characterize abuse rather than therapeutic use, the release of DA is the action that produces rewarding and reinforcing effects.

Stimulants probably increase alertness by increasing monoamine availability at the level of the ascending reticular activating system. Hypothalamic effects are likely responsible for their **appetite-suppressant properties**. Their stimulatory effects on locomotion and their rewarding effects at higher doses are the result of their effects on DA in the nucleus accumbens and prefrontal cortex. Amphetamine and its derivatives are potent stimulants of the sympathetic nervous system because they enhance noradrenergic neurotransmission. The peripheral effects of the amphetamine-like drugs at therapeutic doses include mild increases in both systolic and diastolic blood pressure and often a reflex slowing of the heart rate. With higher doses, the heart rate increases and there may be arrhythmias.

Although the precise mechanism of action of psychostimulants in ADHD is still unknown, as mentioned earlier, their enhancing effect on DA neurotransmission is thought to play a significant role in improving executive function in ADHD. In contrast to sympathomimetic effects and euphoria, tolerance to the therapeutic effects in ADHD appears to be quite rare. A prior hypothesis held that somehow the stimulants paradoxically sedate children with ADHD, but this appears not to be the case because the effects of amphetamine in children with ADHD differ only in degree, not in kind, from its effects in normal children.

Chronic use of high-dose amphetamines and related compounds may produce a psychotic syndrome with prominent paranoid ideation and stereotypic movements. Amphetamine-induced psychosis is likely caused by the facilitation of dopaminergic neurotransmission in the limbic system and prefrontal cortex.

Therapeutic Effects in ADHD

Stimulant drugs are an effective treatment in 70% to 80% of children with ADHD, but are best used as part of a comprehensive treatment program involving behavioral, educational, and/or cognitive interventions. Stimulant drugs improve attention and decrease impulsiveness and hyperactivity. However, they do not help with specific learning disabilities that are often associated with ADHD (e.g., dyslexia). Stimulants are not indicated for "problem children" who do not meet the diagnostic criteria for ADHD.

MPH, DEX, Adderall, and related compounds are all equally effective. Although the overall therapeutic efficacy of stimulants appears to be comparable, there is no complete overlap in therapeutic effects, and patients may respond to one stimulant but not to another. For this reason, many clinicians may try two stimulants before switching to other agents. The therapeutic benefits of stimulants in ADHD are almost immediate when the starting dose is adequate.

Therapeutic Use

Before Starting Psychostimulants

Prior to starting psychostimulants, patients should have a comprehensive clinical assessment and, whenever possible, a thorough physical examination (including, in children, an evaluation of vision and hearing), with attention directed to heart rate, rhythm, and blood pressure. In children, it is helpful to assess intellectual ability and to look for possible comorbid learning disabilities. No specific laboratory tests are required. Psychostimulants should be administered with caution in patients with hypertension, and follow-up monitoring is imperative. Psychostimulants should probably be withheld from patients with tachyarrhythmias. As per the FDA recommendations, Adderall XR should not be given to patients with heart defects. In children, an examination should be performed with attention to the presence of tics and dyskinetic movements (there is a possibility that stimulants may precipitate or worsen Tourette's syndrome and dyskinesias—see later in the chapter). In patients with preexisting liver disease, amphetamine and MPH can be used, but in lower than usual dosages.

Dosing and Prescribing Strategies

The available preparations and dosing of stimulants are listed in Tables 9.2 and 9.3. DEX is usually begun at dosages of 5 to 10 mg twice daily in adults and at 5 mg once or twice daily in children and elderly patients. For children younger

TABLE 9.2 Available Preparations of Stimulants

Drug	Trade Name	Dose Forms
Adderall (mixed salts of dextroamphetamine and amphetamine)	Adderall	5-, 7.5-, 10-, 12.5-, 15-, 20-, 30-mg tablets
	Adderall XR	5-, 10-, 15-, 20-, 25-, 30-mg tablets
Lisdexamfetamine dimesylate	Vyvanse	20-, 30-, 40-, 50-, 60-, 70-mg tablets
Dextroamphetamine	Dexedrine and generics	5-mg tablet
	Dextrostat	5-, 10-mg tablets
	Dexedrine Spansules	5-, 10-, 15-mg tablets
	LiquADD	5 mg/5 mL oral solution
Methylphenidate	Ritalin and generics	5-, 10-, 20-mg tablets
	Ritalin SR	20-mg tablets
	Ritalin LA	10-, 20-, 30-, 40-mg tablets
	Methylin	5-, 10-, 20-mg tablets
	Methylin ER	10-, 20-mg tablets
	Methylin	5 mg/5 mL and 10 mg/5 mL oral solution
	Methylin	2.5-, 5-, and 10-mg chewable tablets
	Metadate CD	10-, 20-, 30-, 40-, 50-, 60-mg tablets
	Concerta	18-, 27-, 36-, 54-mg tablets
	Daytrana	27.5-, 41.3-, 55-, and 82.5-patch (nominal delivered dose: 10, 15, 20, and 30 mg/9 h)
Dexmethylphenidate	Focalin	2.5-, 5-, 10-mg tablets
	Focalin XR	5-, 10-, 15-, and 20 mg capsules

TABLE 9.3	Dosing of Stimulants		
Drug	**Starting Dose**	**Maximum Dose**	**Usual Dosing**
Adderall	5 mg q.d./b.i.d.	1.5 mg/kg/d 40 mg/d (adults)	q.d./b.i.d.
Adderall XR	10 mg q.d.	1.5 mg/kg/d 40 mg/d (adults)	q.d.
Vyvanse	30 mg q.d.	70 mg q.d.	q.d.
Dexedrine and generics	5 mg q.d./b.i.d.	1.5 mg/kg/d 40–60 mg/d (adults)	b.i.d./t.i.d.
Dexedrine Spansules	5 mg q.d.	1.5 mg/kg/d 40–60 mg/d (adults)	b.i.d.
LiquADD	5 mg q.d.	40–60 mg/d	b.i.d./t.i.d.
Ritalin and generics	5 mg q.d./b.i.d./t.i.d.	2 mg/kg/d 40–80 mg/d (adults)	t.i.d.
Ritalin SR	20 mg	2 mg/kg/d 40–80 mg/d (adults)	b.i.d.
Ritalin LA	10 mg q.d.	2 mg/kg/d 40–80 mg/d (adults)	q.d.
Methylin	10 mg q.d.	2 mg/kg/d 40–80 mg/d (adults)	q.d./b.i.d.
Metadate CD	20 mg q.d.	2 mg/kg/d 40–80 mg/d (adults)	q.d.
Concerta	18 mg q.d.	2 mg/kg/d 36–72 mg/d (adults)	q.d.
Daytrana	10 mg/9 h	30 mg/9 h	q.d.
Focalin	2.5 mg b.i.d.	20 mg/d	b.i.d.
Focalin XR	5 mg q.d.	20 mg/d	q.d.

b.i.d., twice a day; q.d., once a day; t.i.d., three times a day.

than 6 years and in debilitated elderly patients, a starting dosage of 2.5 mg once or twice daily is prudent. The dosage is increased until the desired therapeutic effects are achieved. In healthy adults, the usual dosage range is 5 to 40 mg per day, although dosages as high as 60 mg per day may be needed. The dosage for children is 0.25 to 1.5 mg per kilogram per day and can therefore reach 40 mg per day. DEX is usually given two to three times daily (unless a slow-release formulation is used), with the last dose given by late afternoon to avoid insomnia.

MPH is usually begun at 5 to 10 mg two to three times daily in adults; children and elderly patients might be given initially 5 to 10 mg twice daily. The dosage is slowly increased (10 mg every 2 to 4 days) until therapeutic results are achieved. The average daily adult dose is 40 mg, although doses as high as 80 mg may be used. Dosages for children are 0.5 to 2.0 mg per kilogram per day. MPH in its immediate-release formulation is usually given in three or four daily doses to maintain effectiveness and avoid rebound. Dexmethylphenidate (Focalin) is usually begun at 2.5 mg twice daily. The dosage, which is typically half of that used for MPH, is slowly increased until therapeutic results are achieved. The average daily adult dose is 20 mg. The SR or the extended-release formulations of MPH can be given once or twice daily.

Current recommendations support initial use of extended-delivery preparations (i.e., Concerta, Metadate, Ritalin LA, Adderall XR) in clinically appropriate situations in children, adolescents, and adults. In deciding between immediate-release versus extended-delivery preparations, clinicians should consider the amount of time the patient requires coverage. Although all stimulants are indicated up to absolute dosages (i.e., MPH 60 mg per day, Concerta 72 mg per day, Metadate CD 60 mg per day, Ritalin LA 60 mg per day, Adderall XR 40 mg per day), weight is typically used as a guide. As mentioned previously, MPH is typically targeted for 1 mg per kilogram per day, although the range may be 0.5 to 2 mg per kilogram per day, and the amphetamine target is usually 0.5 mg per kilogram per day with a range of 0.25 to 1.5 mg per kilogram per day. The dose is usually given in the morning after breakfast, with the knowledge that for amphetamine and with certain forms of extended-delivery MPH food may delay the T_{max} but not the total area under the curve. The dose may be titrated upward in weekly intervals to the target dose. It is important to recognize that all the stimulants are equally efficacious but they have unequal potency, with **5 mg of amphetamine being equal to 10 mg of MPH**. These differences are likely due to their different pharmacodynamic effects.

As far as lisdexamfetamine dimesylate (lisdexamfetamine) is concerned, in children 6 to 12 years of age or adults who are either starting treatment for the first time or switching from another medication, 30 mg once daily in the morning is the recommended dose. Daily dosage may be adjusted in increments of 10 or 20 mg at approximately weekly intervals to a maximum recommended dose of 70 mg per day.

The daily dose of Adderall in children is 0.3 to 1.5 mg per kilogram per day in split dosing, one in the early morning and the other around noon. The initial dosage can be 5 mg twice daily, with increases over the course of the first week to 20 or 40 mg as needed or tolerated. In adults with ADHD, the dosing can start at 10 mg initially in the morning for several days, then 10 mg in the morning and noon for several days; the ultimate dose over the course of the first 2 weeks may be 20 mg twice daily.

Use in Pregnancy
Psychostimulants are lipophilic and thus cross the placental barrier. For this reason, these drugs should be avoided during pregnancy.

Use in Elderly Patients
These drugs are safe in elderly patients but should be used in lower dosages.

Side Effects and Toxicity
Central Nervous System Side Effects
The major adverse effects of psychostimulants are central, with insomnia (which can often be minimized by administration early in the day) and appetite suppression being certainly the most common. Other adverse events include weight loss, irritability, upset stomach, headache, fatigue, lethargy, changes in arousal (either overstimulated and anxious or alternatively listless and lethargic), and changes in mood (either overly euphoric or occasionally tearful and oversensitive). Dysphoric reactions are more commonly reported in children. These **side effects emerge shortly after starting treatment**, are typically mild in nature, and may be diminished with careful dose titration. As in the case of efficacy, patients who are intolerant to one stimulant may tolerate another one.

Other Side Effects
Patients with underlying fixed or labile hypertension may have mild elevations in blood pressure; rarely, this is severe enough to require discontinuation of the drug,

although risks should be discussed with patients and careful monitoring of blood pressure and coordination with primary care are important. Sinus tachycardia and other tachyarrhythmias rarely occur at standard clinical doses. Another possible side effect is abdominal pain. In addition, intravenous amphetamine abusers have developed necrotizing angiitis affecting the brain.

In children, there has been concern about possible long-term growth and weight suppression, although this problem appears to be mild. Treatment with stimulants in childhood can modestly reduce expected height and weight. Although these effects attenuate over time and some data suggest that ultimate adult growth parameters may not be affected, it has been argued that more work is needed to clarify the effects of continuous treatment from childhood to adulthood. Although physicians should monitor height, deficits in height and weight do not appear to be a clinical concern for most children treated with stimulants. It has been suggested that growth deficits may simply represent a temporary delay (2-year follow-up studies suggest that delay in growth may represent slowing of growth velocity by 1 to 2 cm over a 2-year period) and not a true decrease in growth. Some clinicians give children time off the drug (e.g., during summer vacation) to make up any weight loss and minimize the risk of growth suppression, although 2-year data suggest that medication holidays do not improve growth, but patients often see resumption of their normal appetite. There is no good evidence that this is a necessary approach, and there may be risks of clinical deterioration associated with medication holidays.

Stimulants have been typically viewed as being associated with an increased risk of development of transient motor or vocal tics, resolving on drug discontinuation. In addition, it has been suggested that children with personal or family histories of Tourette's syndrome or other preexisting tic disorders were at greater risk for developing a tic disorder on stimulants, but recent studies have challenged this view.

Pemoline (Cylert), which used to be available in the United States is a stimulant, produces liver function test abnormalities in some patients, and has been associated with fatal cases of hepatotoxicity. The FDA concluded in October 2005 that the overall risk of liver toxicity from Cylert and generic pemoline products outweighs the benefits of this drug, and pemoline was withdrawn from the U.S. market.

Shire Pharmaceuticals—the manufacturer of Adderall—reported 12 child deaths to U.S. and Canadian regulatory agencies between 1999 and 2003. These 7- to 16-year-old boys had been taking Adderall for as little as 1 day or as long as 8 years. Five of the deaths were in children with known heart defects. Many of the other seven children had unusual circumstances that make the link to Adderall hard to interpret. However, on the basis of these reports, in the first quarter of 2005, Canada suspended the sale of the drug, whereas the FDA in August 2004 had simply required a label change for Adderall XR, stating that Adderall XR should not be given to patients with heart defects.

Abuse and Withdrawal

Stimulant Abuse

A major drawback to the use of psychostimulants is their **potential for abuse**, dependence, and addiction, and that is why these are typically schedule II drugs. Amphetamines are abused orally and intravenously, and MPH is typically abused orally. These drugs may produce feelings of euphoria and enhanced self-confidence. In the high doses of abuse, there are often signs of adrenergic hyperactivity (i.e., increased pulse and blood pressure, dry mouth, and pupillary dilatation). High doses of amphetamine may result in stereotyped behaviors, bruxism, formication, irritability, restlessness, emotional lability, and paranoia. With chronic abuse, a paranoid psychosis may develop, characterized by paranoid delusions, ideas/delusions of reference, and auditory, visual, or tactile hallucinations. The phamacodynamic properties of some formulations of MPH (e.g., osmotic-controlled release oral delivery system) and of the prodrug lisdexamfetamine (with the rate-limiting enzymatic conversion to active drug) may lead to a lower ability to abuse.

Withdrawal

Although there are no physical withdrawal symptoms, patients who have used high doses of psychostimulants for prolonged periods may experience a marked central syndrome, including fatigue, hypersomnia, hyperphagia, and severe depression in the short term and anhedonia, dysphoria, and drug craving in the long term. Currently, there is no proven pharmacologic treatment for psychostimulant dependence and withdrawal. Referral to a comprehensive treatment program is usually the best course. Patients should be observed for the emergence of a major depressive syndrome and suicidality or, alternatively, for recurrent drug abuse.

Overdose

Overdose with psychostimulants results in a syndrome of marked sympathetic hyperactivity (i.e., hypertension, tachycardia, hyperthermia), often accompanied by toxic psychosis or delirium. Patients may be irritable, paranoid, or violent. Grand mal seizures may occur. Death may result from hypertension, hyperthermia, arrhythmias, or uncontrollable seizures. Treatment consists of supportive care and blockade of adrenergic receptors. If the patient is unconscious or seizing, the airway must be protected. High fevers should be treated with cooling blankets. Seizures can be controlled with an intravenous benzodiazepine, such as lorazepam (1 to 2 mg) or diazepam (5 to 10 mg), repeated as necessary. Delirium or psychosis usually responds to an antipsychotic agent. Additional sedation can be provided by benzodiazepines, such as lorazepam, 1 to 2 mg orally or 1 mg intramuscularly, or diazepam, 5 to 10 mg orally every 1 to 2 hours as needed. Delirium usually clears in 2 to 3 days, but paranoid psychoses due to long-term, high-dose abuse may take longer to clear. Severe hypertension or tachyarrhythmias can usually be treated with β-blockers, administered intravenously if necessary.

ATOMOXETINE

Atomoxetine is part of the class of drugs called norepinephrine reuptake inhibitors (see Chapter 3). Atomoxetine is indicated by the FDA in doses up to 1.4 mg per kilogram per day or 100 mg total daily dose to treat ADHD in children, adolescents, and adults.

In vitro, ex vivo, and *in vivo* studies have shown that atomoxetine is a selective antagonist of the presynaptic norepinephrine transporter, with little or no affinity for other noradrenergic receptors or other neurotransmitter transporters or receptors [except for a weak affinity for the serotonin (5-hydroxytryptamine) (5-HT) transporter]. In rat microdialysis studies, atomoxetine increased extracellular levels of norepinephrine and DA in prefrontal cortex threefold, but did not alter 5-HT levels and did not alter extracellular DA in striatum or nucleus accumbens.

Atomoxetine is available in the United States with an FDA-approved indication of ADHD. Atomoxetine is rapidly absorbed, with peak plasma concentrations occurring 1 to 2 hours after dosing, and its half-life hovers around 3 to 4 hours. The most common drug-related events reported in trials have been decreased appetite, insomnia, sedation, and an initial period of weight loss, followed by an apparently normal rate of weight gain. Atomoxetine has also been associated with mild increases in blood pressure and pulse that plateau during treatment and resolve on discontinuation. There have been no effects seen on the Q-T interval. There is no evidence of a negative effect of atomoxetine on growth in height or weight. It is a substrate of cytochrome P450 (CYP) 2D6 and its biotransformation involves aromatic ring hydroxylation, benzylic oxidation, and N-demethylation. At high therapeutic doses, atomoxetine inhibits CYP2D6 and CYP3A activity, although *in vivo* studies clearly indicate that atomoxetine administration with substrates of CYP2D6 and CYP3A does not result in clinically significant drug interactions. Although no evidence of liver injury was detected in clinical trials of about 6,000 patients, there have been **rare cases of clinically significant liver injury** that were considered probably or possibly related to atomoxetine use in postmarketing experience. In one patient, liver injury, manifested by elevated hepatic enzymes (up to 40× upper limit of normal) and jaundice (bilirubin up to 12× upper limit of normal), recurred upon rechallenge, and was followed by recovery upon drug discontinuation, providing evidence that atomoxetine likely caused the liver injury. The patient recovered from his liver injury, and did not require a liver transplant. However, severe liver injury due to any drug may potentially progress to acute liver failure resulting in death or the need for a liver transplant. Therefore, atomoxetine should be discontinued in patients with jaundice or laboratory evidence of liver injury, and should not be restarted. Laboratory testing to determine liver enzyme levels should be done upon the first symptom or sign of liver dysfunction (e.g., pruritus, dark urine, jaundice, right upper quadrant tenderness, or unexplained "flulike" symptoms) The FDA has also issued another warning concerning suicidal ideation risk. Atomoxetine was found to increase the risk over placebo of suicidal ideation in short-term studies in children or adolescents with ADHD, with comorbidities occurring with ADHD perhaps being associated with an increase in the risk of suicidal ideation and/or behavior. Patients who are started on therapy should be monitored closely for suicidality (suicidal thinking and behavior), clinical worsening, or unusual changes in behavior. The average risk of suicidal ideation in patients receiving atomoxetine was 0.4% (5 of 1,357 patients), compared to none in placebo-treated patients (851 patients). No suicides occurred in these trials.

Atomoxetine (Strattera) is available in 10-, 18-, 25-, 40-, 60-, 80-, and 100-mg strengths. In children and adolescents, treatment with atomoxetine is typically initiated at a total daily dose of approximately 0.5 mg/kg and increased after a minimum of 4 days to a target total daily dose of approximately 1.2 mg/kg administered either as a single daily dose in the morning or as evenly divided doses in the morning and late afternoon or early evening. The total daily dose in children and adolescents typically does not exceed 1.4 mg per kilogram per day. In adults, treatment with atomoxetine is typically initiated at a total daily dose of 40 mg and increased after a minimum of 3 days to a target total daily dose of approximately 80 to 100 mg administered either as a single daily dose in the morning or as evenly divided doses in the morning and late afternoon or early evening. After 2 to 4 additional weeks, the dose may be increased to a maximum of 120 mg in divided doses among patients who have not achieved an optimal response. Patients must realize that the therapeutic effects of atomoxetine may take a number of weeks. Preliminary evidence suggests that it is relatively safe and effective to use stimulants adjunctively with atomoxetine.

BUPROPION

As mentioned in Chapter 3, bupropion is considered a norepinephrine-DA reuptake inhibitor, because of the evidence for this compound's effects on norepinephrine and DA neurotransmission. Although double-blind, placebo-controlled studies suggest the efficacy of bupropion in ADHD, the use of bupropion for ADHD is off-label. Bupropion is a phenylethylamine compound, structurally related to amphetamine, primarily blocking the reuptake of DA and norepinephrine and with minimal or no affinity for postsynaptic receptors. Thus, it is not surprising that it has been reported to possess some stimulant-like effects when used for

ADHD. Bupropion is rapidly absorbed after oral administration and demonstrates biphasic elimination, with an elimination half-life of 11 to 14 hours. It is converted to three active metabolites, hydroxybupropion, threohydrobupropion, and erythrohydrobupropion.

Patients are generally begun on 100 mg twice daily of the immediate-release or 150 mg once per day of its two extended-release formulations (XR and XL). A significant proportion of patients may respond to the initial dosage, although the dosage is typically increased to 300 mg per day (once daily in the XL formulation or in divided doses) and, in some cases, up to 450 mg per day in divided doses. Although the agent is usually well tolerated, patients may develop agitation, dry mouth, restlessness, diminished appetite, weight loss, headache, constipation, insomnia, and anxiety or gastrointestinal distress soon after initiation of treatment. For those who have significant difficulties tolerating it because of agitation, benzodiazepine augmentation can be considered. Rare adverse events reported with bupropion are blood pressure elevations, cognitive side effects, and dystonias. The major medically important adverse event associated with bupropion is seizure. With the immediate-release formulation the seizure rate is 0.4% (4/1,000) at dosages up to 450 mg per day, whereas with bupropion SR the seizure rate is 0.1% (1/1,000) at doses up to the target antidepressant dosage of 300 mg per day, a rate comparable to those of other antidepressants. Patients who do not improve may have their bupropion dosage increased to as high as 450 mg per day. Because of the risk of seizures, it is recommended that the total daily dose of bupropion be not higher than 450 mg (in any formulation) and that no individual dose of the original bupropion formulation be higher than 150 mg in the immediate-release formulation and 200 mg in the SR formulation, whereas single doses of 300 mg can be administered in the XL extended-release formulation; doses of 150 mg should be given no more frequently than every 4 hours.

Bupropion lacks anticholinergic properties and does not cause postural hypotension or alter cardiac conduction in a clinically significant manner. It is a substrate of CYP2B6 and appears to have CYP2D6 inhibition potential. Bupropion is contraindicated for use in patients with a history of brain injury and anorexia or bulimia because these patients were reported to have a very high incidence of seizures in prerelease studies.

MODAFINIL

Modafinil (Provigil) is a racemic compound that is structurally different from psychostimulants and promotes wakefulness through mechanisms that are still unknown. It has an indication for the treatment of excessive sleepiness associated with narcolepsy, obstructive sleep apnea and hypopnea syndrome, and shift-work sleep disorder. Its use in ADHD is off-label but is partly supported by placebo-controlled studies. Its main advantage over stimulants is that modafinil is a schedule IV drug with relatively low abuse potential. Modafinil has linear pharmacokinetics, with moderate plasma protein binding. Its half-life is approximately 15 hours; therefore, once per day dosing is typical. It is metabolized by the liver and has been shown to slightly induce CYP1A2, CYP2B6, and CYP3A4 in a concentration-dependent manner. There is a positive placebo-controlled study in children supporting the efficacy of modafinil, particularly in dosages of 300 mg per day. The most common side effects are headache, nausea, diarrhea, anorexia, and nervousness. There are no consistent changes in mean heart rate or blood pressure. It is available in 100- and 200-mg tablets. It is usually started at 100 mg daily, with the daily dose quickly raised to 200, 300 (in children and adolescents), and 400 mg (in adults) in the event of nonresponse. Modafinil was not approved by the FDA for the treatment of ADHD based on safety concerns about a rare but potentially serious rash characteristic of Stevens-Johnson syndrome.

TRICYCLIC ANTIDEPRESSANTS

The TCAs (see Chapter 3 for a description of their pharmacologic properties) are considered by many to be second-line agents in the treatment of ADHD and are typically used in patients who have not responded to stimulants and atomoxetine. Their use, as in the case of bupropion, is considered off-label. Although fairly effective in the treatment of behavioral symptoms of ADHD, their efficacy in treating inattentiveness and poor concentration is considered by many to be inferior to that of stimulants. In addition, concerns about the safety of using TCAs in children have limited their use; in particular, unexplained deaths have occurred in children treated with TCAs for ADHD. For this reason, greater than usual monitoring of electrocardiograms is recommended when TCAs are used in children and adolescents. On the other hand, a study estimating the magnitude of desipramine-associated risk of sudden death in children suggested that such risk may not be much greater than the baseline risk of sudden death in this age group.

Oral preparations of tricyclics and related drugs are rapidly and completely absorbed from the gastrointestinal tract; a high percentage of an oral dose is metabolized by the liver as it passes through the portal circulation (first-pass effect). The tricyclics are metabolized by the microsomal enzymes of the liver.

Tricyclic drugs are highly lipophilic, meaning the free fraction passes easily into the brain and other tissues. They are also largely bound to plasma proteins. Given their lipophilicity and protein binding, they are not removed effectively by hemodialysis in cases of overdose. The time course of metabolism and elimination is biphasic, with approximately half of a dose removed over 48 to 72 hours, and the remainder is strongly bound to tissues and plasma proteins, slowly excreted over several weeks. There is considerable variation among individuals in their metabolic rate for TCAs based on genetic factors, age, and concomitantly taken drugs. In fact, when metabolic differences are combined with variation in the degree of protein binding, as much as a 300-fold difference in effective drug levels may be found among individuals.

A medical history and examination are indicated before beginning TCAs, particularly to determine whether the patient has cardiac conduction system disease, which is the major medical contraindication to TCA use. An electrocardiogram should be obtained in all patients, with subsequent frequent monitoring in children and adolescents.

TCAs are started at a low dose with gradual increase until the therapeutic range is achieved. In children and adolescents, the starting dosage is typically 10 mg per day (0.5 mg per kilogram per day for nortriptyline and 1 mg per kilogram per day for imipramine), whereas for healthy adults, the typical starting dose is 25 or 50 mg of imipramine or the equivalent. In some clinical situations, it may be necessary to start with lower doses (as low as 10 mg of imipramine or the equivalent) because of intolerance to side effects.

Generally, imipramine and nortriptyline are probably the TCAs most commonly used in the treatment of ADHD. It is not uncommon to administer them in divided doses to minimize the risk of side effects. The dose can be increased by 50 mg every 3 to 4 days, as side effects allow, up to a dose of 150 to 200 mg of imipramine or its equivalent at bedtime (up to 4 mg per kilogram per day) or 100 to 150 mg of nortriptyline at bedtime (up to 2 mg per kilogram per day). Discontinuation of treatment should be done with a taper over 2 to 4 weeks to minimize the risk of discontinuation symptoms, including gastrointestinal distress and dizziness.

Because of the concerns about toxicity in children and adolescents, routine monitoring of plasma levels is considered to be prudent, although blood levels cannot be used as a guide toward determining the effective dose in ADHD, because the reference range is derived from patients treated for depression. Of the currently available cyclic antidepressants and TCAs, only four drugs have been studied well enough to make generalizations about the value of their blood levels in treatment of depression: imipramine, desipramine, amitriptyline, and nortriptyline.

In general, **the side effects of the TCAs are more difficult for patients to tolerate than the side effects of stimulants, atomoxetine, or bupropion.** Another difficulty with the TCAs lies in their potential for lethality in overdose.

At therapeutic levels, tricyclics may produce sedation, postural hypotension, anticholinergic (antimuscarinic) effects (e.g., dry mouth, dry throat, urinary retention, blurred vision, constipation, diminished working memory, and dental cavities), and quinidine-like effects on cardiac conduction. They may also decrease the seizure threshold and may cause weight gain that may be significant. TCAs may cause sexual dysfunction, most frequently erectile dysfunction in men. In addition, patients may experience excessive sweating, which may interfere with quality of life. Most side effects of cyclic antidepressants worsen with increased doses, although some may manifest even at lower doses (e.g., dry mouth, constipation, postural hypotension). Elderly patients are generally more susceptible to these side effects. The major medical contraindications to the use of cyclic antidepressants are serious cardiac conduction disturbances, narrow angle glaucoma, and prostate hypertrophy.

Acute doses of more than 1 g of TCAs are often toxic and may be fatal. Death may result from cardiac arrhythmias, hypotension, or uncontrollable seizures. Serum levels should be obtained when overdose is suspected both because of distorted information that may be given by patients or families and because oral bioavailability with very large doses of these compounds is poorly understood. Nonetheless, serum levels of the parent compound and its active metabolites provide less specific information about the severity of the overdose than one might hope. Serum levels of greater than 1,000 ng/mL are associated with serious overdose as are increases in the QRS duration of the electrocardiogram to 0.10 seconds or greater. However, serious consequences of a TCA overdose may occur with serum levels less than 1,000 ng/mL and with a QRS duration of less than 0.10 seconds. For a description of TCA overdoses and their management, see Chapter 3.

α_2-ADRENERGIC AGONISTS

As with the TCAs, α_2-adrenergic agonists are typically used as **second- or third-line treatment of ADHD,** although they have been particularly appealing to clinicians as a treatment of ADHD in patients with tic disorders, because this class of drugs can be helpful in treating tics as well. There have been reports of severe toxicity (and even death) when the α_2-agonist clonidine (Catapres) has been combined with stimulants such as MPH. Two controlled studies with daily doses of clonidine up to 4 to 5 µg/kg (average dose: 0.2 mg per day) have supported its beneficial effect on the behavioral aspects of ADHD, but not all studies have been supportive of its usefulness. Clonidine is available in 0.1-, 0.2-, and 0.3-mg tablets. Similarly, following two small, positive, open trials, a double-blind, placebo-controlled, crossover study showed that guanfacine (Tenex) (average dose: 1.1 mg per day) was better than placebo in treating ADHD symptoms, and a placebo-controlled study of guanfacine provided support for the efficacy of this agent in the treatment of children with tic disorders and ADHD. Guanfacine (Tenex) is available in 1- and 2-mg tablets. An extended-release formulation of guanfacine (Intuniv) has received an approvable letter from the FDA at doses of 1, 2, 3, and 4 mg. Common side effects of clonidine and guanfacine are **drowsiness, dizziness, dry mouth,** confusion, depression, and sedation.

SELECTIVE SEROTONIN REUPTAKE INHIBITORS, SEROTONIN-NOREPINEPHRINE REUPTAKE INHIBITORS, AND MONOAMINE OXIDASE INHIBITORS

Some studies have suggested the potential usefulness of selective serotonin reuptake inhibitors (SSRIs), serotonin-norepinephrine reuptake inhibitors (SNRIs), and MAOIs in ADHD, but the lack of supportive placebo-controlled studies for SSRIs and SNRIs and the safety concerns about MAOIs markedly limit the use of these drugs in this condition. For a description of the pharmacology and clinical uses of SSRIs, SNRIs, and MAOIs, see Chapter 3.

OTHER DRUGS

Cholinesterase inhibitors (e.g., donepezil at dosages between 5 and 15 mg per day) and antipsychotic drugs have been used in ADHD, particularly in the treatment of patients with tic disorders or severe behavioral problems. The serotonin 5-HT_{1A} partial agonist buspirone (Buspar) (in two open trials—dosage: 15 to 30 mg per day in divided doses) and the serotonin 5-HT_{1A} antagonist pindolol (in one double-blind, placebo-controlled study—dosage: 20 mg twice daily) have shown some modest benefit in the treatment of ADHD, although their use is limited.

TREATMENT RESISTANCE IN ADHD

Although the treatments available are fairly effective in ADHD, a significant proportion of patients may not respond at all or may respond only partly to treatment. In these cases, clinicians, in addition to reevaluating the patients diagnostically, may use polypharmacy as a way of addressing incomplete responses. The polypharmacy may involve using two or more drugs that have shown some benefit in the treatment of ADHD or the use of drugs targeting comorbid psychiatric disorders, such as anticonvulsant drugs in patients with bipolar disorder or antidepressants in patients with major depressive disorder.

Bibliography

ADHD

Adesman AR. The diagnosis and management of attention-deficit/hyperactivity disorder in pediatric patients. *Prim Care Companion J Clin Psychiatry* 2001;3:66.

Biederman J. Attention-deficit/hyperactivity disorder: a life-span perspective. *J Clin Psychiatry* 1998;59(suppl 7):4.

Deutsch CK, Dube WV, McIlvane WJ. Attention deficits, attention-deficit hyperactivity disorder, and intellectual disabilities. *Dev Disabil Res Rev.* 2008;14(4):285–292.

Mannuzza S, Klein RG, Bessler A, et al. Adult outcome of hyperactive boys: educational achievement, occupational rank, and psychiatric status. *Arch Gen Psychiatry* 1993; 50:885.

Wender PH, Reimherr FW, Wood DR. Attention deficit disorder ("minimal brain dysfunction") in adults. *Arch Gen Psychiatry* 1981;38:449.

Epidemiology

Mayes R, Bagwell C, Erkulwater J. ADHD and the rise in stimulant use among children. *Harv Rev Psychiatry* 2008;16(3):151–166.

Pastor PN, Reuben CA. Diagnosed attention deficit hyperactivity disorder and learning disability: United States, 2004–2006. *Vital Health Stat 10* 2008;(237):1–14.

Neurobiology and Genetics

Faraone SV, Perlis RH, Doyle AE, et al. Molecular genetics of attention-deficit/hyperactivity disorder. *Biol Psychiatry* 2005;57:1313–1323.

Spencer TJ, Biederman J, Wilens TE, et al. Overview and neurobiology of attention-deficit/hyperactivity disorder. *J Clin Psychiatry* 2002;63(suppl 12):3.

Brain Imaging Studies

Casey BJ, Epstein JN, Buhle J, et al. Frontostriatal connectivity and its role in cognitive control in parent–child dyads with ADHD. *Am J Psychiatry* 2007;164:1729–1736.

Durston S. Converging methods in studying attention-deficit/hyperactivity disorder: what can we learn from neuroimaging and genetics? *Dev Psychopathol* 2008;20(4):1133–1143.

Krause KH, Dresel SH, Krause J, et al. The dopamine transporter and neuroimaging in attention deficit hyperactivity disorder. *Neurosci Biobehav Rev* 2003;27:605.

Sowell ER, Thompson PM, Welcome SE, et al. Cortical abnormalities in children and adolescents with attention-deficit hyperactivity disorder. *Lancet* 2003;362:1699.

Treatments

Biederman J, Spencer TJ. Psychopharmacological interventions. *Child Adolesc Psychiatr Clin N Am* 2008;17(2):439–458.

Spencer TJ, Biederman J, Wilens TE, et al. Novel treatments for attention-deficit/hyperactivity disorder in children. *J Clin Psychiatry* 2002;63(suppl 12):16.

Psychosocial Treatments

Knouse LE, Cooper-Vince C, Sprich S, Safren SA. Recent developments in the psychosocial treatment of adult ADHD. *Expert Rev Neurother* 2008;8(10):1537–1548.

Psychostimulants

Faraone SV, Biederman J, Morley CP, et al. Effect of stimulants on height and weight: a review of the literature. *J Am Acad Child Adolesc Psychiatry* 2008;47(9):994–1009.

Howland RH. Lisdexamfetamine: a prodrug stimulant for ADHD. *J Psychosoc Nurs Ment Health Serv.* 2008;46(8):19–22.

Mattes JA, Boswell L, Oliver H. Methylphenidate effects on symptoms of attention deficit disorder in adults. *Arch Gen Psychiatry* 1984;41:1059.

Pelham WE, Aronoff HR, Midlam JK, et al. A comparison of Ritalin and Adderall: efficacy and time course in children with attention-deficit/hyperactivity disorder. *Pediatrics* 1999;103:43.

Pliszka SR. The use of psychostimulants in the pediatric patient. *Pediatr Clin North Am* 1998;45:1085.

Spencer T, Wilens TE, Biederman J, et al. A double-blind, cross-over comparison of methylphenidate and placebo in adults with childhood onset attention deficit hyperactivity disorder. *Arch Gen Psychiatry* 1995;52:434.

Swanson J, Wigal S, Greenhill L, et al. Objective and subjective measures of the pharmacodynamic effects of Adderall in the treatment of children with ADHD in a controlled laboratory classroom setting. *Psychopharmacol Bull* 1998;34:55.

Wallace LJ, Connell LE. Mechanisms by which amphetamine redistributes dopamine out of vesicles: a computational study. *Synapse* 2008;62(5):370–378.

Wender PH, Reimherr FW, Wood D, et al. A controlled study of methylphenidate in the treatment of attention deficit disorder, residual type, in adults. *Am J Psychiatry* 1985;142:547.

Wilens TE. Effects of methylphenidate on the catecholaminergic system in attention-deficit/hyperactivity disorder. *J Clin Psychopharmacol* 2008;28(3 suppl 2):S46–S53.

Atomoxetine

Biederman J, Heiligenstein JH, Faries DE, et al. Atomoxetine ADHD Study Group. Efficacy of atomoxetine versus placebo in school-age girls with attention-deficit/hyperactivity disorder. *Pediatrics* 2002;110:e75.

Bymaster FP, Katner JS, Nelson DL, et al. Atomoxetine increases extracellular levels of norepinephrine and dopamine in prefrontal cortex of rat: a potential mechanism for efficacy in attention deficit/hyperactivity disorder. *Neuropsychopharmacology* 2002;27:699.

Carlson GA, Dunn D, Kelsey D, et al. A pilot study for augmenting atomoxetine with methylphenidate: safety of concomitant therapy in children with attention-deficit/hyperactivity disorder. *Child Adolesc Psychiatry Ment Health* 2007;1(1):10.

Michelson D, Adler L, Spencer T, et al. Atomoxetine in adults with ADHD: two randomized, placebo-controlled studies. *Biol Psychiatry* 2003;53:112.

Spencer T, Heiligenstein JH, Biederman J, et al. Results from 2 proof-of-concept, placebo-controlled studies of atomoxetine in children with attention-deficit/hyperactivity disorder. *J Clin Psychiatry* 2002;63:1140.

Bupropion

Daviss WB, Bentivoglio P, Racusin R, et al. Bupropion sustained release in adolescents with co-morbid attention-deficit/hyperactivity disorder and depression. *J Am Acad Child Adolesc Psychiatry* 2001;40:307.

Kuperman S, Perry PJ, Gaffney GR, et al. Bupropion SR vs. methylphenidate vs. placebo for attention deficit hyperactivity disorder in adults. *Ann Clin Psychiatry* 2001;13:129.

Wilens TE, Haight BR, Horrigan JP, et al. Bupropion XL in adults with attention-deficit/hyperactivity disorder: a randomized, placebo-controlled study. *Biol Psychiatry* 2005;57(7): 793–801.

Wilens TE, Spencer TJ, Biederman J, et al. A controlled clinical trial of bupropion for attention deficit hyperactivity disorder in adults. *Am J Psychiatry* 2001;158:282.

Modafinil

Biederman J, Pliszka SR. Modafinil improves symptoms of attention-deficit/hyperactivity disorder across subtypes in children and adolescents. *J Pediatr* 2008;152(3):394–399.

Rugino TA, Samsock TC. Modafinil in children with attention-deficit hyperactivity disorder. *Pediatr Neurol* 2003;29:136.

TCAs

Spencer T, Biederman J, Coffey B, et al. A double-blind comparison of desipramine and placebo in children and adolescents with chronic tic disorder and comorbid attention-deficit/hyperactivity disorder. *Arch Gen Psychiatry* 2002;59:649.

Wilens TE, Biederman J, Prince J, et al. Six-week, double-blind, placebo-controlled study of desipramine for adult attention deficit hyperactivity disorder. *Am J Psychiatry* 1996;153:1147.

Note: Page numbers followed by "f" indicate a figure; page numbers followed by "t" indicate a table.

Confusional states
treatment with antipsychotics, 36–37
Corgard. *See* Nadolol (Corgard)
Creatinine clearance
with lithium, 128
Cutaneous side effects
due to antipsychotics, 45
Cycloplegia
due to antipsychotics, 44
Cylert. *See* Pemoline (Cylert)
Cymbalta. *See* Duloxetine (Cyrnbalta)

D
Daxolin. *See* Loxapine (Loxitane,
Daxolin)
Dehydroepiandrosterone (DHEA)
and testosterone, 83
Delirium
due to anticholinergic drugs, 37
due to psychostimulant overdose, 277
in alcohol withdrawal, 204
medical causes of, 23
treatment benzodiazepines for, 206
treatment with antipsychotics, 37
Delusional disorders
treatment with antipsychotics, 6
Dementia
differential diagnosis of, 255t
drug for treatment of, 254
frontotemporal, 254
treatment with antipsychotics, 25
vascular, 262
Depakene. *See* Valproate; Valproic acid
(Depakene)
Depakote, 211t
Depression
acute unipolar, 111
anxious, 56
atypical, 56–57
carbamazepine for, 139
central nervous system, 98
comorbid conditions with, 60
drugs for treatment of, 54–107
due to grief, bereavement, and loss, 58
major, 1, 54–55
melancholic, 56
minor, 55
nicotine dependence in, 223
nonpsychotic, 21
psychostimulants in, 269
resistant
antidepressants in, 68
tricyclic antidepressants for, 281
with anger attacks, 57

with psychotic features, 22t, 58–59
with substance abuse, 60
Depressive disorders
continuation and maintenance
treatment in, 67–68
subtypes of, 56–60
Dermatologic reactions
to carbamazepine, 140
to lithium, 127
Desipramine (Norpramin)
blood levels of, 94
dosage of, 70t
side effects of, 71t
SSRIs and, 84
use of
in ADHD, 280
in chronic cocaine use, 221
in panic disorder, 182
in resistant depression, 67
Desmethyldiazepam, 206
Desyrel. *See* Trazodone (Desyrel)
Detoxification, 204
inpatient, 205–206
outpatient, 205
Dexedrine. *See* Dextroamphetamine
(Dexedrine)
Dexmethylphenidate (Focalin), 270
dosage of, 273t, 274
Dextroamphetamine (Dexedrine)
dosage of, 269, 273t
pharmacology of, 269
use of
in ADHD, 269, 273t
in narcolepsy, 250
in primary hypersomnia, 250
with tricyclic antidepressants, 96
Diazepam (Valium), 211t
elimination half-life of, 206–207
loading method for, 206
lorazepam versus, 206–207
use of
in alcohol withdrawal, 205
in generalized anxiety disorder, 165t
in psychostimulant overdose, 277
in situational or stress related
anxiety, 175
Dibenzodiazepine(s), 9, 11t
preparations of, 12t
Dietary restrictions
with MAOls, 102, 104
Diphenhydramine (Benadryl)
use of
in antipsychotic overdosage, 47
in disulfiram-alcohol reaction, 215

Ocular pigmentation
  due to antipsychotics, 44–45
Ocular side effects
  of topiramate, 218
Olanzapine (Zyprexa), 7, 9, 10, 13t, 31, 81
  in bipolar disorder, 147
  mechanism of action of, 32
  preparations of, 13t
  use of
    in acute psychosis, 24
    in dementia, 261
    in depression with psychotic
      features, 7, 58
    in insomnia, 249
    in nonpsychotic depression, 7
    in schizophrenia, 31
  weight gain from, 44
Ondansetron
  dose forms of, 217
  mechanism of action of, 216–217
  method of use of, 217
  naltrexone plus, 220
  pharmacology of, 216–217
Opiates
  SSRIs and, 83
  use of
    in restless legs syndrome, 235
Opioid dependence, 196
  chronic
    treatment of, 197
Opioid withdrawal, 194, 196
  clonidine for, 194–195
Orap. *See* Pimozide (Orap)
Oros-methylphenidate (Concerta), 270
Orthostatic hypotension. *See* Postural
      hypotension
Overdosage
  of antipsychotics, 47
  of tricyclic antidepressants, 93
  of valproate, 144
Oxazepam (Serax), 240t
  pharmacokinetics of, 241t
  use of
    in insomnia, 244t
    in situational or stress related
      anxiety, 175
Oxoquazepam, 245

P
Pamelor. *See* Nortriptyline (Pamelor)
Panic disorder, 1, 181–184
  antidepressants for, 182
  comorbid disorders associated with,
    184

diagnosis, 181
  pharmacologic treatment of, 181–184
  psychotherapy in, 184
Paradoxical intention
  in insomnia, 238–239
Paranoid disorders
  treatment with antipsychotics, 6
Parasomnias, 252
Parkinsonism
  from antipsychotics, 34
Parkinson's disease
  clozapine in, 27
  psychotic symptoms with, 27
  with dementia, 254
Parnate. *See* Tranylcypromine
      (Parnate)
Paroxetine (Paxil), 79
  dosage of, 69t
  use of
    in obsessive-compulsive disorder,
      185
    in panic disorder, 182
    in social phobia, 176
Pemoline (Cylert), 276
  before starting, 276
  pharmacology of, 276
Pergolide
  use of
    in periodic limb movements in
      sleep, 235
Periodic limb movements in sleep
      (PLMS), 235
Permitil. *See* Fluphenazine (Prolixin,
      Permitil)
Perphenazine (Trilafon)
  potency and side effects of, 11t
  preparations of, 12t
Personality disorders
  lithium for, 113
  treatment with antipsychotics, 42
Phenelzine (Nardil)
  dosage of, 70t
  side effects of, 71t
  use of
    in panic disorders, 182
    in posttraumatic stress disorder,
      187–188
    in social phobia, 176
Phenothiazine(s)
  aliphatic side chains of, 9
  derivative, 7
  potency and side effects of, 11t
  preparations of, 12t
  subtypes of, 9